# GERIATRIC DENTISTRY
## AGING AND ORAL HEALTH

# GERIATRIC DENTISTRY
## AGING AND ORAL HEALTH

**ATHENA S. PAPAS, D.M.D., Ph.D., F.A.C.D.**

Associate Professor and Co-head, Division of Geriatric Dentistry
Tufts University School of Dental Medicine
Boston, Massachusetts

**LINDA C. NIESSEN, D.M.D., M.P.H., M.P.P., F.A.C.D.**

Associate Professor
Department of Community and Preventive Dentistry
Baylor College of Dentistry, Dallas;
Veterans Affairs Medical Center
Dallas, Texas

**HOWARD H. CHAUNCEY, Ph.D., D.M.D., F.I.C.D.**

Associate Chief of Staff for Research and Development
Department of Veteran Affairs Outpatient Clinic
Boston, Massachusetts

*with **27** contributors*

*with **207** illustrations*

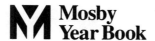

**Mosby Year Book**

St. Louis  Baltimore  Boston  Chicago  London  Philadelphia  Sydney  Toronto

 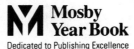

**Mosby**
**Year Book**
Dedicated to Publishing Excellence

Editor: Robert W. Reinhardt
Assistant Editor: Susie H. Baxter
Project Manager: Mark Spann
Manuscript Editor: Carl Masthay
Interior and Cover Design: Gail Morey Hudson
Production: Kathleen L. Teal

Mosby–Year Book, Inc.
11830 Westline Industrial Drive
St. Louis, MO 63146

**Library of Congress Cataloging in Publication Data**

Geriatric dentistry : aging and oral health / [edited by] Athena S.
  Papas, Linda C. Niessen, Howard H. Chauncey ; with 27 contributors.
      p.     cm.
    Includes index.
    ISBN 0-8016-5790-3
    1. Aged—Dental care. 2. Mouth—Aging. I. Papas, Athena S.
  II. Niessen, Linda C. III. Chauncey, Howard H.
    [DNLM: 1. Aging—physiology. 2. Dental Care for Aged. 3. Oral
  Health.     WU 490 G3693]
  RK55.A3G46  1991
  618.97'76—dc20
  DNLM/DLC
  for Library of Congress                                          91-10567
                                                                       CIP

GW/MY  9  8  7  6  5  4  3  2  1

# Contributors

**DAVID W. BANTING, D.D.S., Ph.D.**

Associate Dean, Faculty of Dentistry
University of Western Ontario
London, Ontario, Canada

**BRUCE J. BAUM, M.D., Ph.D.**

Clinical Director and Chief
Clinical Investigations and Patient Care Branch
National Institute of Dental Research
Bethesda, Maryland

**DOUGLAS B. BERKEY, D.M.D., M.P.H., M.S.**

Acting Chairman, Department of Applied
  Dentistry and Director of Clinical Geriatrics
University of Colorado School of Dentistry
Denver, Colorado

**ANTHONY J. CARUSO, Ph.D.**

Associate Professor
Department of Speech Pathology and Audiology
Kent State University,
Kent, Ohio

**†HOWARD H. CHAUNCEY, Ph.D., D.M.D.,
  F.I.C.D.**

Associate Chief of Staff for Research and
  Development
Department of Veteran Affairs Outpatient Clinic
  Boston;
Research Professor
Department of Oral Pathology
Tufts University School of Medicine
Boston, Massachusetts

**SIDNEY EPSTEIN, D.D.S.**

Clinical Professor
University of California School of Dentistry
Department of Public Health and Oral Hygiene
San Francisco;
Clinical Professor, Department of Dermatology
Stanford University of Medicine
Stanford, California

**RONALD L. ETTINGER, B.D.S., M.D.S.**

Professor, Department of Prosthodontics and
  Dows Institute for Dental Research
College of Dentistry, University of Iowa
Iowa City, Iowa

**DENISE J. FEDELE, D.M.D., M.S.**

Director, Geriatric Dental Program
Veterans Administration Medical Center;
Assistant Clinical Professor
Department of Oral Health Care Delivery
University of Maryland at Baltimore
Perry Point, Maryland

**CHARLES M. GOLDSTEIN, D.D.S., M.P.H.**

Clinical Professor and Chairman
Section of Community Dentistry and Public Health
University of Southern California School of Dentistry
Los Angeles, California

**S. MICHAL JAZWINSKI, Ph.D.**

Department of Biochemistry and Molecular Biology
Louisiana State University Medical Center
New Orleans, Louisiana

**JUDITH A. JONES, D.D.S., M.P.H.**

Director, Geriatric Dental Program
Veterans Affairs Medical Center
Bedford; Assistant Professor
Harvard School of Dental Medicine
Boston, Massachusetts

**H. ASUMAN KIYAK, M.A., Ph.D.**

Professor, Department of Oral and
    Maxillofacial Surgery and Psychology
University of Washington
Seattle, Washington

**BARNET M. LEVY, A.B., D.D.S., M.S.**

Clinical Professor, School of Medicine
University of California at San Diego
La Jolla, California;
Professor Emeritus, Oral Pathology
University of Texas at Houston, Dental Branch
Houston, Texas

**ROSEANNE MULLIGAN, D.D.S., M.S.**

Associate Professor and Chairwoman
Department of Dental Medicine and Public Health
University of Southern California School of Dentistry
Los Angeles, California

**LINDA C. NIESSEN, D.M.D., M.P.H., M.P.P.,
    F.A.C.D.**

Associate Professor, Department of Community and
    Preventive Dentistry
Baylor College of Dentistry
Dallas;
Veterans Affairs Medical Center
Dallas, Texas

**LONNIE H. NORRIS, D.M.D., M.P.H.**

Associate Professor of Oral and Maxillofacial Surgery
Tufts University School of Dental Medicine;
Surgical Staff, New England Medical Center Hospital
Boston, Massachusetts

**CAROLE A. PALMER, Ed.D., R.D., A.C.D.**

Associate Professor
Tufts University School of Dental Medicine
Boston, Massachusetts

**ATHENA S. PAPAS, D.M.D., Ph.D., F.A.C.D.**

Assistant Professor and Co-head, Division of Geriatric
    Dentistry
Tufts University School of Dental Medicine
Boston, Massachusetts

**CATHY A. PAVLATOS**

Formerly Manager
Department of Marketing and Seminar Services
American Dental Association
Chicago, Illinois

**HENRY ROTHSCHILD, M.D., Ph.D.**

Department of Medicine
Louisiana State University Medical Center
New Orleans, Louisiana

**MAUREEN C. ROUNDS, M.Ed., R.D.H.**

Assistant Clinical Professor
Tufts University School of Dental Medicine
Boston, Massachusetts

**JOSEPH M. SCAVONE, M.S., Pharm.D.**

Assistant Clinical Professor of Psychiatry
Tufts University School of Medicine;
Associate Professor of Clinical Pharmacy
Massachusetts College of Pharmacy and Allied Health
    Professions;
Assistant Professor of Community Medicine and
    Sociomedical Sciences
Boston University School of Medicine
Boston, Massachusetts

**ADRIANNE SCHMITT, M.Sc., D.D.S.**

Assistant Professor, Department of Prosthodontics
Faculty of Dentistry, University of Toronto
Toronto, Ontario, Canada

**DAVID SCHWAB, Ph.D.**

Marketing Consultant, David Schwab and Associates
Evanston; Formerly Director of Marketing
American Dental Association
Chicago, Illinois

**JONATHAN A. SHIP, D.M.D.**

Senior Investigator
Clinical Investigations and Patient Care Branch
National Institute of Dental Research
Bethesda, Maryland

**JON B. SUZUKI, D.D.S., Ph.D.**

Dean, School of Dental Medicine
University of Pittsburgh
Pittsburgh, Pennsylvania;
Clinical Professor
Department of Periodontics and Microbiology
University of Maryland
Baltimore, Maryland

**JOSEPH I. TENCA, A.B., D.D.S., M.A.**

Professor and Chairman, Department of Endodontics
Tufts University School of Dental Medicine
Boston, Massachusetts
Diplomate, American Board of Endodontics

**THOMAS J. VERGO, Jr., D.D.S.**

Professor and Division Head, Maxillofacial Prosthetics
Tufts University School of Dental Medicine
Boston, Massachusetts

**ANDY WOLFF, D.M.D.**

Lecturer, Department of Prosthetic Dentistry
Tel-Aviv University, School of Dental Medicine
Ramat Aviv, Israel

**GEORGE A. ZARB, B.Ch.D. (Malta), D.D.S., M.S. (Michigan), M.S. (Ohio State), FRCD (Canada), Dr. Odont. (H.C.)**

Professor and Chairman, Department of Prosthodontics
Faculty of Dentistry, University of Toronto
Toronto, Ontario, Canada

*"It is not enough for a great nation to have added new years to life. Our objective must be to add new life to those years."*

**John F. Kennedy**

*In memory of*
**Dr. Maury Massler**
a mentor to us all.

*In memory of*
**Dr. Elias Stavropoulos Stevens**
my father, who inspired me to enter the field of dentistry.

*To my husband*
**Dr. Arthur Papas**
for his support, patience, and understanding.

A.S.P.

*To*
**John, Devin, and Owen**
for adding lots of life to the years.

*To*
**Nan**
for sharing the joy of her years during my life.

L.C.N.

*With deep appreciation to my colleagues in*
**the Department of Veterans Affairs and the
National Institute of Dental Research**
for their continued encouragement and assistance.

H.H.C.

# In Memoriam
# HOWARD H. CHAUNCEY, PhD, DMD

The untimely death of Dr. Howard Chauncey reminded all involved in the preparation of this text of the fragility of life. Sudden death causes one great pause, and in the reflection after such an occasion, one often takes inventory of the daily gifts life offers. The life of Dr. Howard Chauncey offered many gifts.

Bostonians always like to regard themselves as pioneers. Dr. Chauncey was no exception. However, in his case the perception and the reality were consonant. He was a pioneer. He entered dentistry with a PhD first and then pursued his DMD. His gift to dentistry was his love of dental research. His gift to colleagues and students was his ability to serve as friend, mentor, teacher, and advisor. To the editors and many contributors of this textbook, Dr. Chauncey served in one or all of these roles.

To those of us in the VA, Dr. Chauncey was a pioneer in VA research. His stewardship of the "Dental Longitudinal Study" of the VA's Normative Aging Study gained him prominence both nationally and internationally. He was one of the first dentists to serve as Associate Chief of Staff for Research. His understanding of the VA as an organization was impressive to those both inside and outside of the VA. He had a remarkable facility for making the organization work and viewed the bureaucracy as an opportunity, never an obstacle. His gift of sharing that knowledge and expertise readily with any who would ask and listen benefited many investigators new to the VA. He leaves behind a national treasure in the Dental Longitudinal Study, which will continue to expand our horizons in the understanding of oral health and aging for years to come.

As a dental educator, Dr. Chauncey was a pioneer at two of the schools of dental medicine in Boston, Tufts, where he received his dental training and started his dental career, and Harvard, where he served as a faculty member. His gift to students at all levels was his willingness to share his dedication and commitment to dental research.

As a pioneer and senior statesman in geriatric dentistry, Dr. Chauncey did much to encourage, support, nurture, cajole, and humor this developing field. His advice, both sought and unsought, was given graciously. His purple pen (affectionately known to Dr. Chauncey by his coeditors and contributors as *"Howard and His Purple Crayon"* from the children's book) equally frustrated the new investigator and the seasoned investigator. But it always improved the manuscripts and grant proposals of both.

Dr. Chauncey's dedication to dentistry, particularly dental research, will serve as his legacy. For Dr. Chauncey, his family included his many friends and colleagues in dental education and in the VA and the NIDR, as evidenced by his dedication in this textbook. The publication of this textbook is a testimonial to Dr. Chauncey's pioneering spirit in the field of geriatric dentistry and his gift to friends, colleagues, and students—past, present and future.

LCN
ASP

# Preface

*One of the best ways to assess the overall quality
of a nursing home would be to determine the
proportion of residents who have properly fitted
dentures or the proportion needing them who
have dentures at all.*

BRUCE VLADECK: *Unloving Care,*
New York, 1980, Basic Books

Older Americans are healthier, wealthier, and more dentate than previous generations were. This statement by Bruce Vladeck in 1980 addressed the relationship of oral health to nursing home quality. However the majority of older adults do not live in nursing homes and now have some natural dentition. Examining a proportion of nursing home residents to determine their denture status will no longer serve as the quality assurance indicator that it once would have. Oral health for older adults has now come to represent maintenance of one's natural dentition throughout one's lifetime.

This book is about people—those who are aging, particularly people over the arbitrary age of 65 years, and those who in the course of daily living will visit their dental hygienists and dentists. Like the specialty of pediatric dentistry, geriatric dentistry focuses on the individual patient, not a specialized set of dental techniques or procedures.

This book is for people—the oral health practitioners who will be caring for patients in the next century.

This change in society's expectations about oral health and aging is but one of the changes expected to occur over the next 40 years. By 2030, or the practicing life span of dental students reading this book, one fourth of the US population is estimated to be over 65 years. Robert Butler, former director of the National Institute on Aging, estimated that three fourths of the practice of today's medical students will be composed of older adults. Similarly the majority of patients in a general dental practice in the twenty-first century will consist of older adults.

The challenges of caring for an aging population are many and varied. This book addresses the oral health issues that dental professionals will face as they care for this aging population. The purpose of this book is to serve as a starting point for dental practitioners interested in aging and its implications for oral health. The contributors to this book have been most perceptive regarding future needs and demands of older adults. The contributors have focused on subjects that encompass a spectrum of information relevant to the etiology, diagnosis, prevention, and management of oral diseases in older adults.

The book is divided into three sections. Part One provides an overview of the aging process and how it affects oral health. Part Two addresses issues concerned with providing oral health care to older adults. This part reflects the wide array of services that older adults will need and demand as they maintain their natural dentitions for a lifetime. Part Three addresses management issues that arise in caring for this population. It is our hope that this book will improve dental professionals' knowledge and interest in oral health and aging and ultimately improve the oral health care provided to patients.

• • •

The editors would like to thank all the contributors to this textbook. Without their willingness to participate and to share their expertise, this book could not have come to fruition.

The editor (ASP) is grateful to Susan Sharp for her support and typing while this book was being prepared.

The editor (LCN) would like to thank Ms. Shirley Scott and Dr. Philip Levinson at the VA Medical Center in Perry Point, Maryland, and Drs. Warren Parker and Dominick DePaola at the Baylor College of Dentistry for their support during the preparation of this textbook. The editor would also like to thank Dr. John Lipkin for his encouragement in this endeavor.

The editors would like to acknowledge Sandy Reinhardt, Susie Baxter, and Carl Masthay of Mosby–Year Book, Inc., and Dr. Sidney Epstein for their efforts in bringing this manuscript from an idea to a reality. There are few rewards for the editorial staff, but expertise and friendship are the gifts they provided to us.

**Athena S. Papas**
**Linda C. Niessen**
**Howard H. Chauncey**

# Contents

# PART ONE

# Overview of Aging

# 1

# Facing the Challenge: The Graying of America

*Linda C. Niessen*
*Judith A. Jones*

The United States is undergoing a major demographic change—the aging of its population. There are more Americans today over 60 years of age than under 10.[10] The average American now has more parents than children. How will this demographic change affect dental practice in the future?

The approaching turn of the millennium presents many tough new challenges in health care and dentistry. How to identify and meet the health care needs of the elders of tomorrow is not the least of these. Because a dramatic increase is expected in both the number and percent of Americans 65 years of age and older over the next three decades, health practitioners from all disciplines must be cognizant of special problems presented by this segment of the population. Dr. Robert Butler, former director of the National Institute on Aging, noted that when today's medical students reach the prime of their careers they will find themselves spending as much as 75% of their practice time with older people.[10] This will also be true of dentists, nurses, pharmacists, and health administrators.[32]

Before one considers the problems of clinical care and even concepts of normal versus pathologic aging, however, it is important to understand why so much attention is currently being focused on the older segments of our population. This chapter delineates the demographic changes in our society that compel us to focus our attention on the older generations. It then presents the principles of geriatric medicine and their implications for dental care delivery to elders. Finally, it explores the concepts of normal, usual, and successful aging as a guiding paradigm for future research in geriatric dentistry.

## DEMOGRAPHICS

The past 90 years have borne witness to a dramatic increase in the older segment of American society. At the turn of the twentieth century, 3.1 million Americans were 65 years of age and older.[1] By 1980, 25.5 million (11.3%) Americans were 65 years of age and older (Table 1-1).[33-37] Over the next three decades elder segments of American society are expected to continue to grow. The percent of the population who are 65 and above is expected to peak between 2030 and 2040, when the post–World War II baby-boom generation will compose the eldest segments of the population.

What factors have contributed to these dramatic changes that span this century? Declines in infant mortality, mortality associated with childbirth, and deaths attributable to infectious diseases have had a significant impact on life expectancy.[14] Thus life expectancy at birth has increased from 54 years in 1920 to 75 years in 1985 (Table 1-2).[34] Improvement in nutrition, health care, and life-styles have similarly made a contribution, such that not only has there been an increase in life expectancy at birth but also at 65 years of age (Table 1-3).[14,35] These changes in life expectancy and population

3

**Table 1-1** Persons 65 years of age and older by race, national origin, and year, USA, 1980-2020
Number of persons in millions (percentage of population of all ages per race in parentheses)

| Years | All races | Black | White | Hispanic |
|---|---|---|---|---|
| 1980 | 25.5 (11.3%) | 2.1 (7.8%) | 22.9 (12.1%) | 0.7 (4.9%) |
| 1990 | 31.6 (12.6%) | 2.6 (8.4%) | 28.3 (13.5%) | 1.1 (5.7%) |
| 2000 | 34.9 (13.0%) | 3.1 (8.9%) | 30.8 (13.9%) | 1.7 (6.8%) |
| 2010 | 39.4 (13.9%) | 3.9 (9.9%) | 34.0 (14.8%) | 2.5 (8.0%) |
| 2020 | 52.1 (17.7%) | 5.6 (13.3%) | 44.1 (18.8%) | 3.9 (10.6%) |

**Table 1-2** Life expectancy at birth

| Year | Females | Males | Total |
|---|---|---|---|
| 1920 | 54.6 | 53.4 | 54.1 |
| 1940 | 65.2 | 60.8 | 62.9 |
| 1960 | 73.1 | 66.6 | 69.7 |
| 1980 | 77.5 | 70.0 | 73.7 |
| 1985 | 78.8 | 71.2 | 74.7 |

Data from US Bureau of Census, Gregory Spencer: Current Population Reports, series P-25, no. 995, Projections of the Hispanic population: 1983-2080, Washington, DC, 1986, US Government Printing Office.

**Table 1-3** Life expectancy at 65 years of age

| Year | Female | Male |
|---|---|---|
| 1949-1951 | 15.0 | 12.8 |
| 1959-1961 | 15.9 | 13.0 |
| 1970 | 16.9 | 13.0 |
| 1980 | 18.5 | 14.2 |

Data from the National Center for Health Statistics: US Tables and Actuarial Tables 1949-51 and 1959-61; Vital Statistics of the United States, annual; and unpublished data.

**Table 1-4** Median age of population by race, national origin, and year, USA, 1980-2020

| Year | All | Black | White | Hispanic |
|---|---|---|---|---|
| 1980 | 30.0 | 24.9 | 30.9 | 23.2 |
| 1990 | 33.0 | 28.1 | 33.9 | 26.3 |
| 2000 | 36.4 | 30.7 | 37.5 | 28.0 |
| 2010 | 39.0 | 32.8 | 40.3 | 29.3 |
| 2020 | 40.2 | 35.2 | 41.5 | 31.2 |

structure will result in the median age of the population increasing over the next 50 years (Table 1-4).[33-37]

**Young-old, old, and old-old**

Gerontologists separate persons who are 65 and older into three categories: the young-old (65-74), the old (75-84), and the old-old (85 and over). The old-old cohort is not only the fastest growing segment of the elderly, but also of the entire United States population. In 1980, 1% of the population, or 2.2 million people, were 85 and over. By the year 2030, persons 85 and older will comprise 2.9% of the population, or 8.8 million people.[20]

**Gender**

The aging of the population has been described as a "women's issue." The increased life expectancy of women at virtually every age (Tables 1-2 and 1-3) contributes to the gender gap. Table 1-5 lists the number of men for every 100 women at 55, 65, and 75 years of age and illustrates the extent of the gender gap.[26]

**Race**

Approximately 90% of older persons in the USA are white, 8% are black, and 2% are of other races, such as American Indians and Asians.[17] Three percent of the population are Hispanics, who may be of any race. As blacks, Asians, and Hispanics age, their numbers are expected to increase in the future (Table 1-1).

**Marital status**

In 1987, 51% of women over 65 years of age were widows. The number of widows is about five times

**Table 1-5** The gender gap

| Age | Men | Women |
|-----|-----|-------|
| 55 | 100 | 100 |
| 65 | 100 | 123 |
| 75 | 100 | 246 |

Data from the National Institute on Aging: Publication no. 88-2899, Washington, DC, 1988.

the number of widowers (8.1 million compared to 1.6 million). Older men are twice as likely to be married as older women (77% of men compared to 41% of women).[2]

**Geographic distribution**

Florida leads the nation in the percentage of older Americans with 17.8% of its population over 65 years of age. About half of older Americans live in eight states: California, New York, Florida, Illinois, Michigan, Ohio, Pennsylvania, and Texas (also the states with the largest populations). Although dental practitioners in these states can expect to see a certain percentage of older patients, states such as Alaska, Nevada, Hawaii, Arizona, New Mexico, South Carolina, Delaware, Utah, and North Carolina have the fastest rate of increase in the older population. For example, Alaska, though a small state populationwise, has experienced a 63% increase in its older adults in the past decade.

**Living arrangements**

The majority (67%) of older Americans live in a family setting in the community. Approximately 60% of women and 80% of men live in family arrangements: these percentages decrease with age. Of the 19 million households headed by older persons, 75% are owners whereas 25% are renters. Of home owners, approximately 80% owned their home free of any mortgage payment.

Women are more likely than men to be living alone, with 41% of older women compared to 16% of older men. Women are also more likely than men to be living with another, that is, not a spouse. Twenty percent of women and 10% of men live with a person other than a spouse.

Although one in four elders will spend some part of their life in a nursing home, another 10% are estimated to be homebound.[14] Only 5%, or 1 million, older adults live in nursing homes or long-

term care institutions.[13] This proportion varies by age, with 2% of the 65 to 74, 6% of the 75 to 84, and 22% of persons 85+ living in nursing homes. For those elders in a nursing home or homebound, access to dental care may be difficult. However, for the majority of the elderly, dental care will continue to be provided as it has in the past, on an outpatient basis in private dental offices.

**Income and education**

The median income of older men was $11,854 and $6,734 for women in 1987. Blacks had approximately half the income of whites. Median personal income of the 65+ population varies by age group with the 65 to 69 year olds having the highest median income and those over 80 years having the lowest.[16] Income of the elderly is expected to continue to increase as those 55 to 64 year olds prepare for their retirement years. In addition, 30 to 50 year olds are preparing financially for retirement with IRAs, Keoughs, and other retirement plans. Resultant increases in median income should translate into a higher disposable income, eliminating for some the financial barrier to receiving needed dental care.

Social Security payments have had a major impact on the income of the elderly for two reasons. First, more elderly are receiving payments, and second, the average of payment has increased in real terms. In 1984, 91% of aged household units (couples or single persons) received benefits compared to 69% in 1962.[20] In addition, the average monthly benefit in constant 1984 dollars for retired workers increased from $257 in 1960 to $461 in 1984.[41]

Social Security benefits, however, were never intended to be the sole source of income in retirement. Rather, they were designed to supplement pensions and assets accrued during one's lifetime. Over time, private pensions and assets have become an increasingly important source of income for the elderly.

Although financial status of older adults is improving, poverty is still a problem for certain segments of older adults. Although the white population has a poverty rate of 11%, older Hispanics have a poverty rate of 21%, and older blacks, 32%.

As income of the elderly increases, so will the education levels of the elderly. In a recent survey in Iowa, the so-called new elderly (age 60-64) had higher educational levels than the old elderly (age 75 and over).[17] The educational level of the elderly will continue to increase as each succeeding cohort is better educated than its predecessors.[15] Since income and education levels are highly related to one's dental expectation and use of care, future cohorts of elders will expect to maintain their natural dentition throughout their life and be more likely to seek dental services.

### Use of dental services

Although the elderly had the lowest rate of dental visits of any age group from 1963-1964 to 1984, the use of dental services by the elderly has increased more than any other age group during that period. In 1963, the elderly averaged 0.8 visits per person per year, with the visits made by only 20% of the elderly.[25] By 1983, the rate had increased to 1.5 visits per person, with 43% of the elderly having visits.[24] The use rate of the elderly will continue to increase in the coming years as middle-age adults with higher income and education levels and consequently higher dental care expectation levels reach 65 years of age.

In summary, the US population is aging rapidly. As the population ages, each age cohort will bring a different set of expectations about oral health to the dental practitioner. Although their expectations cannot be predicted and will vary from person to person, as a group, these people will (1) be better educated than previous generations of older adults; (2) have higher expectations about maintaining and preserving their natural dentition, and (3) have the financial resources to meet their expectations. They will, however, be variable in their oral health needs and their demands; thus the desire to stereotype them will do a disservice to you and to them.

## MEDICAL IMPLICATIONS OF AN AGING POPULATION: PRINCIPLES OF GERIATRIC MEDICINE

As the population ages, more people will suffer from any number and combination of acute and chronic diseases. Geriatric medicine has provided a foundation for addressing the medical conditions of this population, sometimes referred to as the "principles of geriatric medicine" (see box). This section is a discussion of each issue and its implications for dental care for older adults.

---

### PRINCIPLES OF GERIATRIC MEDICINE

Age-related changes
Disease-related changes
Atypical presentation of disease
Multiple pathologic conditions
Underreporting of disease
Importance of functional status
Role of interdisciplinary team

---

### Age-related changes

Gerontology is the study of aging in all its aspects: biologic, physiologic, sociologic, psychologic. Aging refers to the irreversible and inevitable changes that occur with time. Before understanding the pathogenesis and etiology of disease one must first understand the normal aging process. Gerontologic studies or studies of normal aging allow one to distinguish healthy aging from the effects of disease. This is essential to avoid confusing aging with disease.

Perhaps the most common (mis)perception of the aging oral cavity centered on the issue of whether tooth loss was part of the normal aging process. For generations, indeed centuries, people believed that tooth loss was inevitable in advanced age. Distinguishing between aging and disease has enabled dental practitioners to explain to patients that tooth loss is the sequela of oral diseases, not merely a result of the aging process.

Past studies on oral changes with age were often conducted using small numbers of subjects or subjects who were medically compromised, without describing their medical conditions.[5] Studies that compared nursing home residents with dental students often attributed the changes to aging and not medical status. Dental students were young and *healthy*, whereas nursing homes residents were not only old, but also *sick*. Thus observed differences were not necessarily the result of age but rather differences between healthy and sick sample populations. Longitudinal studies contribute to a better understanding of the differences between age-related and disease-related changes.

An example of an oral physiologic change with age that has benefited from improvements in research design is that of salivary gland function with age. At one time, salivary flow was believed to decrease as a result of aging. It is now generally accepted that in healthy, nonmedicated persons, parotid salivery flow rates do not decrease as a result of normal aging.[4,6] A decrease in functional reserve capacity of the salivary glands has been hypothesized to account for the contrast between morphologic changes with age and the lack of functional change.[29] This decrease in functional reserve capacity is noted in virtually all organ systems and accounts for the reason physiologic decreases are observed in organ systems yet individuals remain functioning even in late life.

Changes in the appearance of teeth occur with age. In the later decades of life enamel appears darker, thus increasing the desire for older adults to have tooth-whitening procedures. Additionally, tooth wear in response to use may result in clinical crowns shortening and a change in appearance. Alternatively, gingival recession or periodontal disease results in teeth increasing in size, the so-called "long of tooth" of literary note. Both short or long clinical crowns can be altered to improve a person's appearance. The cosmetic dentistry revolution is rapidly approaching the older population in an effort to alter these effects of aging on the dentition.

### Disease-related changes

Geriatric medicine refers to social, psychologic, and clinical aspects of disease in older adults. Table 1-6 lists the leading causes of death for men and women, from 35 to 75+ years of age. For men and women over 75, heart disease, cancer, cerebrovascular disease, and pneumonia with influenza are the top four causes of death.[31]

Chronic disease is defined as any condition lasting more than 3 months.[21] The frequency of chronic conditions increase with advancing age. Table 1-7 lists the proportion of the middle-aged and older adult population with various conditions. For the 65+ population, arthritis is twice as common as in the 45 to 65 year group and affects over half the population. The proportion of persons with chronic disabilities is 14% for all ages and increases to 39% for those 65 to 74 and to 66% for those 85+.[28]

Arthritis, hypertension, and heart disease affect at least one third or more of older adults. These chronic conditions, which have implications for dental practice, are common in the elderly. Knowledge of the pathophysiology of chronic diseases will be critical to the dental practitioners of the future. In addition, consultation with a patient's physician will be more common as dentists treat many more people with an array of chronic diseases.

People with chronic diseases are likely to be taking medications. Data from the National Center for Health Services Research show that the percentage of the population with at least one prescription medicine increases with age.[23] The mean number of prescriptions also increases with age from five in 19 to 24 year olds to a staggering 14 for the 65-and-over age group (Table 1-8). Knowledge of the medications used in the treatment of chronic diseases and an adequate medication history are critical to providing dental care to the aging population. Over 400 medications are known to have oral side effects. In fact, the standard of dental care will require that in addition to a thorough medical history the dentist should record all the prescribed and over-the-counter medications a patient of record is taking.

### Oral disease–related changes

The major oral disease–related change occurring in the United States population is the decline of edentulism. A recent survey by the National Institute of Dental Research (NIDR) of employed adults and senior citizens found that only 4% of employed adults and 41% of seniors were edentulous.[27] There are now more older adults with teeth than without teeth. This decline in tooth loss, however, results in an increasing number of seniors with natural dentition who will be at risk for caries, either coronal, recurrent, or root, and periodontal diseases.

Dental caries has not traditionally been perceived as a problem for the elderly. However, recent statewide surveys have found that decay rates were higher in some adult groups than in children.[7,18] The Iowa survey found that 30% of the dentate elderly had untreated coronal decay.[7]

Root caries is believed to be a greater caries problem in older persons. In fact, several small studies confirm this viewpoint.[3,38] More recently, the NIDR Adult Oral Health Survey found that 63% of men and 53% of women had evidence (either a decayed or filled root surface) of root caries.[27]

Although the prevalence of periodontal diseases

**Table 1-6** Mortality, 10 leading causes of death by age group and sex, USA, 1985

| | Ages 35-54 | | Ages 55-74 | | Ages 75+ | |
|---|---|---|---|---|---|---|
| | Male<br>All causes<br>116,814 | Female<br>All causes<br>65,635 | Male<br>All causes<br>460,728 | Female<br>All causes<br>308,728 | Male<br>All causes<br>421,525 | Female<br>All causes<br>566,374 |
| 1 | Heart diseases 35,091 | Cancer 27,001 | Heart diseases 181,126 | Cancer 106,299 | Heart diseases 177,192 | Heart diseases 258,426 |
| 2 | Cancer 25,733 | Heart diseases 11,530 | Cancer 136,869 | Heart diseases 100,642 | Cancer 79,220 | Cancer 78,921 |
| 3 | Accidents 12,875 | Accidents 4238 | Chronic obstructive lung diseases 21,465 | Cerebrovascular diseases 19,887 | Cerebrovascular diseases 34,934 | Cerebrovascular diseases 68,278 |
| 4 | Suicide 6053 | Cerebrovascular diseases 3360 | Cerebrovascular diseases 21,378 | Chronic obstructive lung diseases 12,795 | Pneumonia and influenza 21,483 | Pneumonia and influenza 27,518 |
| 5 | Cirrhosis of liver 5616 | Cirrhosis of liver 2463 | Accidents 10,800 | Diabetes 8712 | Chronic obstructive lung diseases 21,366 | Arteriosclerosis 13,265 |
| 6 | Homicide 4202 | Suicide 2105 | Cirrhosis of liver 9014 | Accidents 5965 | Accidents 7685 | Chronic obstructive lung diseases 12,201 |
| 7 | Cerebrovascular diseases 3686 | Diabetes 1377 | Pneumonia and influenza 8805 | Pneumonia and influenza 5153 | Arteriosclerosis 6607 | Diabetes 11,296 |
| 8 | Diabetes 1779 | Chronic obstructive lung diseases 1231 | Diabetes 7266 | Cirrhosis of liver 4906 | Diabetes 5829 | Accidents 8703 |
| 9 | Pneumonia and influenza 1712 | Homicide 1207 | Suicide 5302 | Nephritis 3181 | Nephritis 5808 | Nephritis 6874 |
| 10 | Chronic obstructive lung diseases 1441 | Pneumonia, influenza 958 | Aortic aneurysm 5271 | Septicemia and pyemia 2424 | Aortic aneurysm 4424 | Septicemia and pyemia 5,935 |

Data from Silverberg E and Lubera JA: Cancer statistics 1989, CA 39(1):9, 1989.

increases with age, it is not clear that the severity of the diseases increases in older adults. The Iowa and North Carolina state surveys suggest that the prevalence of advanced periodontal disease in the white population may be lower than previously believed.[18-19] Data from North Carolina on the black population are showing periodontal disease to be more prevalent and the extent and severity of the disease also to be greater than in the white population.*

Data from the NIDR Adult Oral Health Survey[27] found that 66% of seniors had subgingival calculus and 47% had at least one site of bleeding gingiva.

---

*James D. Beck, personal communication, Chapel Hill, N.C., 1990.

**Table 1-7** Frequency of common chronic conditions in middle-aged and older persons in the USA

| Chronic condition | Ages 45-64 | 65+ |
|---|---|---|
| Arthritis | 25.0% | 53.0% |
| Hypertension | 24.0% | 42.0% |
| Hearing impairment | 14.0% | 40.0% |
| Heart conditions | 12.0% | 34.0% |
| Visual impairment | 5.5% | 23.0% |
| Diabetes | 5.7% | 8.3% |

Data from American Association of Retired Persons: A profile of older Americans, 1988, Washington, DC, 1989, the Association.

Ninety-five percent of seniors had attachment loss (defined as 2 mm or greater) with a mean attachment loss of 3.2 mm. Twenty-one percent of seniors had mesial pockets of 4 mm or greater.

With caries and periodontal disease occurring throughout life preventive efforts will continue to be indicated. Brushing and flossing techniques will need to be reinforced throughout one's lifetime and modified in cases of physical or mental disabilities that cause loss of neuromuscular or cognitive function such as stroke, arthritis, or dementia (see Chapter 17). New devices such as rotary electric toothbrushes, standard electric toothbrushes, or other oral hygiene aids will be indicated for these persons.

Self-applied fluorides are indicated for those elders with high coronal, root, or recurrent caries rates. The choice of fluoride, sodium fluoride versus stannous fluoride, and the vehicle, rinse versus gel, will be a decision best made by the dental team in consultation with the patient. The use of other antimicrobials, such as chlorhexidine and Listerine Antiseptic will also be indicated for selected patients.

Oral cancer is primarily a disease of the older adult. The estimated incidence rate for oral cancer is about 4% for males and 2% for females.[30] The incidence rates for oral cancer increases with age.[12] If incidence rates stay the same as the older population increases, oral cancer will become a more significant problem. The risk factors for oral cancer are tobacco and alcohol use. Educating patients about the signs and symptoms of oral cancer, its risk factors, and screening for early diagnosis will continue to be a priority of the dental team.

**Table 1-8** Percentage of people with prescribed medicines and mean number of prescribed medicines per person with at least one prescribed medicine, USA, 1977.

| Age | Percentage with at least one prescribed medicine | Mean number of prescribed medicines per person with at least one prescribed medicine |
|---|---|---|
| 19-24 | 53 | 5 |
| 25-54 | 59 | 7 |
| 55-64 | 69 | 12 |
| 65+ | 75 | 14 |
| TOTAL (ALL AGES) | 58 | 8 |

Data from the National Center for Health Services Research, National Health Care Expenditures Study: Prescribed medicines: use, expenditures and source of payment, PHS publ. 82-3320, 1980.

## Altered presentation of disease

Geriatric medicine has categorized diseases of older adults as (1) those diseases occurring more frequently in older adult and (2) those diseases that occur in patients of all ages but present unusually in older adults. This second group is the larger of the two categories.

Almost any disease that has a classic array of symptoms or signs will show few or even none of the characteristic findings. Symptoms in older adults often become vague and nonspecific. They include refusing to eat or drink, falling, incontinence, acute confusion, worsening dementia, weight loss, and failure to thrive.[9] Any of these symptoms may be suggestive of the worsening of disease and should never be attributed to aging. Examples of diseases that are likely to present nonspecifically include depression, drug intoxication, and myocardial infarction. The silent (presenting without chest pain) myocardial infarction (MI) is of grave concern in the dental office. It means that diagnosing an acute MI in the dental office will be considerably more difficult unless dental practitioners are trained to understand that an altered presentation of disease occurs in older adults.

Altered presentation of oral disease in older adults also occurs. The signs include altered appearance of phenytoin-induced gingival overgrowth, any combination of diseased teeth with or without replacement, or an array of oral lesions. Gingival overgrowth secondary to phenytoin use in young adults results in pink, firm, fibrous gingival tissue. In older adults the gingival tissue appears much more edematous and erythematous.

In addition, the acute exacerbation of a periapical infection appears to occur much less frequently in older adults, being replaced by a more chronic infection.

## Multiple pathologic conditions

Just as chronic disease increases with increasing age, the prevalence of multiple disease processes occurring in the same person also increases with age. An early Scottish study of adults over 65 years of age found on average they had 3.5 conditions per person.[39] Among older adults being admitted to the hospital, six conditions per person were identified.[40] The box lists the most common coexisting conditions in an American nursing home.[8]

For dental practitioners, the presence of multiple

| COMMON COEXISTING CONDITIONS IN THE ELDERLY | |
| --- | --- |
| Congestive heart failure | Urinary incontinence |
| Depression | Vascular insufficiency |
| Dementia | Constipation |
| Chronic renal failure | Diabetes |
| Angina pectoris | Sensory deficits |
| Osteoarthritis | Sleep disturbance |
| Osteoporosis | Adverse drug reactions |
| Gait disorders | Anemia |

Data from Besdine RW: Clinical evaluation of the elderly patient. In Hazzard WR, Andrus R, Bierman EL, and Blass JP, editors: Principles of geriatric medicine and gerontology, ed 2, New York, 1990, McGraw-Hill Book Co.

medical conditions warrants a thorough medical history and medication history. Often the best medication history is obtained when one asks the patient to bring all his or her prescription and over-the-counter medications to the dental office for the initial appointment. Additionally, it is essential to update the medical history at frequent intervals, such as every 3 months, since the medical history can change in short periods of time.

The presence of multiple diseases will make history taking more complex and more time consuming. The history should be taken in a quiet place with the patient comfortably seated. If the patient is an unreliable historian, the dental team will then need to rely on another, such as a spouse or caregiver for a medical history. One of the advantages of a dental practice located in a nursing home or hospital is that the patient's medical records are available to the dental treatment team. Consultation with the patient's physician or physicians is warranted if there is any question about the patient's ability to tolerate certain dental procedures.

Because of dentistry's role in the past, patients may not understand why the dentist needs to know about a person's medical status. A polite explanation of how oral diseases can affect systemic diseases and vice versa can answer the patient's inquiry and allay any fears.

In the case of diagnosing oral diseases, like medical conditions, it is not uncommon to treat an older adult who had multiple oral diseases, such as root caries, type III periodontal disease, and oral candidiasis. A thorough regular oral examination evaluating oral soft tissue and hard tissues and documenting periodontal status must accompany the medical and medication history.

### Underreporting of disease

Although older adults have often been deemed as chronic complainers by their family members, studies of symptom reporting by older people living in the community repeatedly show that older adults minimize their symptoms and do not report those symptoms to their physician.[22] Although older adults perceive and comprehend pain, often they do not report symptoms and subsequently do not receive timely treatment for their problems. One explanation for such behavior is that by underreporting symptoms, older adults are denying that disease may be occurring. Unfortunately, symptoms often portend serious disease, and the sooner it is treated, the better the prognosis may be.

Similarly patients may be reluctant to report symptoms to their dentists. Since oral cancer is a disease occurring primarily in older adults, persons must learn the warning signs of oral cancer and report any symptoms of these conditions to their dentists or dental hygienists. Patients also may be reluctant to express their desire for esthetic oral changes to improve their appearance. With this in mind, treatment planning should involve consideration of esthetic needs and where feasible offer such options to older adults.

Elder abuse is a condition that will always be underreported. Continual trauma to head and neck areas may occur but may not necessarily cause the person to come into contact with the health care system. Like child abuse, fractured teeth may precipitate a visit to the dental office. Depending on state laws, dentists may be required to report suspected cases of elder abuse.

### Importance of functional status

Functional loss means the person's ability to meet his or her daily needs and is measured by assessment of the activities of daily living (ADL). Activities of daily living include mobility, eating, toileting, dressing, bathing, and transferring. The instrumental activities of daily living measure a person's ability to function independently and include housekeeping, cooking, shopping, banking,

driving, or using public transportation.

An ADL of most concern to the dental team is the ability to eat. If a person can eat, it usually indicates that the person has sufficient upper arm mobility to perform oral hygiene procedures on a daily basis.

Instrumental activities of daily living of concern to the dental team include the person's independence in transportation. Does the person drive or must he or she take public transportation to the dental office? Does he or she rely on another for transportation? Time of day in scheduling the dental appointment may depend on transportation arrangements or the patient's medical condition. For example, diabetics are best scheduled in the morning, whereas arthritic patients may prefer afternoon appointments.

### Role of the interdisciplinary team

Caring for an aging population requires the dental team to become a member of the array of health care professionals who play a role in geriatric medicine. Although the extent of the interdisciplinary team can be experienced in private dental practice, nowhere can this be better accomplished than in a hospital or nursing home setting where the dental professional plays an active role in the overall health care treatment plan.

Consultations with physicians, nurses, pharmacists, physical therapists, and nutritionists may be required to meet the oral health needs of older adults. Conversely, these practitioners may seek consultation from you regarding conditions they observe in their patients. You should always answer consultations from other health care professionals in a timely manner and in legible writing, clearly indicating your objective findings, assessment, and plan.

### SUMMARY

Providing dental care to older adults will be a challenging and rewarding component to dental practice. It will include understanding normal aging, the pathophysiology of chronic diseases commonly seen in the elderly, and the pharmacology of various medications used in the treatment of these diseases. It will include understanding the interaction of systemic illnesses on oral health status, adequate diagnosis of oral diseases, and appropriate treatment planning. It will include the preventive dentistry emphasis that has decreased caries in children and the esthetic dentistry emphasis that has changed smiles in middle-aged adults. It may include practicing dentistry in a nursing home or making housecalls for a homebound patient. It will include working as part of the team of health care professionals, physicians, dentists, podiatrists, ophthalmologists, nurses, social workers, and nutritionists, all of whom provide a comprehensive array of services. Finally, it will include the compassion and kindness that is offered to all patients.

# REFERENCES

1. American Association of Retired Persons: A profile of older Americans, 1988, Washington, 1989, the Association.
2. American Geriatric Society: Geriatric review syllabus, Washington, 1988, the Society.
3. Banting D, Ellen RP, and Fillery ED: The prevalence of root surface caries among institutionalized older persons, Community Dent Oral Epidemiol 8(2):84, 1980.
4. Baum BJ: Evaluation of stimulated parotid saliva flow rate in different age groups, J Dent Res 60(7):1291, 1981.
5. Baum BJ: Research on aging and oral health: an assessment of current status and future needs, J Spec Care Dent 1(4):152, 1981.
6. Baum BJ: Salivary gland function during aging, Gerodontics 2:61, 1986.
7. Beck JD, Hunt RJ, Hood JS, and Field HM: Prevalence of root and coronal caries in a non-institutionalized older population, J Am Dent Assoc 111:964, 1985.
8. Besdine RW: Approach to the elderly patient. In Rowe JW and Besdine RW editors: Geriatric medicine, ed 2, Boston, 1988, Little, Brown & Co.
9. Besdine RW: Clinical evaluation of the elderly patient. In Hazzard WR, Andrus R, Brerman EL, and Blass JP, editors: Principles of geriatric medicine and gerontology, ed 2, New York, 1990, McGraw-Hill Book Co.
10. Butler R: Gerontology—a long neglected part of medicine, Forum Med 3:139, 1980.
11. Butler RN: Why survive: being old in America, New York, 1975, Harper & Row.
12. Cutler SJ and Young JL: Third National Cancer Survey: incidence data, National Cancer Institute monograph, Bethesda, Md, 1975.
13. Department of Health, Education & Welfare—National Center for Health Statistics: The National Nursing Home Survey, 1977. Summary for the US DHEW publ no (PHS) 79-1794, Hyattsville, Md, 1979, Public Health Service.
14. Department of Health and Human Services: Health—United States, 1982, DHHS publ no (PHS) 83-1232, Hyattsville, Md, 1982, Public Health Service.
15. Ettinger RL and Beck JD: The new elderly: What can the dental profession expect? Special Care in Dent 2(2):62, 1982.
16. Grad S (Department of Health and Human Services, Social Security Administration): Income of the population 55 and over, 1980, SSA publ no 13-11871, Washington, DC, 1983, US Government Printing Office.
17. Hooyman NR and Kiyok HA: Social gerontology, Boston, 1988, Allyn & Bacon, pp 474-498.
18. Hughes JT, Rozier RG, and Ramsey DL: The natural history of dental diseases in North Carolina, 1976-77, Durham NC, 1982, Carolina Academic Press.
19. Hunt RJ, Field HM, and Beck JD: The prevalence of periodontal conditions in a non-institutionalized elderly population, Gerodontics 1:176, 1985.
20. Institute of Medicine: America's aging: health in an older society, Washington, DC, 1985, National Academy Press.
21. Jack S and Ries P, editors: Current estimates from the National Health Interview Survey, United States, 1979, DHHS (PHS) 81-1564, Washington, DC, 1981, National Center for Health Statistics.
22. Leventhal EA, and Prohaske TR: Age, symptom interpretation and health behavior, J Am Geriatr Soc 34:185, 1986.
23. National Center for Health Services Research, National Health Care Expenditures Study: Prescribed medicines: use, expenditures and source of payment, PHS publ no 82-3320, Hyattsville, Md, 1982, Public Health Service.
24. National Center for Health Statistics: Current estimates from the National Health Interview Survey, United States, 1981, series 10, no 141, PHS publ no 82-1569, Hyattsville, Md, 1982, Public Health Service.
25. National Center for Health Statistics: Dental visits: volume and interval since last dental visit, United States, 1978 and 1979, series 10, no 138, PHS publ no 82-1566, Hyattsville, Md, 1982, Public Health Service.
26. National Institute on Aging: Publication no 88-2899, Washington, DC, 1988, the Institute.
27. National Institute of Dental Research: Oral health of United States adults: the national survey of oral health in U.S. employed adults and seniors: 1985-86, national findings, National Institutes of Health NIH publ no 87-2868, Hyattsville, Md, August 1987, US Dept. of Health and Human Services, Public Health Service.
28. Rabin DL: Waxing of the gray, waning of the green. In Institute of Medicine: America's aging: health in an older society, Washington, DC, 1985, National Academy Press.
29. Scott J: Structure and function in aging human salivary glands, Gerontology 5:149, 1986.
30. Silverberg E: Cancer statistics, CA 38:5, 1988.
31. Silverberg E and Lubera JA: Cancer statistics, 1989, CA 39(1):9, 1989.
32. Somers A and Fabian D: The geriatric imperative, New York, 1981, Appleton-Century-Crofts.
33. US Bureau of the Census: 1980 census of the population, vol 1, Characteristics of the population, PC80-1 United States summary, pp 91, 147, Washington, DC, US Government Printing Office.
34. US Bureau of the Census, Gregory Spencer: Current population reports, series P-25, no 995, Projections of the Hispanic population: 1983-2080. Washington, DC, 1986, US Government Printing Office, pp. 41, 43, 44.
35. US Bureau of the Census: 1980 Census of the population, vol 1, Chapter B (PC80-1-B); Current population reports,

series P-20, no 416; and unpublished data as presented in US Department of Commerce's Statistical abstract of the United States, 1988, ed 108, pp 14-17, Washington, DC, 1987, US Government Printing Office.

36. US Bureau of the Census: Current population reports, series P-25, no 1017, Projections of the population of states, by age, sex and race: 1988-2010, Washington, DC, 1988, US Government Printing Office, pp 29, 94, 95, 97, 99, 100, 101, 103, 105.

37. US Bureau of the Census, Gregory Spencer: Current population reports, series P-25, no 1018, Projections of the population of the United States, by age, sex and race: 1988-2080, Washington, DC, 1989, US Government Printing Office, pp 42, 43, 62, 63, 82, 83, 86, 87.

38. Vehkalahati M, Rajala M, Tuominen R, and Paunio L: Prevalence of root caries in the adult Finnish population, Community Dent Oral Epidemiol 11(3): 188, 1983.

39. Williamson J et al: Old people at home: their unreported needs, Lancet 1:1117, 1964.

40. Wilson LA et al: Multiple disorders in the elderly, Lancet 2:841, 1962.

41. Ycas MA and Grad S: Income of retirement-aged persons in the United States, Social Security Bull 50(7):5, 1987.

# 2

# Psychologic Aspects of Aging:

## Implications for dental care of the older patient

*H. Asuman Kiyak*

Age-related changes in sensory and cognitive functioning as well as the psychosocial changes and role losses that accompany aging are the focus of this chapter. In these functions, pathologic changes that impair an older person's ability to perform activities of daily living and may adversely affect his or her self-esteem, self-confidence, and coping abilities are addressed. Finally, the implications of these changes for communicating with elderly patients and their caregivers in the dental setting are emphasized. Through a better understanding of normal psychologic changes and potential impairments in these areas, the dental team can assist older persons in obtaining appropriate oral health care and can manage frail older patients with greater empathy and psychosocial skills.

## SENSORY CHANGES

There is a popular belief that, as we get older, we cannot see, hear, touch, taste, or smell as well as we did when we were younger, and it appears to be true. The decline in all our sensory receptors with aging is normal; in fact, it begins relatively early. We reach our optimum capacities in our twenties, maintain this peak for a few years, and

gradually experience a decline, with a more rapid rate of decline after 45 to 55 years of age. On the other hand, a few older persons may have better visual acuity than most 25 year olds; there are many 75 year olds who can hear better than younger persons. Changes in different senses occur at varying rates and degrees. Thus the person who experiences an early and severe decline in hearing acuity may not have any deterioration in visual functioning. Some sensory functions, such as hearing, may show an early decline. Yet others, such as taste and touch, change little until well into advanced old age. Over time, however, sensory changes affect older people's ability to negotiate with their social and physical world.

### Vision

Although the proportion of blind persons in old age is not significantly higher than among younger persons, the rates of impairments that affect some aspects of visual functioning increase with age. Vision problems increase with age; even when we compare 55 to 64 year olds with those over 85, there is a fourfold increase in the rate of visual impairments, from 55 per 1000 people to 225 per 1000.[2] As a result, older persons are more likely to experience problems with daily tasks that require good visual skills. Such tasks as reading small print or signs on moving vehicles, locating signs, or

This chapter was adapted from Hooyman N and Kiyak HA: Social gerontology: a multidisciplinary perspective, Needham Heights, Mass, 1988, Allyn & Bacon.

14

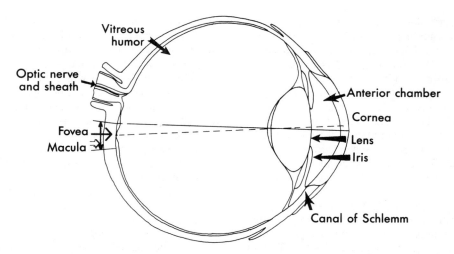

**Fig. 2-1** The eye. (From Hooyman N and Kiyak HA: Social gerontology: a multidisciplinary perspective, Needham Heights, Mass, 1988, Allyn & Bacon.)

adapting to sudden changes in light level can become extremely difficult.

Most age-related problems in vision are attributable to changes in parts of the eye. However, there is growing evidence that these problems are aggravated by changes in the central nervous system that block the transmission of stimuli from the sensory organs.[89,127] Changes in the visual pathways of the brain and in the visual cortex may be a possible source of some of the alterations that take place in visual sensation and perception with age (Fig. 2-1).

The cornea is usually the first part of the eye to be affected by age-related changes. The surface of the cornea thickens with aging, and the blood vessels become more prominent. The smooth, rounded surface of the cornea becomes flatter and less smooth and may take on an irregular shape. The older person's eye appears to lose its luster and is less translucent than it was in youth. In some cases, a fatty yellow ring, known as the *arcus senilis,* may form around the cornea. This is not a sign of impending vision loss; in fact, it has no impact on vision. It is sometimes associated with increased lipid deposits in the blood vessels.

At its optimal functioning, the pupil is sensitive to light levels in the environment. With aging, the pupil appears to become smaller and more fixed in

size. The maximum opening of the pupil is reduced in old age, commonly to about *two thirds* the original maximum. That is, the older person's pupil is less able to respond to low light levels by dilating or opening to the extent needed. The eye also responds more slowly to changes in light conditions. This problem is compounded by a slower shift from cones to rods under low-light conditions. As a result, the older person may have considerable difficulty functioning in low-light situations, or in adjusting to significant changes in ambient light. In fact, older people may need *three times more light* than young persons to function effectively.[93]

Problems in rod and cone function may be related to a reduced supply of oxygen in the retina; oxygen is necessary for the production of *rhodopsin,* which is a critical element in the functioning of rods. Some researchers have suggested that the slowing of rhodopsin production may be attributable to a deficiency of vitamin A. However, there is little research evidence to indicate that increased intake of vitamin A in old age can improve visual functioning under low-light conditions.

Perhaps the greatest age-related changes in the eye occur in the lens. With normal aging, the lens becomes less elastic, thereby reducing its ability to change form (that is, from rounded to elongated and flat) as it focuses from near to far. Muscles that help stretch the lens also deteriorate with age, thereby compounding the problem of changing the shape of the lens. Therefore *accommodation* begins to deteriorate in middle-age and is manifested in increasing problems with close vision. As a result, many persons in their forties may need to use reading glasses or bifocals. By 60 years of age accommodative ability is significantly deteriorated.[16] Decrements in accommodation may cause difficulties for the older person when shifting from near to far vision; for example, when looking across a room, walking up or down stairs, and when reading and looking up.

The hardening of the lens caused by changes in collagen tissue does not occur uniformly. Rather, there is differential hardening, with some surfaces allowing more light to enter than others. This results in uneven refraction of light through the lens and onto the retina. When combined with poor refraction of light through the uneven, flattened surface of the cornea, extreme sensitivity to glare often results. This problem becomes particularly acute in environments with a single source of light aimed at a shiny surface, such as a large window at the end of a long, dark corridor with highly polished floors, occasional street lights on a rain-slicked highway, or a bright, single, overhead incandescent light shining on a linoleum floor. These conditions may contribute to older people's greater caution and often anxiety while driving or walking. This also raises the need for greater caution in the dental practice with the use of dental lamps. It is critical to avoid aiming the light at the older patient's eyes. It is also important to position older patients so that they are not looking directly into a window in the dental operatory, especially on bright, sunny days.

Untreated glaucoma is the third leading cause of blindness in the United States, the United Kingdom and Canada,[1,62,68] and increases in frequency with age, from a rate of 1.4 per 100 at 52 to 64 years of age to 7.2 at 75 to 85.[57] This disease is caused by problems in the drainage of aqueous humor from the anterior chamber of the eye.

Unlike the aqueous humor, which drains and is replenished throughout life in healthy persons, the vitreous humor remains constant. With aging, it may thicken and shrink. Lumps of collagen, the primary content in this fluid, may be formed. Older persons who complain of "floaters" in the eye are responding to these free-floating formations in the front part of the eye. These changes, which cannot be prevented or treated, are often upsetting to those who experience them. Such persons should be assured that floaters do not cause blindness. Frequent examinations by an ophthalmologist are useful in the later years to check for such conditions and to determine if they may be caused by other diseases.

The lens is a transparent system through which light can easily enter. With normal aging, however, the lens becomes more opaque, and less light passes through, compounding the problems of poor vision in low light that were described earlier. Some older persons experience a more severe opacification to the point that the lens prevents light from entering. This condition, known as a "cataract," is the second leading cause of blindness in the United States.[62] Its incidence increases significantly with age. Thus, for example, in the Framingham Eye Study,[57] 4.5% of the sample 52 to 64 years of age had at least one senile cataract. Among those 75 to 85, 45.9% had a cataract in one or both eyes; this represents a tenfold difference between the two age groups. If the lens becomes totally opaque, cataract surgery may be required to extract the lens. One of the most frequently performed types of eye surgery, it carries relatively little risk, even for very old persons. Indeed, this is the most common surgical procedure performed on people over 65 years of age.[120] Researchers have found that patients who receive a lens implant show improvement not just in visual function, but also in objective assessments of ADL and manual function within 4 to 12 months.[4]

Depth and distance perception also deteriorate with aging because of inadequate convergence of images formed in the two eyes. This is caused by differential rates of hardening and opacification in the two lenses, uneven refraction of light onto the retina, and reduced visual acuity in aging eyes. (The problem of depth perception becomes compounded for people who have had cataract surgery and must use contact lenses or cataract glasses.) As a result, there is a rapid decline after 75 years of age in the ability to judge distances and depths, particularly in low-light situations and in the absence of orienting cues. Examples of situations with inadequate cues include stairs with no color distinctions at the edges, and pedestrian ramps or curb cuts with varying slopes and no cues to guide the user. The older driver who is undergoing changes in depth perception experiences increased problems when driving behind others, approaching a stop sign, or parking between other cars.

Loss of the central visual field occurs with macular degeneration. The macula is that point in the retina with the best visual acuity because it has the highest concentration of cones. *Macular degeneration,* the fourth major cause of blindness in the United States, occurs if the macula receives less oxygen than it needs, resulting in destruction of the existing nerve endings in this region. The incidence of macular degeneration, like cataracts, increases with age but even more dramatically. Of those persons 52 to 64 years of age in the Framingham study, 1.6% had signs of macular degeneration, compared to 27.9% of those in the 75 to 85 age group.[57]

### Hearing

In terms of survival, vision and hearing are perhaps our most critical links to the world. Whereas vision is important for getting around in the physical environment, hearing is vital for communication. Because hearing is closely associated with speech, its loss disrupts a person's understanding of others and even the recognition of one's own speech.

How does a person function if these abilities gradually deteriorate? Clearly, an older person who is experiencing hearing loss learns to adapt and make changes in behavior and in social interac-

tions, so as to reduce the detrimental social impact of hearing loss. Many younger hearing-impaired persons learn sign language or lip reading. But these are complex skills requiring extensive training and practice and are less likely to be learned by those who experience gradual hearing loss late in life (Fig. 2-2).

The supporting walls of the external auditory canals deteriorate with age, as is true for many muscular structures in the human body. Arthritic conditions may affect the joints between the malleus and stapes, making it more difficult for these bones to perform their vibratory function. *Otosclerosis* is a condition in which the stapes becomes fixed and cannot vibrate. It is sometimes found in young persons but more frequently occurs in the later years.

The greatest decline with age occurs in the cochlea, where structural changes result in *presbycusis,* or age-related hearing loss. Changes in auditory thresholds can be detected by 30 years of age or even younger, but the degeneration of hair cells and membranes in the cochlea is not observed until much later.[89] It is estimated that 13% of the population 65 and older in the United States suffer from advanced presbycusis. Another 40% to 50% have mild to moderate loss of hearing.[27,101,119] Both structural changes in the auditory system and those in the central nervous system appear to be responsible for the deterioration in auditory functioning. These may include cellular deterioration and vas-

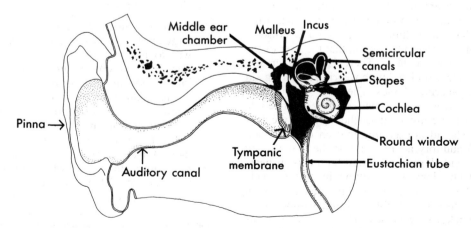

**Fig. 2-2** The ear. (From Hooyman N and Kiyak HA: Social gerontology: a multidisciplinary perspective, Needham Heights, Mass, 1988, Allyn & Bacon.)

cular changes in the major auditory pathways to the brain.[27] Hearing loss may also be caused by excess earwax, which seems to accumulate more rapidly in some older people. A thorough audiology exam should be done after a physician removes the earwax in these cases.

*Tinnitus* is another problem that affects hearing in old age. This is a high-pitched "ringing" that is particularly acute at night or in quiet surroundings. It may occur bilaterally or in one ear only. The incidence increases from 3% for younger adults to 9% for middle-aged persons and 11% among those 65 to 74 years of age.[101] Tinnitus is generally not associated with other types of hearing impairments; it cannot be "cured," but people suffering from tinnitus can learn to manage to tolerate or even ignore it. At times it may abate.

Hearing loss can be of several types, involving limited volume and range or distortion of sounds perceived. Older persons who have lost hearing acuity in the range of speech (250 to 3000 Hz) have particular difficulties distinguishing the sibilants or high-frequency consonants such as *z, s, sh, f, p, k, t,* and *g.* Their speech comprehension deteriorates as a result, which may be the first sign of hearing loss. In contrast, low-frequency hearing loss has minimal impact on speech comprehension.

Although hearing aids can assist many older persons with hearing impairments, hearing aids cannot completely obliterate the problem of presbycusis. In fact, they often result in such major adaptation problems that many older persons stop wearing them after several months of frustrated attempts to adjust to the device. A major difficulty with hearing aids is that the volume of background noise is raised, in addition to the sound that the user of the device is trying to hear. There is also a greater social stigma associated with wearing a hearing aid than with wearing glasses. These are undoubtedly some of the reasons why relatively few older people who are hearing-impaired use them. Hence the dental team should *not* assume that an older person has good auditory acuity if he or she is not using a hearing aid. Fortunately, developments in hearing-aid technology are resulting in custom-made designs that amplify only those frequencies that an individual user has trouble hearing, without magnifying background noises. These newer designs also are less obtrusive and fit well inside the ear. Unfortunately, however, their cost is also much higher, making them inaccessible to many low- and middle-income elderly persons.

There is a popular belief that hearing-impaired elderly tend to become more isolated and paranoid. In fact, researchers have found *no* association between hearing disorders and emotional distress in independent elderly.[79,124] Social involvement also does not appear to be impaired as a function of hearing disorders.[87,97] That is, older people with significant hearing loss are just as likely to remain active and socially integrated as their peers with less impairment in this area.

### Implications for communicating with elderly patients

Communication is the process of transmitting, perceiving, and interpreting information through verbal and nonverbal channels. Both the sender and the receiver of a particular message must possess certain skills. Verbal skills include the ability to express oneself both through the semantics and nuances of a language and the corresponding ability to perceive and correctly interpret the message. The receiver must also possess intact auditory and visual skills as a first step in perceiving the message accurately. We have seen, however, that older persons with hearing and visual declines may not be able to receive verbal messages accurately, thereby compromising the communication between dentists and patients. In this section I offer some recommendations* to the dental team to improve their communication skills, so that at least their ability as senders is enhanced:

1. When writing down a message, use bold, large print. This is a simple yet very effective way to assist the older person's visual function. But it is amazing how often oral health information aimed at the older person is written in small, illegible type or is even handwritten. The use of a bold, large print will necessitate condensing messages; this is an indirect benefit because it makes it more likely for the message to be read!

2. Use contrasting colors when preparing written messages. Blue letters against a pale yellow background are particularly effective.

---

*From Kiyak HA: Communication in the practitioner−aged patient relationship. In Holm-Pedersen P and Löe H, editors: Geriatric dentistry, Copenhagen, 1986, Munksgaard.

Even if black print is used, it can be effective as long as color contrasts are strong.

3. When speaking with aged patients, one can aid the patient's use of compensatory mechanisms by facing the patient directly and maintaining eye contact. This will permit older persons who have severe hearing loss to read lips if they have that skill and to block out extraneous sounds. It will also aid in orienting the person with poor visual function.

4. Standing closer to older patients than with younger patients may also aid their reception of information through auditory and visual channels. However, the dental practitioner must be sensitive to the fact that some older persons may react negatively to reduced distance between themselves and the dentist. The dentist must exercise good judgment in selecting the appropriate communication distance with aged patients.

5. Touch can be a valuable form of communicating with older persons in general but especially with people who are experiencing significant hearing and visual declines. It allows interpersonal barriers to be reduced and increases empathy between the speaker and the listener. As with reduced communication distances, however, touch may create discomfort for some older persons. To the extent that both the patient and the dental practitioner are comfortable with tactile contact during discussions, it is an excellent aid to communication.

6. The pattern and volume of speech must also be considered. Thus it will aid the older person's comprehension if the dentist and staff speak more slowly and clearly but of course without exaggerating each syllable. Speaking more distinctly will reduce the possibility of losing parts of speech or confusing some consonant phonemes such as *z, s, sh, t, th, f, p,* and *k*. Raising one's voice slightly may be helpful, *but there is no need to shout!*

7. For severely hearing impaired (but not deaf ) older persons, the dental team may choose to use a special device that allows older persons to place a receiver directly into their ears. The speaker then speaks directly into a microphone-like unit that blocks extraneous sounds.

8. Discussions with aged patients should be held in a quiet, unhurried environment. Thus, for example, the dentist's private office is a better environment in which to obtain the patient's health history, to listen to dental complaints, and to discuss treatment plans than the waiting room or the dental operatory is. A private office generally has fewer background noises and fewer conversations that can divert the patient's attention and allows greater privacy for older persons to express their thoughts in confidence.

9. Finally, it helps to avoid any physical barriers such as a desk between the patient and dentist. These obstacles increase the physical distance between the listener and speaker, as well as creating a psychological barrier, which may make it difficult for older persons who are unfamiliar with dental environments to express their concerns and questions.

## Taste and olfaction

Although older people may complain that food does not taste as good as it once did, these complaints are probably *not* attributable to an age-associated generalized loss of taste sensitivity. It was once believed that age brought dramatic decreases in the number of taste buds on the tongue, that this loss of receptor elements led to a functional loss that was experienced as a dulling of taste sensation, and that these changes account for older people's reduced enjoyment of food.[78] Recent studies, however, have challenged each link in this chain of reasoning.

Early research on taste anatomy reported taste bud loss,[5] but more recent studies show that the number of taste buds does not decline with age.[6,76] In addition, recent studies have also found less change in taste thresholds than previously believed.[10,28,128] Moreover, using sophisticated measurement techniques that control for differences between generations in the way they respond to an experimental task, researchers have found that threshold increases almost never involve more than one of the four basic taste qualities.

Thresholds reflect the ability of the sensory system to detect weak stimuli, but this aspect of taste function may be less relevant to the enjoyment of food than the ability to appreciate taste intensity. For example, older people with decreased taste-threshold sensitivity will require more salt to know if there is any salt on their vegetables. But to determine *how* salty the vegetables are requires a different taste mechanism that may still be functioning. This ability to appreciate the strength of a taste stimulus has been assessed by modern direct-scaling techniques; these studies have demonstrated that taste-intensity perception is remarkably robust with age.[125]

The notion that various functions decline differentially has replaced the belief that older people experience a generalized taste loss. The research task now is to specify which aspects of taste function remain intact and which decline with normal aging or disease.

One's appreciation of food does not depend on taste acuity alone. The sense of smell clearly is involved. We have all experienced changes in the way food "tastes" during a head cold with a stuffy nose. These changes indicate that sensitivity to airborne stimuli may play a key role in the perception of foods. Unlike taste acuity, there is considerable evidence for age-related declines in the sense of smell. When parallel assessments are made in the same older person, age-related declines for smell are greater than for taste. Older people perceive airborne stimuli as less intense than younger persons do, and they do less well on odor identification.[30,118] This finding indicates that one way to increase older people's enjoyment of eating may be to provide them with enhanced food odors.[105]

### Tactile sensitivity

Somesthetic receptors detect temperature, pressure, position, or movement and include also touch sensitivity, which deteriorates with age. This decline is partially attributable to changes in the skin and partially to a loss with age in the number of nerve endings. Reduced touch sensitivity is especially prevalent in the fingertips and palms and in the lower extremities.[56,126,130] An important aspect of touch sensitivity is pain perception. The elderly tend to be less able to discriminate among levels of perceived pain than young respondents. Studies of age differences in threshold levels of pain, however, have produced mixed results.[47]

It is important to distinguish between pain perception and pain behavior. Tolerance for pain is a subjective experience, which may be related to cultural and personality factors. In older people, increased complaints of pain may be a function of depression and psychosomatic needs. On the other hand, some people may attempt to minimize their pain by *not* reporting above-threshold levels of unpleasant stimuli. This is consistent with a frequently observed attitude among many older persons that pain, illness, and discomfort are necessary corollaries of aging. If fact, most elderly probably underreport actual pain experienced. For example, an older person may not report symptoms of a heart attack unless or until it is severe. These age differences in pain behavior are probably likely for differences in the clinically observed phenomenon among elderly dental patients that they are likely to tolerate painful dental procedures better than younger patients, sometimes even opting not to use a local anesthetic. It appears that older persons have similar thresholds for pain as younger persons have, but they can *tolerate* higher levels of pain.

The kinesthetic system lets the person know his or her position in space; adjustments in body position become known through kinesthetic cues. Because of age-related changes in the central nervous system, which controls the kinesthetic mechanism, as well as in muscles, older people demonstrate a decreased ability to orient their bodies in space and to detect externally induced changes in body position. Other physiological and disease-related changes, such as damage to the inner ear, may exacerbate this problem.

Not surprisingly, these changes in the kinesthetic system result in greater caution among older persons. They may take slower, shuffling, and more deliberate steps. Older people are more likely to seek external spatial cues and supports while walking. As a result, they are less likely to go outside in inclement weather for fear of slipping or falling. Some may complain of dizziness and vertigo, especially if they suffer from hypertension as well. These changes combine with the problems of slower reaction time, muscle weakness, and reduced visual acuity to make it far more likely for older people to fall and injure themselves. This makes it imperative for the dental team to look for signs of disorders in the kinesthetic system in their older patients and to assist these patients into and out of the dental chair. Because sudden shifts in body position can produce orthostatic hypotension, the dental team must also be cautious in the rate at which they raise or lower the dental chair.

## COGNITIVE CHANGES WITH AGING

One of the most important and most studied aspect of aging is cognitive functioning, that is, learning, memory, and intelligence. These are critical to a person's performance in every aspect of life, including work and leisure activities, relationships with family and friends, and ability to perform activities of daily living. Older people who have problems in cognitive functioning will eventually experience stress in these other areas as well, along with an increasing incongruence between their competence levels and the demands of their environments. Researchers have attempted to determine whether normal aging is associated with a decline in these three areas of cognitive functioning and, if so, to what extent such a decline is attributable to age-related physiological changes. Other studies have been undertaken in response to concerns expressed by many older persons or their families that they cannot learn as easily as they used to or that they have more trouble remembering names, dates, and places than previously. In this section some of the normal age-related changes in learning abilities and memory are examined.

### The process of learning and memory

Learning and memory are two cognitive processes that must be considered together. That is, learning is assumed to have occurred when a person is able to retrieve information from his or her memory store. On the other hand, if a person cannot retrieve information from memory, it is assumed that learning has not adequately taken place. Thus learning is the process by which new information (verbal or nonverbal) or skills are encoded or put into one's memory. Memory, in turn, is the process of retrieving or recalling the information stored in the brain when needed. Memory also refers to a part of the brain that retains what has been learned throughout a person's lifetime. For example, a person may have learned many years ago how to ride a bicycle. If this skill has been encoded well through practice, the person can retrieve it many years later from his or her memory store, even if he or she has not ridden a bicycle in many years. Although the exact location in the brain where memories are stored cannot be identified, research-

ers have attempted to distinguish among types of memory such as primary, or short-term, memory and secondary, or long-term, memory.

*Primary memory* is a temporary stage of holding and organizing information and does not necessarily refer to a storage area in the brain. Despite its temporary nature, primary memory is critical for our ability to process new information. We all have experienced situations where we heard or read a bit of information such as a phone number or someone's name, used that name or number immediately, and then forgot it. In fact, most adults can recall seven, plus or minus two, pieces of information (such as digits, letters, words) for 60 seconds or less. It is not surprising therefore that local phone numbers in most countries are seven digits or less! In order for this information to be retained in our permanent memory store (secondary memory), it must be rehearsed actively. In contrast, if we are distracted while trying to retain the information for the 60 seconds that it can last in short-term memory, we immediately forget it, even if it consists of only two or three bits of information. This happens because the rehearsal of such material is interrupted by the reception of newer information in our sensory memory.

As Poon[95] notes in a recent review of memory function with age, most studies of primary memory have found minimal age differences. For example, people 20 to 30 years of age have been found to recall 6 or 7 letters presented auditorily, compared with 5.5 letters by subjects in their seventies.[19] Differences that exist may be attributable more to increased reaction time with age than to a reduced capacity of primary memory.

True learning implies that the material we have acquired through our primary memories has been stored in *secondary memory.* This is the part of the memory store in which everything we have learned throughout our lives is kept; unlike primary memory, it has an unlimited capacity. Age differences in secondary memory appear to be more pronounced than in primary memory and are often frustrating to older people and their families. Indeed, there appears to be a widespread concern among middle-aged and older people that they cannot remember and retrieve information from secondary memory.[95] This perception that one has poor memory can seriously harm an older person's self-concept and his or her performance on many tasks, and it may even result in depression.[58,88] Such concern is generally out of proportion to the actual level of decline. These concerns often stem from fear of dementia, including Alzheimer's disease, that dramatically impair cognitive functions. Older people consistently recall less information than younger people do in tests with retention intervals as brief as 1 hour or as long as 8 months. However, older persons *can* benefit significantly from methods to help organize their learning, such as imagery and the use of mnemonics.

The learning process may be disrupted because of the inability to retrieve information efficiently from secondary memory. For example, a person may associate a newly heard name with someone known in the past. If he or she has difficulty retrieving the stored name from secondary memory however, this may be so frustrating as to redirect that person's attention from the new name to the old one. Aging appears to reduce the efficiency of processing information in primary memory and to reduce retrieval from secondary memory. It does *not* influence the storage capacity of primary or secondary memories. That is, contrary to popular opinion, these memory stores are not physical spaces that become overloaded with information as we age.

### Factors that affect learning in old age

One problem with assessing learning ability is that it is not possible to measure the process that occurs in the brain while a person is acquiring new information. Instead, one must rely on a person's performance on tests that presumably measure what was learned. This may be particularly disadvantageous to older persons, whose performance on a test of learning may be poor because of inadequate or inappropriate conditions for expressing what was learned.[18]

Time constraints are particularly detrimental to older people. Although the ability to encode new information quickly is a sign of learning ability, it is difficult to measure this ability. Instead, response time is generally measured, but psychomotor and sensory slowing with age has a significant impact on the older person's speed in responding. Researchers have shown that older persons make more *errors of omission* than *errors of commission*.[17,23] That is, older persons are more likely not to give

an answer than to guess and risk being wrong. This phenomenon was first recognized in middle-aged and older adults in tests of psychomotor functioning. The older the respondent in that study, the more likely he or she was to work for accuracy at the expense of speed. This occurs even when the older learner is encouraged to guess and told that it is acceptable to give wrong answers (that is, commission errors). This problem is particularly noteworthy in the dental setting when obtaining health and social histories of older patients. They are more likely to omit a medication from their list of current medications because they cannot remember its name or purpose and less likely to mention a drug they believe they are using but whose name they cannot recall. They also are less likely to risk guessing the dates of major surgery and to omit these and other health variables.

Verbal ability and educational level are important factors in learning verbal information.[50] Studies that entail learning prose passages have shown age deficits among those with average vocabulary abilities and minimal or no college education. In contrast, older persons with high verbal ability and a college education perform as well as younger subjects in such experiments. This may be attributable to greater practice and facility with such tasks on the part of more educated persons and those with good vocabulary skills. In fact, education and vocabulary skills are generally correlated and emerge as better predictors of performance in studies of prose learning than chronological age does.[74,98-99]

It is helpful to pace the information so that it is presented at a rate suitable to older learners and to give them opportunities to practice the new information. Another condition that supports learning is the presentation of familiar and relevant material compared to material perceived by the older learner to be unimportant. Recall of recently acquired information has been found to be worse in older persons than in younger when the new information is unfamiliar or confusing.[9,49] Similarly, greater age differences have been identified when the material to be learned was low in meaning and personal significance.[37] These characteristics of the learning condition make it imperative for the dental team to provide new information to older patients at a slower pace, integrating the new knowledge with the patient's existing store of dental information (such as linking flossing with toothbrushing, comparing fluoride rinse procedures with use of mouthwash). In all cases, it is crucial to provide information that has high significance to the older person; for example, it may not be appropriate to emphasize flossing with a frail older person who has never before flossed.

### Age-related changes in memory

As we have seen, learning involves encoding information and storing it into secondary or long-term memory, so that it can be retrieved and used later. Studies of this process have focused on two types of retrieval: recall and recognition. *Recall* is the process of searching through the vast store of information in secondary memory, perhaps with a cue or a specific, orienting question (for example, "List all the medications you are taking," "Describe how you do daily oral hygiene"). *Recognition* requires less search. The information in secondary memory must be matched with the stimulus information in the environment (for example, "Which of these three medications for depression are you using?"). Recall is demanded in essay exams, recognition in multiple-choice tests. Not surprisingly, most researchers have found age-related deficiencies in recall, but few if any differences in recognition.[52]

An area of considerable controversy in aging and memory function is the question of whether older people have better recall of events that occurred in the distant past than recent situations. Many events are firmly embedded in secondary memory because they are unique or so important that subsequent experiences do not interfere with the ability to recall them. The birth of a child, one's wedding ceremony, or the death of a parent, spouse, or sibling are events that most people can recall in detail 40 to 50 years later. This may be because the situation had great private significance or, in the case of world events, such as the bombing of Hiroshima or John F. Kennedy's assassination, had a profound impact on world history. Some distant events may be better recalled because they had greater personal relevance for the individual's social development than recent experiences or because they have been rehearsed or thought about more. Another possibility is that cues that helped the other person recall events in the past are less

effective in recalling recent occasions because of "cue overload."[107] That is, the same cues that were once helpful in remembering certain information are also used to recall many recent events. But the cues are so strongly associated with one's earlier life experiences that the newer information becomes more difficult to retrieve. For example, older people may have difficulty memorizing new phone numbers because the cues that helped them recall phone numbers in the past may be so closely associated with previous ones that they confuse recent phone numbers with old ones.

One problem in determining whether recall of distant events is really better than recall of recent events is the difficulty in validating an older person's memories. In many cases, there are no sources that can be checked to determine the accuracy of an older person's recollections.

Several theories have been offered to explain why older people may have problems with retrieving information from secondary memory. One explanation is that not using the information results in its loss (the disuse theory). This theory is the supposition that information can fade away or decay unless it is exercised, as in the old adage, "Use it, don't lose it." However, this explanation fails to account for the many facts that are deeply embedded in a persons's memory store and that can be retrieved even after years of disuse.

A more widely accepted explanation is that new information interferes with the material that has been stored over a period of many years. As noted earlier, interference is a problem in the learning or encoding stage. When the older person is distracted while trying to learn new information, it may not become stored in memory. Poor retrieval may be attributable to a combination of such distraction during the learning stage and interference by similar or new information with the material being searched in the retrieval stage. Although researchers in this area have not conclusively agreed on any of these explanations, the interference theory appears to hold more promise than others for explaining observed problems with retrieval.

Researchers have begun to examine older people's feelings about their memory failures and how they cope with these. For example, participants in a recent longitudinal study kept diaries of their experiences with memory. Older adults described more incidents in which they forgot names, objects, locations, and appointments, especially in nonroutine tasks. They also reported feeling more frustrated with a memory failure than younger people did.[24] This frustration may impair the older person's confidence in a learning or test situation, thereby negatively affecting performance in these cases. Indeed, older persons have been found to express less confidence in their response than the young in tests of recognition and recall.[8]

### Implications for communicating with elderly patients

The normal, age-related changes in learning and memory have numerous consequences for dental communication with and management of older patients. With greater awareness of declines in learning efficiency, especially among the less educated older persons, and with greater sensitivity to problems in recall and recognition memory on the part of their older patients, the dental team can provide more appropriate dental care and avoid misunderstandings in treatment and inaccurate health histories. The following recommendations may assist the dental team in enhancing their communication with the older person who is experiencing some problems with learning and memory. These techniques may also be helpful in communicating with elderly who are in the *early* stages of Alzheimer's or other irreversible dementias:

1. Structure the message being presented. It is important to organize information given to aged patients. Thus one may explain procedures for home care chronologically or in a step-by-step manner (for example, "Remove your dentures at night, brush them with nonabrasive toothpaste and a medium brush, place the dentures in a cup of tepid water overnight, and rinse your mouth"). Dental treatment planning may best be explained by procedure (for example, "We will first extract these teeth and then design a partial denture for them. We will begin to repair your lower denture at your next visit on March 21").

2. Do not present too much information at once. In an attempt to reduce information overload, the dental team must avoid the tendency to give all home care instructions and proce-

dures at one visit. The older person has a greater chance of retaining the information in secondary memory if the technique of successive approximations is used. Using this approach, one could explain procedures for home care of dentures first, followed by a description of care for natural teeth at the next visit. At a subsequent visit, one could review dietary habits and counsel the patient regarding nutritional deficiencies.

3. Take more time to listen to the older patient's complaints, to discuss dental procedures, and even to repeat the message. It is essential to allow more time to explain dental procedures to aged patients. This should include time for clarifying technical terms (note that "technical" often includes words such as "denture," "extract," and "mandible" for this generation of patients), for allowing the patient to ask questions at each step and even for asking the patient to recount specific points. This method of *active inquiry* has proved successful in the classroom; unfortunately, it is underused in the dental care setting.

4. Finally, it is useful to use multiple modes of communication. Information that is presented in a written format and reviewed orally by the dentist with the patient will be retained longer than talking to patients or giving them a written message "to read when you get home." This approach is also useful for alleviating the problem of reduced information retention caused by visual and auditory deterioration with age.

### PERSONALITY AND COPING

*Personality* may be defined as a set of innate and learned traits that influence the manner in which each person responds and interacts with the environment. A person may be described in terms of several personality traits, such as passive or aggressive, introverted or extroverted, independent or dependent. Personality may be evaluated with regard to particular standards of behavior; for example, an individual may be described as adapted or maladapted, adjusted or maladjusted.

Personality styles influence how we cope with and adapt to the external and internal changes we experience as we age. The process of aging involves numerous stressful life experiences. How an older person responds to these experiences in an attempt to alleviate such stress has an influence on that person's long-term well-being. In this section the life events that occur more frequently in old age and how older people have been found to cope with them are examined also.

### Erikson's psychosocial model

Most theories of personality have emphasized the developmental stages of personality and imply that the social environment influences development. However, there has been disagreement about whether this development continues through adulthood. Sigmund Freud's focus on psychosexual stages of development through adolescence has had a major influence on developmental psychology. In most of his writings, Freud suggests that a personality achieves stability by adolescence. Some personality theorists have agreed that personality traits remain stable after the teen years.[132] In contrast, Erik Erikson, who was trained in psychoanalytic

theory, moved away from this approach and focused on psychosocial development throughout the life cycle. According to his model, a person undergoes eight stages of development of the ego, with the final stage occurring in mature adulthood. At each stage a person experiences a major crisis or conflict; the conflicts of each stage of development are the foundations of successive stages. Depending on the outcome of the crisis associated with a particular stage, a person proceeds to the next stage of development in alternative ways (Table 2-1).

As shown in Table 2-1, a person in the last stage of life is confronted with the crisis of ego integrity versus despair. According to Erikson,[34] a person at this stage of development accepts the inevitability of mortality, achieves wisdom and perspective, or despairs because he or she has not come to grips with death and lacks ego integrity. A major task associated with this last stage is to integrate the experiences of earlier stages and to realize that one's life has had meaning, whether or not it was

**Table 2-1** Erikson's psychosocial stages*

| | Stage | Goal |
|---|---|---|
| I | Basic trust versus mistrust | To establish basic trust in the world through trust of the parent |
| II | Autonomy versus shame and doubt | To establish a sense of autonomy and self as distinct from the parent; to establish self-control versus doubt in one's abilities |
| III | Initiative versus guilt | To establish a sense of initiative within parental limits without feeling guilty about initiating |
| IV | Industry versus inferiority | To establish a sense of industry within school setting; to learn necessary skills without inferiority or fear of failure |
| V | Ego identity versus role diffusion | To establish identity, self-concept, and role within larger community, without confusion about the self and about social roles |
| VI | Generativity versus stagnation | To establish a sense of care and concern for well-being of future generations; to look toward the future and not stagnate in the past |
| VII | Ego integrity versus despair | To establish a sense of meaning in one's life versus despair or bitterness that life was wasted |

*Adapted from Hooyman N and Kiyak HA: Social gerontology: a multidisciplinary perspective, Needham Heights, Mass, 1988, Allyn & Bacon.

"successful" in a socially defined sense. Older people who achieve ego integrity feel a sense of connectedness with younger generations and need to share their experiences and wisdom with them. This may take the form of face-to-face interactions with younger people, counseling, sponsoring a young person or group of younger people, or writing memoirs or letters. Life satisfaction, or the feeling that life is worth living, may be achieved through these tasks of adapting a wider historical perspective upon one's life, accepting one's mortality, sharing experiences with the young, and leaving a legacy to future generations.

### Jung's psychoanalytic perspective

Carl Jung's model of personality also assumes changes throughout life, as expressed in the following statement from one of his early writings:

We cannot live the afternoon of life according to the program of life's morning, for what was great in morning will be little at evening, and what in the morning was true will at evening have become a lie (p. 108).[54]

Jung's model emphasizes stages in the development of consciousness and the ego, from the narrow focus of the child to the other-worldliness of the older person. But the development of personality need not always imply maturation and increased wisdom. As Jung[54] suggests, "The wine of youth does not always clear with advancing years; oftentimes it grows turbid" (p. 105).

Like Erikson, Jung examined the individual person's confrontation with death in the last stage of life. He suggested that life for the aging person must naturally contract, that the person in this stage must find meaning in inner exploration and in an afterlife. In contrast to the young, older persons have "a duty and a necessity to devote serious attention to (themselves). After having lavished its light upon the world, the sun withdraws its rays in order to illuminate itself" (p. 109).[54] Jung also focused on changes in archetypes with age. That is, according to Jung, all humans have both a feminine and a masculine side. An archetype is the feminine side of a man's personality (the anima) and the masculine side of a woman's personality (the animus). As they age, people begin to adopt psychological traits more commonly associated with the opposite sex. For example, older men may show more signs of passivity, whereas women may be-

come more assertive as they age, a change that has been confirmed through studies with diverse populations of elderly.

### Measuring personality across the life span

Researchers who have systematically examined personality in middle and old age have found support for Jung's observations regarding decreased sex-typed behavior in old age. David Gutmann,[43-44,46] who has studied personality across the life span in diverse cultures from a psychoanalytic perspective, has found a shift from active mastery to passive mastery as men age. In contrast, women appear to move from passive to active mastery. That is, in most cultures examined by Gutmann, young adult males tend to be more achievement-oriented and concerned with controlling their environments, whereas young adult women tend to be more affiliative and expressive. Gutmann found greater expressiveness, nurturance, and need for affiliation among older males than in younger men, whereas older women tended to be more instrumental and to express more achievement-oriented responses than young women.

Longitudinal research by Neugarten, Havighurst, and Tobin[85] among community-dwelling elderly is consistent with Gutmann's findings and has contributed to our understanding of many other age-related changes in personality and coping. Neugarten found that older men became more accepting of their affiliative, nurturant, and sensual side, whereas women learned to display the egocentric and aggressive impulses that they had always possessed but had not displayed during their younger years. Neugarten, similar to Jung, has suggested that these characteristics always exist in both sexes, but social pressure and societal values encourage the expression of more sex-typed traits in youth.

Contrary to popular stereotypes, aging is also associated with greater differences (individuation) among individuals; as persons age, they appear to develop unique styles of interaction. Neugarten and colleagues[85] suggested that people do not resemble each other more in old age but in fact become more differentiated because they grow less concerned about societal expectations.

Other age-related changes observed in these studies included shifts toward greater cautiousness and interiority, that is, a preoccupation with one's inner life and less extroversion. The movement toward interiority does not mean, however, that older persons become more religious. There is very little research evidence that we become *more* religious as we age. It may be that the current cohort of people over 70 years of age have always been more religious than younger cohorts.

Decreased impulsiveness and a movement toward using more sophisticated ego defense mechanisms with age have also been observed. For example, older persons tended to use less denial and more sublimation. Attitudes toward the world were also likely to change with age, but these were found to relate closely to personal experiences. For example, people do not necessarily become more conservative as they age. Based on generational (cohort) differences and personal experiences, some persons have become more liberal in their social perspective during the later years. Others have been more conservative than younger cohorts throughout their lives. These age-related changes in impulsiveness, types of defense mechanisms used, and attitudes have been supported in studies of personality by researchers examining a diverse variety of cultural and ethnic groups.[113,123]

### Self-concept and self-esteem

A major adjustment required in old age is the ability to redefine one's self-concept or one's image of the self as social roles shift and as new roles are assumed. For example, how does a retired dentist identify himself or herself upon giving up the work that has been that person's central focus for the past 40 to 50 years? How does a woman whose self-concept is closely associated with her role as a wife express her identity after her husband dies?

Many older persons continue to identify with the role that they have lost. Others experience role confusion, particularly in the early stages, when cues from other people are inconsistent with a person's self-concept. Still others may undergo a period of depression and major readjustment to the changes associated with role loss. These persons generally have not established independent self-concepts. To the extent that a person's self-concept is defined independently of particular social roles, one adapts more readily to the role losses that may accompany old age.

For an older person whose self-concept is based on social roles and others' expectations, role losses have a particularly significant impact on that person's self-esteem, that is, evaluation or feeling about his or her identity relative to some ideal or standard. *Self-esteem* is based on an emotional assessment of the self, whereas *self-concept* is the cognitive definition of one's identity. The affective quality of self-esteem makes it more dynamic and more easily influenced by such external forces as retirement, widowhood, health status, and reinforcements (both positive and negative) from others (such as respect, deference, ostracism). As a result, alterations in social roles and the loss of status that accompanies some of these changes often have a negative impact on an older person's self-esteem. Think, for example, of an older person whose "ideal self" is an independent individual. If this person is forced to rely on others for care because of a major debilitating illness such as a stroke or dementia, such a person is unwittingly robbed of this ideal, and self-esteem may suffer.

A person who experiences multiple role losses not only must adapt to the life-style changes associated with aging (such as financial insecurity, shrinking social networks), but must also integrate the new roles with his or her "ideal self" or learn to modify this definition of "ideal." Older persons who are experiencing major physical and cognitive disabilities simultaneously with role losses or, worse yet, whose role losses are precipitated by an illness (such as early retirement because of stroke or institutionalization because of Alzheimer's disease) must cope with multiple problems at a time in their lives when they have the fewest resources to resolve them successfully. Depression is not an uncommon reaction in these cases, as we will see in the next section. Other older persons may not experience such major emotional upheavals; nevertheless, their self-esteem may be affected. Some studies have shown a generalized decrease in self-esteem from 50 to 80 years of age, though others have found considerable variability in patterns of self-esteem.[61,69]

One method of overcoming these pitfalls is for the older person to learn to accept the aging process, its limitations and possibilities. That is, persons who realize that they have less energy and respond more slowly than in the past but that they can still participate in life will adapt more readily to the social and health losses of old age. It is critical to achieve this level of awareness without giving up on life, as some older persons do. Unfortunately, socialization into old age is not so easy as socialization into other stages because most people have few appropriate role models that they can emulate.[103] As a result, environmental feedback in the form of television advertising and negative remarks of family and friends may reinforce a person's internal slowing process and suggest that the older person must withdraw. It therefore appears important for the media and society to provide role models of older people who have adapted successfully to their aging and how they have done so. All too often, however, the images of "successful" aging are persons who have unusual athletic, intellectual, or artistic abilities or who have achieved extreme longevity in isolated societies. The typical older person often cannot identify with such people; hence, these "exceptional" people are not used by most individuals as role models of how *they* can adapt to old age.

**Stress, coping, and adaptation**

The process of aging entails numerous life changes. These changes, both positive and negative, place demands on the aging person's abilities to cope with and adapt to new life situations. Together with health and cognitive functioning, personality characteristics influence coping responses. Self-concept and self-esteem are two important elements that play a role in coping styles and may help explain why some older people adjust readily to major life changes, whereas others have difficulty with such transitions. Indeed, self-esteem, health, and cognitive skills all contribute to a person's sense of competence. Major life events and situations represent environmental stressors that place demands on a person's competence. These and other factors that influence adaptation in old age are discussed next.

The concept of cognitive appraisal is an assumption that a person who perceives a particular situation as a challenge (that is, a positive stressor) copes with it differently from one who views it as a threat (that is, a negative stressor). For example, an older woman who moves voluntarily to a retirement home may view it as an exciting and much-needed change in her life-style (a positive stressor) or she may resent the change as too demanding and disruptive (a negative stressor). In the former case, she will adapt more readily and will experience less negative stress than in the latter. On the other hand, if this person views the move as totally benign and does not expect it to place any demands on her, she will probably be unpleasantly surprised by the level of stress that she eventually encounters, no matter how minimal.

There has been much discussion among researchers about the nature of life events in the later years, the older person's ability to cope with them, and whether old age is associated with more or fewer life events than youth. Admittedly, many significant life events tend to occur more often in old age, such as widowhood, retirement, and relocation to a nursing home. Numerous other events generally take place in people's lives during youth and middle age. As noted earlier, many of these represent role gains or replacement, such as the role of student, voter, homeowner, marital partner, and worker. Both the nature of such roles and the novelty associated with assuming a social role for the first time result in major changes in a person's daily functioning and demand adaptation to the new situation. Table 2-2, adapted from the work of Pastalan,[92] illustrates the ages when many social roles are generally gained or lost. Some of the role losses that may occur with aging, such as retirement, are associated with a decline in social status. It would be worthwhile to examine the recent role losses of an older person who is experiencing a decline in self-esteem or a change in self-concept (Table 2-2).

The degree to which a person can anticipate an event may influence the stress produced by it and the ability to cope with it. Life events that are "on time" or are expected (such as death of a spouse after a long illness) are less stressful than unexpected events.[83-84] On the other hand, the loss of a spouse after a long illness has been found to result in more medical problems of the widowed spouse than sudden death or chronic illness of shorter duration.[39] This may be attributable to the cumulative effects of other stressors (such as the demands of caregiving) associated with the terminal illness that the surviving spouse could not resolve during the caregiving and anticipatory grieving stages. Thus the evidence is mixed regarding older people's ability to cope with on-time events. It may be that anticipatory coping does not take the place of coping with an event *after* it occurs. In addition, a

**Table 2-2** Continuum of role gains and losses

| Age | Event | |
| --- | --- | --- |
| 0 ---- | | |
| | Student | + |
| 10 ---- | | |
| | Consumer | + |
| | Driver | + |
| | Adult | + |
| | Voter | + |
| 20 ---- | | |
| | Worker | + |
| | Marital partner | + |
| 30 ---- | Parent | + |
| | Home owner | + |
| 40 ---- | | |
| | Auditory decline | − |
| 50 ---- | Empty nest | − |
| | Visual decline | − |
| 60 ---- | Grandparent | + |
| | Widowhood | − |
| | Tactile decline | − |
| | Taste decline | − |
| | Retirement | ± |
| 70 ---- | | |
| | Olfactory decline | − |
| | Motor function | − |
| 80 ---- | Give up driving | − |
| | Health | − |
| | Institutionalization | − |
| 90 ---- | | |

Adapted from Pastalan LA: J Architectural Educ 31:11, 1977.

person must cope with other stressors that were not part of the anticipated event.

It is still unclear whether older persons experience more stress in a given period than the young do. Some studies provide evidence that older persons are indeed confronted with more stressful life events.[26,51,67,69] Others have found the same distribution of such events in young, middle-aged, and older persons, though none of these studies has compared people across a wide age range.[66,70,91] Still others have argued that older people experience *fewer* stressful life events in a given time period than the young do.[33]

It has been argued that the cohort of people over age 65 today have experienced more traumatic life events than younger age groups because they lived through the Depression, World War II, and the Korean and Vietnam Wars. These events, however, do not necessarily have long-term effects on a person's adaptation and psychologic well-being, unless a person has experienced them directly (for example, posttraumatic stress disorder has been identified in some veterans of the Vietnam War).

Although researchers have focused on the stress produced by major life events, Lazarus and Cohen[65] have suggested that most people experience stress as a result of "chronic daily hassles." Their "hassles scale" measures such day-to-day problems as feelings of loneliness, lack of energy, regrets over past decisions, and concerns about one's current situation. Other emotions that may produce stress for a person include feelings of powerlessness, normlessness, and social isolation.[111] These are generally not specific events with a beginning or end point but are chronic and may occur simultaneously with other "hassles." A person must cope with these emotions, just as with discrete life events. To the extent that an older person feels powerless, lonely, and regretful, feelings of stress will increase, with a corresponding need to adapt to the situation in some way.

The manner in which we respond to life events, role changes, and chronic daily hassles depends on many internal and external factors. Internal factors include the person's interpretation of the situation. The cognitive appraisal of a situation by a person as being stressful or not has already been noted to be important. In addition, an event's relative desirability or undesirability and whether it is anticipated and a person's previous experiences with similar events may determine how he or she responds to the situation. An important external factor is the availability of a strong social network that can provide emotional support. An older person who must face all challenges alone may use coping strategies differently from one who has family and friends to turn to in times of crisis.

Personality styles also may influence how people respond to stress. Gutmann's research[43-45] on active and passive mastery styles is described earlier. A person with a passive style does not feel powerful enough to directly influence his or her fate, whereas one with an active style tends to rely more on personal abilities and less on others. Differences in responses to stress by older people with these different styles would be expected.

## Aging and coping styles

The question of whether coping styles change with age has not been extensively researched. Some studies of coping among young and middle-aged persons have reported few significant differences, whereas others have found that older persons use more mature coping styles (such as problem solving and seeking the advice of family, friends, and professionals). Other studies have reported major age differences. For example, older persons are less likely than the young to use confrontive coping, especially when the stressor could be defined as a threat. They are more likely to use distancing techniques and to reappraise the situation in a positive light.[36,53]

Religious coping has also been found to be an important coping strategy in several studies of older persons.[60,71-72] For example, in one study 45% of the respondents 55 to 80 years of age mentioned trust and faith in God, prayer, and seeking help from God as coping strategies for at least one of the three major life events they had experienced. In most cases, these styles are appropriate for the problem at hand and result in successful adaptation. Only in the case of significant cognitive deterioration is there a restriction in the range of a person's coping responses and a tendency to resort to more primitive reactions, such as denying or ignoring the problem. Nevertheless, the majority of older people appear capable of using a wide repertoire of coping responses and can call upon the most effective ones for a given situation. In sum, the available research indicates that most people maintain their coping styles into old age and use appropriate responses for the problem at hand.

## Adaptation to aging

To conclude this section, it is important to discuss the implications of older persons' coping responses for their long-term adaptation. *Adaptation* refers to the adjustments that people make in response to changes in themselves or their environments in order to fit themselves to their new conditions and to maintain their self-esteem, even after numerous role losses and changes. Given older people's numerous experiences with life events, role loss, and environmental changes throughout life, it would appear that adaptation in old age should occur with relative ease. Indeed, in one sense, a person who has reached 75 or 80 years of age has proved to be the most adaptable of his or her generation, since the ultimate proof of adaptation is survival. As we have seen thus far, older people continue to face challenges to their well-being in the form of personal and family illnesses, age-related declines in sensory and physiological functions, and changes in their social and physical environments. To the extent that older people are capable of using coping skills that were effective in youth and middle age, they will continue to adapt successfully, thereby maintaining their self-esteem and life satisfaction.

## Implications for the dental team

Dental practitioners recognize the value of healthy teeth for maintaining one's self-concept and sense of attractiveness. But what is the impact of aging on a person's need for attractiveness, especially for those who can no longer manage their personal oral hygiene? There is considerable evidence that aging itself does not result in a loss of this need for attractiveness; therefore it is important to help older patients maintain and even enhance their oral health status, with restorations of existing teeth, fixed and removable prostheses if needed, and even cosmetic dentistry. It is not unusual today to find patients in their fifties seeking orthodontics and orthognathic surgery for esthetic reasons. Just as plastic surgery is becoming more acceptable for people in their sixties and seventies, orthognathic surgery may also assume greater importance for older persons in the future. We have already seen the tremendous growth of dental implants for older patients in the past 10 years; a major motive for both young and older patients is to improve their appearance.[59] Hence, it is important not to discourage an older person who seeks the dentist's advice regarding cosmetic dentistry or surgery.

The dental team can gauge the older person's self-concept and self-esteem from the importance they place on dental care. For example, an older woman who perceives herself as young, healthy, and active is more likely to use dental services regularly and perhaps to seek the type of procedures described above, whereas an older man who views himself as near death just because he is 75 years old may neglect his oral health altogether and reject any dental treatments beyond emergency care. The latter is much more of a challenge to the dental team and requires patience and the ability to convince the patient that old age does not preclude good oral health. Similarly, the patient with low self-esteem will be less motivated to maintain good oral health than one who has high self-esteem. Indeed, if the dental team observes signs of declining oral hygiene in their elderly patients, these signs may point to a more severe loss of self-esteem as in depression or may indicate dementia. These conditions and their impact on dental care are discussed in the next section.

Finally, coping with new situations may require more effort by older persons, as noted earlier in this section. For this reason, an elderly person who is making his or her first visit to a dentist in more than 20 years (not an unusual situation for this cohort of elderly) may experience tremendous stress during the dental visit. This feeling of stress may be manifested as anxiety about dental care, reluctance to comply with treatment recommendations, and problems in the dental chair (including gagging while trying to place a rubber dam or refusing to have the chair in a prone position), giving the appearance of a difficult or obstinate patient. The dental team must therefore take the time to walk a new older patient through the operatory, explaining all the equipment, the staff, and the steps involved in providing dental care. This may require an extra 15 minutes of a staff person's time, but the savings in terms of treatment time and patient cooperation will make the effort worthwhile.

## MENTAL HEALTH IN AGING

It should be apparent to the reader by now that old age is accompanied by some deterioration in sensory and cognitive functions, but personality remains relatively stable in normal aging. Nevertheless, personality disorders and psychiatric symptoms may emerge among some older persons who showed no signs of a psychopathosis earlier in their lives. In some persons the stresses of old age may compound any existing predisposition to a psychopathosis. In other older persons, mental disorders may represent a continuation of a lifelong psychopathosis.

The primary affective or emotional disorder of

old age is depression, accounting for a significant number of suicides, especially among older men. Alzheimer's disease and other dementias are cognitive disorders that are far more likely to affect the elderly than the young. Alcoholism and drug abuse are less common in older persons, though their effect on the physical health and cognitive functioning of older people is more detrimental than on younger persons. Paranoid disorders and schizophrenia are even less likely to begin in old age; the majority of persons who have either of these conditions were first diagnosed in youth or middle age. In this section these conditions are discussed briefly.

### Epidemiology of mental disorders

The prevalence of psychiatric disorders among older persons who are living in the community ranges from 5% to 45%, depending on the population studied and the categories of disorders examined. Even higher rates can be expected in institutionalized elderly, with estimates of 10% to 40% of people with mild to moderate impairments and another 5% to 10% with significant impairments.[12] One study found that 22% of older persons admitted to a Veterans Administration hospital in 1 year for acute medical or surgical reasons were also suffering from some form of a mental disorder. The rate was even higher (30%) among those admitted to cardiac care units.[108]

### Depression

The three most prevalent forms of late-life psychopathosis are depression, dementia, and paranoia. Of these, depression is the most frequently diagnosed. Epidemiologic surveys have found that 15% to 22% of community elderly report depressed moods; 10% to 15% have depressions that require clinical interventions.[41-42] Women tend to report more symptoms of depression in middle age and early old age, but it may be that more men have clinically diagnosable depression at 80 years of age and beyond.[42]

It is important to distinguish *major depression* from bipolar disorders (that is, ranging from a depressed to a manic state), sadness, grief reactions, and other affective disorders.[3] Most of the depressions of old age are unipolar; manic-depressive disorders are rare.[96] Still other cases in late life are *secondary* or *reactive depressions,* which arise in response to a significant life event with which the person cannot cope. This type of depression is a common reaction to the life stressors associated with aging, as described in the previous section. For example, physical illness and the loss of loved ones through death and relocation may trigger depressive reactions in the elderly.[94] Although depression usually does not result from any one of these alone, the combination of several losses in close sequence is a risk factor for reactive depression.

For this reason, the dental team must be sensitive to signs of depression in their older patients whose recent social history (that is, within the past year) includes multiple major life events. What are some of these signs? According to the 1987 *Diagnostic and Statistical Manual of Mental Disorders* of the American Psychiatric Association,[3] if a patient displays or reports any five of the following symptoms with a duration of 2 or more weeks, they are diagnosed as depressed:

1. Depressed moods
2. Greatly diminished interest or pleasure in activities, apathy
3. Significant weight loss or weight gain, or appetite change
4. Sleep disturbance (awakening early or insomnia)
5. Agitation or slowing down of activity
6. Reduced energy level or fatigue
7. Self-blame, guilt, worthlessness
8. Poor concentration, indecisiveness
9. Recurrent thoughts of death, suicide

The vegetative signs, suicidal thoughts, weight loss, and mood variations from morning to night that are observed in major depression are not found in reactive depression.

Some of the most obvious signs of depression are reports or evidence of sadness and feelings of emptiness or detachment. Also common are expressions or anxiety or panic for no apparent cause, loss of interest in the environment, and neglect of self-care, as well as changes in eating and sleeping patterns. The depressed person may complain of vague aches and pains, either generally or in a specific part of the body. Occasional symptoms are not problematic, however. Only when multiple symptoms appear together and persist *for at least 2 weeks* should a person and his or her family suspect a depressive episode, especially if an older person speaks frequently of death or suicide.

One problem with detecting depression in the elderly is that older persons may be more successful than their younger counterparts at masking or hiding symptoms of depression. In fact, many cases of depression in older people are not diagnosed because the patient either does not express changes in mood or denies them in the clinical interview.[40,106] *Masked depression* is one in which few mood changes are reported. Instead, the patient complains of atypical pain and bodily discomfort, is apathetic, and withdraws from others.[41,75]

Health care professionals and family members need to distinguish depression from medical conditions and changes attributable to normal aging. For example, an older woman with arthritis who complains of increasing pain may actually be seeking a reason for vague physical discomfort that is related to a depressive episode. Similarly, it is important not to dismiss an older person's complaints of increasing sleep disturbance with the assumption that older people merely need less sleep.[112] People with masked depression are more likely to complain of problems with memory or problem solving. Their denial or masking of symptoms may lead health professionals to assume that the person is experiencing dementia, a condition that is generally irreversible. It is for this reason that depression in older persons is often labeled *pseudodementia*.[129]

Because of such likelihood of denial, an older patient who has vague somatic complaints should be referred to a geriatric medicine specialist for a thorough physical exam and lab tests to determine if a person is depressed or has a physical disorder or symptoms of dementia. If the cognitive dysfunction is attributable to depression, this will improve when the depression is treated. On the other hand, some medical conditions, including Parkinson's, rheumatoid arthritis, thyroid dysfunction, and diseases of the adrenal glands, may produce depressive symptoms. Certain medications may also produce feelings of depression; these include antihypertensives, digoxin, L-dopa, corticosteroids, estrogens, and some antipsychotic drugs. In fact, any medication that has a depressant effect on the central nervous system can produce depressive symptoms in older patients, specifically lethargy and loss of interest in the environment.[103] For these reasons, it is important for older persons to be examined thoroughly for underlying physical illness and reactions to medications. Physicians must frequently conduct medication reviews to determine if their older patients begin to show side effects to a drug, even after using it for several months or years. Dentists should also be alert to the potential depressive side effects of medications an older person is using and be particularly cautious when prescribing pain medications to such patients; some of these can exaggerate the patient's depressive symptoms.

### Suicide among depressed elderly

Death rates appear to be greater among elderly with a diagnosis of depression; in one 3-year follow-up study, 60% of depressed patients had died, compared with only 32% among those with no psychiatric diagnosis.[110] Some specialists have suggested that older persons with depression are more apathetic, less interested in their environments, and more likely to entertain thoughts of suicide than younger depressives.[14,75,134]

It has been estimated that 25% of all reported suicides occur in persons 65 years of age and older.[13,21] In 1980, the national rate was 11.9 suicides per 100,000 population. The rate for persons over 65 years of age was 17.7.[82] It is noteworthy that the highest suicide rates in the United States are found among older white males. The prevalence of suicide in this population rises linearly after 65 years of age; almost three times as many suicides occur in white males 85 years of age and over as in all other subgroups of elderly combined.[11] According to data compiled by the National Center for Health Statistics,[82] white males over 85 years of age completed 50 suicides per 100,000 in 1980. In contrast white females completed 7; nonwhite females 2; and nonwhite males 15 suicides per 100,000 in the same year. Since there are probably a significant number of suicides that appear to be accidents or natural deaths (such as starvation, gas poisoning), these statistics may *underrepresent* the actual incidence of the problem.

There are fewer nonfatal suicide attempts in older men compared to the young. That is, the rate of completed suicides is far greater among older men, 4:1 versus 200:1 in the young.[73,117] This difference may be attributable to the use of more lethal methods of suicide such as shotguns and a lower likelihood of survival from serious injury.

One explanation for the higher rates of suicide

among elderly white males is that they generally experience the greatest incongruence between their ideal self-image (that of worker, decision-maker, holder of relatively high status in society) and the realities of advancing age.[22,77] With age, the role of worker is generally lost; chronic illness may diminish one's sense of control, and a person may feel a loss of status. The risk of suicide is greater for people experiencing social isolation. This is an important factor in the lives of older white widowed males, who are most likely to lack supportive social networks.[48,117] Nonwhite elderly males in the United States may be less likely to commit suicide because of more extensive family support systems.

Because attempts at suicide are more likely to be successful in older men, it is important for health professionals to be sensitive to clues of an impending suicide. Risk factors include social isolation, serious physical illnesses that are accompanied by severe pain, the sudden death of a loved one, a major loss of independence, or financial inadequacy. Statements that indicate frustration with life and a desire to end it, a sudden decision to give away one's most important possessions, and a general loss of interest in one's health and well-being must be attended to closely by health professionals. Clearly, not all older people displaying such symptoms will attempt suicide, but the recognition of changes in an older person's behavior and moods can alleviate a potential disaster.

### Implications for the dental team

Dentists, hygienists, and especially the office staff must be tuned into any signs and symptoms of depressed mood and thoughts of suicide among their elderly patients. The best way to assure this is to establish rapport with these patients, so that older persons can trust the dental team. Thus they can feel comfortable expressing grief and sadness over life stressors, including declines in their own health, in that of their spouse or other close relative, and grief over the death of a loved one. This is particularly true for older persons who are isolated and have few friends and family members remaining. For these reasons, it is imperative for the dental team to allow more time to obtain social and medical histories from their older patients. This should not be a cursory checklist but a discussion of the patient's recent social and medical problems, their reactions to those experiences, and any lasting effects they have produced. Perhaps even more important, these questions need to be repeated in detail at each annual or semiannual visit by the patient. The dental team must avoid the potential complacency of assuming that older people's lives do not change much, and therefore a quick question such as, "Any changes in your health or living situation since we last saw you?" may be a callous and inappropriate strategy for interacting with aged patients!

### Dementia

As I have described in the section on cognitive changes, normal aging does not result in significant declines in memory and learning ability. Mild impairments do not necessarily signal a major loss but often represent a mild form of memory dysfunction known as "benign senescent forgetfulness." Only in the case of the diseases known collectively as the "dementias" does cognitive function show pronounced deterioration. Dementia, also referred to as "organic brain syndrome" or "senile dementia," actually includes a variety of conditions that are caused by or associated with damage of brain tissue, resulting in impaired cognitive function and, in more advanced stages, impaired behavior and personality. Such changes in the brain result in progressive deterioration of a person's ability to learn and recall items from the past. Until recently, it was assumed that all these syndromes were associated with cerebral arteriosclerosis ("hardening of the arteries"). It is now known that some of these conditions occur independently of arteriosclerosis. Some features are unique to each type of dementia, but all dementias have in common a change in a person's ability to recall events in recent memory and problems with comprehension, attention span, judgment, and orientation to time, place, and person. The person with dementia may experience increased concreteness of thought (that is, be unable to understand abstract thought or symbolic language; for example, he or she cannot interpret a proverb), particularly in the later stages of the disease.

Although not part of normal aging, the likelihood of experiencing dementia does increase with advancing age. Approximately 3 million persons over 65 years of age experience some degree of cognitive loss,[20,100] and up to 50% of institutionalized elderly are estimated to have mild to moderate levels of dementia. A recent epidemiological study in East Boston revealed that up to half of the people they examined over 85 years of age could be diagnosed with dementia.[35] As more people live to be age 85, the number of persons with dementia is expected to increase by 44% in whites and 72% in blacks between 1980 and 2005.[63] This difference by ethnic minority status is attributed to the more rapid growth of blacks living beyond 70 years of age. However, just as aging and disease are not synonymous, dementia is not inevitable with age.

The major types of dementias are shown in Table 2-3. Notice the distinction between *reversible* and *irreversible* dementias. The first refers to cognitive decline, which may be caused by drug toxicity, hormonal or nutritional disorders, and other diseases that may be reversible. Sources of potentially reversible dementias include tumors in and trauma to the brain, toxins, metabolic disorders such as hypothyroidism or hyperthyroidism, diabetes, hypocalcemia or hypercalcemia, infections, vascular lesions, and hydrocephalus. Severe depression may produce confusion and memory problems in some older people. Some medications may also cause dementia-like symptoms. This problem is aggravated if the person is taking multiple medications or is on a dosage that is higher than what the older kidney or liver can metabolize. A person who ap-

**Table 2-3** Major dementias of late life

| Reversible | Irreversible |
| --- | --- |
| Drugs | Alzheimer's |
| | Multi-infarct |
| Nutritional deficiencies | Huntington's chorea |
| Normal pressure hydrocephalus | |
| Brain tumors | Pick's disease |
| Hypothyroidism or hyperthyroidism | |
| Neurosyphilis | Creutzfeldt-Jakob |
| Depression (pseudodementia) | Kuru |
| | Wernicke-Korsakoff |

Adapted from Hooyman N and Kiyak HA: Social gerontology: a multidisciplinary perspective, Needham Heights, Mass, 1988, Allyn & Bacon.

pears to be suffering from such reactions should be referred promptly for medical screening.

Irreversible dementias are those that have no discernible environmental cause and cannot yet be cured. Although there is considerable research on the causes and treatments for these conditions, they must be labeled irreversible at the present time. Some of these are more common than others; some have identifiable causes, whereas others do not. Pick's disease is one of the rarest; in this type, the frontal lobes of the brain atrophy. Of all the dementias, it is most likely to occur in younger persons and to result in significant personality changes. Creutzfeldt-Jakob disease and kuru have been traced to a slow-acting virus. In the former type of dementia, decline in cognitive abilities occurs quite rapidly. The latter type is quite rare and has been found among some cannibalistic tribes of New Guinea. Huntington's chorea is a genetically transmitted condition that usually appears in people in their thirties and forties. It results in more neuromuscular changes than the other dementias do.

Multi-infarct dementia has been estimated to represent 15% to 20% of all nonreversible dementias.[122] This is the form of dementia that in the past was identified as "senility." In this type, several areas of the brain show infarcts or small strokes that result in damage to one or more blood vessels feeding those areas of the brain. Older people with this condition often have a history of hypertension, strokes, and blackouts. Although multi-infarct dementia may be diagnosed without such a history, such cases are relatively rare and may indicate another type of dementia, most likely Alzheimer's disease.

Senile dementia of the Alzheimer's type (SDAT, or Alzheimer's disease) is the most common irreversible dementia in late life, accounting for 50% to 70% of all dementias. Incidence figures are difficult to obtain, but it has been estimated that 5% to 15% of all persons over 65 years of age and over 25% of elderly in nursing homes have symptoms of SDAT. The prevalence of Alzheimer's disease appears to increase with age; less than 2% of the general population under 60 years of age are affected, whereas rates of 20% have been estimated for the population over 80 years of age.[31,41] Although a distinction was made in the past between presenile (that is, before age 65) and senile de-

mentia, there is now common agreement that these are the same disease.

Alzheimer's disease is characterized by deficits in attention, learning, memory, and language skills. A person with this condition may also have problems in judgment, abstraction, and orientation. In the earlier stages of the disease, a person may have difficulties with attention span and with orientation to the environment, increased anxiety and restlessness, and unpredictable changes in mood. Family members may complain that the older person has become more aggressive or, in some cases, more passive than in the past. Depression may set in as the person realizes that he or she is experiencing these problems. In the more advanced stages of the disease, there may be noticeable aphasia (that is, problems recalling appropriate words and labels), perseveration (that is, repeating the same phrase and thought many times), apathy, and problems with comprehension, such that Alzheimer's victims may not recognize their spouse, children, and long-time friends. However, it is not unusual for some patients in the moderate to advanced stages of SDAT to describe quite articulately and vividly events that took place many years ago. The advanced patient often needs assistance with bodily functions such as eating and oral hygiene. At autopsy, there is a generalized deterioration of cortical tissue, which appears to be tangled and covered with plaque.

Because of recent attention by the media and by researchers on Alzheimer's disease, there is some tendency to overestimate its occurrence and to assume that it is the cause of all dementias. In many ways, it has taken on the role that multi-infarct dementia had several years ago; that is, the label has been given without a thorough diagnosis. Unfortunately, the most confirmatory diagnosis of Alzheimer's disease may be made only at autopsy, when the areas and nature of damaged brain tissue can be identified. However, several psychologic measures of cognitive functioning and a thorough physical exam can provide clues to its existence in the earlier stages or may indicate that the observed changes in behavior or personality are attributable to a reversible condition. Early diagnosis can be made with some certainty with an extensive series of tests. These measures include a medical and nutritional history; laboratory tests of blood, urine, and stool; tests for thyroid function; a thorough physical and psychologic examination; and, in some cases, extensive radiologic studies, including a CAT scan or magnetic resonance imaging.[32,115] In fact, it is primarily through a process of elimination of other conditions that some dementias such as SDAT may be diagnosed. In such diagnoses, it is particularly important to detect depression, drug toxicity, and nutritional deficiencies because, as stated earlier, these conditions may be treated.

### Implications for the dental team

There have been few published reports discussing the dental problems of elderly with Alzheimer's disease and the role of dental teams in caring for these patients. An excellent discussion of this disease from a dental perspective is presented by Niessen and Jones.[86] This chapter emphasizes some of the issues raised by these authors and offers additional recommendations for the dental management of Alzheimer's disease.

Perhaps most important for the patient and family is to recognize that Alzheimer's disease has a downward course and that the patient will gradually deteriorate in cognitive function and self-care skills. This is important from a dental management perspective because any major dental procedure needed by these patients should be completed in the early stages of the disease. It is especially important to construct new dentures while the older person can still adapt to new situations and can express any problems with the fit of these dentures. In more advanced cases, complex dental restorations and new prostheses should be avoided though it may be necessary to reline dentures as the patient's oral musculature deteriorates.

It is also crucial to avoid new situations such as a new dentist or a new office, since the Alzheimer's patient may even have problems recognizing familiar people and places. Each time the dental team meets the patient, even if only 2 or 3 days have elapsed, they must introduce themselves by name *and* role (for example, "Hi, I'm Dr. Smith, your dentist, and today I will examine your mouth"). To the extent possible, background noise and level of activity in the office and the operatory should be kept to a minimum, and so it is suggested that appointments for Alzheimer's patients should be scheduled for times when few others are around. However, late afternoons are not good, especially toward dusk when the patient is generally more fatigued and may show signs of "sundowning," that is, exaggerated confusion and disorientation as light levels change and fatigue sets in.

Families play a critical role in caring for the patient with Alzheimer's disease, providing a familiar and constant link to the outside and serving as a liaison between the patient and health care providers. It is important that they accompany the patient to the dental office and especially into the operatory, to alleviate any stress and anxiety experienced by the patient and, if necessary, to translate for the dentist what the patient needs or wants to express. Family caregivers also are important in providing daily oral hygiene for advanced Alzheimer's patients. But dentists must recognize the tremendous burdens on caregivers and avoid overloading them further with extensive oral hygiene tasks. Finally, when communicating with these patients, family caregivers should always be present, but even with advanced Alzheimer's patients, it is valuable to address the patient directly, making occasional eye contact with the caregiver.

### Alcoholism and drug abuse

It is difficult to obtain accurate statistics on the prevalence of alcoholism in older people because of the stigma associated with this condition among this cohort. Estimates vary, from 10% to 15% of all people over 55 years of age living in the community[133] to less than 10%.[114] Surveys of elderly outpatients in general medical hospitals estimate that 15% to 30% show symptoms of alcoholism.[80,109] A review of national surveys of drinking patterns among women conducted between 1971 and 1982 concluded that women over 65 years of age report the lowest incidence of alcohol consumption in general and the lowest incidence of heavy drinking, with 26% to 40% stating that they consume any alcohol and less than 5% indicating high consumption.[131] In contrast, widowers and men who have never married are at greater risk for alcoholism.[114]

Alcoholics are less likely to be found among the ranks of persons over 60 years of age because of higher death rates at a young age among alcoholics.[7] Nevertheless, surveys of alcoholism rates among older person have revealed approximately equal proportions of those who began to drink heavily before 40 years of age and those who began in old age. In one study, more than two thirds of elderly alcoholics had had this problem for many years; others had increased their drinking in response to age-related stressful events.[102] This is consistent with the findings of Zimberg.[133]

It is important to distinguish lifelong abusers of alcohol from those who began drinking later in life, often as a reaction to losses and isolation experienced by some older people. Some older persons who are diagnosed as alcoholics have had this problem since middle age, but increasing age may exacerbate the condition for two reasons. First, the central nervous system, liver, and kidneys become less tolerant of alcohol with age (such as loss of muscle tissue, reduction in body mass, reduced efficiency of liver and kidney functions). For these reasons, smaller doses of alcohol can be more deleterious in the later years. Second, a person who has been drinking heavily for many years has already produced irreversible damage to the central nervous system, liver, and kidneys, creating more problems than those attributable to normal aging alone. It is difficult to determine the incidence of alcoholism among older persons who have no previous history of alcoholism. Physiologic evidence is lacking, and drinking is often hidden from friends, relatives, and physicians. The elderly person may justify overconsumption of alcohol on the grounds that it relieves sadness and isolation. Even in cases where family members are aware of the situation, they may minimize it by rationalizing that it is one of the older person's few remaining pleasures.

Physicians may overlook the possibility that alcohol is creating a health problem for the older person because the adverse effects of alcohol resemble some physical diseases or psychiatric and cognitive disorders that are associated with old age. Older alcoholics may complain of confusion, disorientation, irritability, insomnia or restless sleep patterns, heart palpitations, or a dry cough.[116] Beliefs held by health care providers that alcoholism does not occur in older people may also prevent its detection.

Older alcoholics are less likely than young alcoholics to demonstrate a serious personality disorder[102] but are more likely to have symptoms of dementia.[38,104] Indeed, middle-aged alcoholics have been found to show significant impairments in learning and memory that are more common in advanced old age, suggestive of a premature aging phenomenon attributable to long-term alcohol abuse.[104] Creutzfeldt-Jakob disease is a form of dementia that is sometimes found in long-term alcoholics. Alcoholism and depression may occur together in the same person. Heavy drinkers in all age groups have been found to report more depressive symptoms.[131]

Older persons use a disproportionately large number of prescription and over-the-counter drugs, representing approximately 25% of all medication costs. In particular, older people are more likely than the young to be using tranquilizers, sedatives, and hypnotics, all of which have potentially dangerous side effects. The use of such medications is even greater in long-term care settings. In a survey of elderly persons residing in the community, 83% of the respondents were using two or more medications; the average was 3.8 per person.[25] Older persons have been found to abuse aspirin compounds,[81] laxatives,[29] and sleeping pills,[121] often because of misinformation about the adverse effects of too high a dosage or too many pills. It is not unusual to hear older patients state that they took twice or three times as much aspirin as they were prescribed because they did not feel their pain was being alleviated with the lower dose. Yet, because of changes in body composition and renal and liver functions with age, combined with the use of multiple medications, older persons are more likely to experience adverse drug reactions. Fortunately there is a growing awareness of the effects of "polypharmacy" among health care providers and among older people themselves. On the other hand, there is very little evidence that older persons abuse drugs to the extent that younger populations do, or use illicit drugs such as heroin, cocaine, and marijuana.

## Paranoid disorders and schizophrenia

Paranoia, defined as an irrational suspiciousness of other people, actually takes several forms. In older persons, paranoia may be attributable to social isolation, a sense of powerlessness, progressive sensory decline, and problems with the normal "checks and balances" of daily life.[32] Still other changes in the aging person, such as problems with memory, may result in paranoid reactions.

Although the foregoing conditions may produce a genuine paranoid state, some of the suspicious attitudes of older persons may represent accurate readings of their experiences. For example, an older person's children may in fact be trying to institutionalize him or her in order to take over the estate, or a nurse's aide may really be stealing from an older patient. It is therefore important to distinguish actual threats to the person from unfounded suspicions. The diagnosis of paranoid disorders in older people is similar to that in younger patients; the symptoms should have a duration of at least 1 week, with no signs of schizophrenia, no prominent hallucinations, and no association to an organic mental disorder.[3]

Schizophrenia is much less prevalent than depression or dementia in old age. It has been estimated that only 1% of the population over 60 years of age living in the community are schizophrenic.[15] Most elderly persons with this condition were first diagnosed in adolescence or in middle age and continue to display behavior symptomatic of schizophrenia though the severity of symptoms appears to decrease with age.[55,64] Late-onset schizophrenia with paranoid features has been labeled *paraphrenia* by some psychiatrists, especially in Europe and in Great Britain.[22]

Many of the current cohort of elderly chronic schizophrenics residing in the community were deinstitutionalized during the early 1960s as part of the national Community Mental Health Services Act of 1963. After spending much of their youth and middle age in state hospitals, these patients were released with the anticipation that they could function independently in the community with medications to control their hallucinations and psychotic behavior. Although this approach has proved effective for many former schizophrenic inpatients, some have not adjusted successfully to deinstitutionalization, as witnessed by the number of older schizophrenics seen on the streets in most major cities.

### Implications for the dental team

The dental team is far less likely to have contact with a schizophrenic older patient than with a paranoid older person, unless they have significant contact with institutionalized elderly. Schizophrenic older persons are generally not difficult to manage dentally, though long-term use of psychotropic drugs in these patients may result in tardive dyskinesia, a condition that makes it difficult to keep the jaw stable during dental procedures. Nevertheless, these patients can and should be treated.

Likewise, the paranoid older person should not be a problem once dental treatment begins, but these patients may be difficult to get into the dental office at all! It is not unusual for paranoid elderly to believe that dentists are overcharging them and performing unnecessary dental procedures just so they can take all the patient's remaining financial resources. Even mildly paranoid elderly, especially those who have not seen a dentist in many years, may suspect the first dentist who gives them a high estimate for a proposed dental treatment of cheating them because they are old and naive! It is therefore crucial to explain immediately to these persons how extensive their dental needs are, to offer them *alternative* treatment plans with wide variations in cost, and to describe the pros and cons of each. It may even be useful to encourage such older persons to seek a second opinion and explain your fee schedule and how it compares with other practitioners in the community.

Paranoid patients, especially if they are hearing impaired, can become very suspicious of the dentist if the dentist speaks to an accompanying spouse or other family member, rather than to the patient directly. For this reason, it is imperative that all communications regarding diagnosis, treatment, and scheduling be directed at the older patient who is to recevie care, even if that person is hearing impaired, blind, or even mildly demented.

### SUMMARY

This chapter is focused on normal and pathologic changes in sensory functioning, learning and memory, and in personality, coping, and adaptation. Affective and cognitive disorders associated with aging have also been presented. Throughout the chapter, I have emphasized the distinction between normal declines in psychologic functioning and rapid deterioration or dysfunctional behavior secondary to disease. It is important for dental practitioners to recognize this distinction; aging in itself does not result in major losses of sensory, cognitive, and emotional skills. Where such changes are observed, the dental team must question the older person, his or her family members, and in many cases his or her primary physician to determine the underlying cause for any changes observed in the older person.

The section on sensory functioning highlights some normal declines in vision and hearing. These include deteriorating visual accommodation, depth and distance perception, poorer response to glare, and difficulty with speech comprehension in high noise environments. These normal changes with aging demand greater awareness on the part of the dental team in presenting written and verbal information to their elderly patients. Both the style and format of communication and the environment in which communication takes place may need to be modified with elderly patients. Touch can be a valuable form of communication with some older persons, especially those who are cognitively impaired. Research findings on taste perception with aging also indicate that complaints by older patients that food no longer tastes good should not be dismissed as a necessary corollary of aging but that the older person may be experiencing taste loss secondary to some other general or oral disease or because of some medications. Taste perception does not appear to change with aging, but olfactory sensitivity does. Research on tactile acuity also indicates that pain perception may not necessarily change with aging; instead, many older people seem to accept pain as an inevitable part of aging and tolerate higher levels of painful stimuli than younger persons do. Nevertheless, the dental team should not assume that all elderly can tolerate more pain but should ask each patient whether he or she wants an anesthetic, so long as his or her medical and medication history does not contraindicate the need for anesthetics.

In the area of cognitive functioning, older people take longer to respond to any new stimulus or task. They have more difficulty retrieving information from their memory store, even what was learned as recently as 1 hour before. There is some question about older people's ability to recall information accurately from the distant past, and so it may not be worthwhile to inquire in depth about the patient's dental history from 20 to 30 years before. Researchers have demonstrated that older people can benefit from methods to enhance learning, including the use of mnemonics, linking new information with old, and active inquiry techniques to test for learning. In dental practice this might in-

clude the development of a mnemonic to look for signs of oral cancer, linking flossing skills with toothbrushing, and active question-and-answer sessions on how to maintain dental and denture care at home.

The section on personality provides considerable evidence for stability, as well as some changes in personality style and coping with aging. Changes include a reduction of sex-typed behavior (for example, men become more accepting of their need for affiliation and nurturance, women of their aggressive or egocentric needs). This change in their elderly patients should not be seen as a harmful process by the dental team, but it may result in problems dealing with the increased demands of some older women patients. Older people may also display greater caution and appear to become more introverted. This may result in a need for more time to make decisions about dental treatment, a need to reject extensive and costly dental procedures, and in some cases a decision to avoid dental care altogether.

In the case of older persons experiencing major life events, especially the loss of loved ones through death or institutionalization or their own loss of independence, sudden decisions to postpone dental treatment and a deterioration in oral home care may signal a reactive depression accompanied by loss of self-esteem. The dental team must be sensitive to such changes in their elderly patients, especially isolated older white males, who are most at risk for suicide as a result of severe depression. Since depression is the most common affective disorder in older persons, it behooves the dental team to be aware of the signs of depression. For those whose depression is being managed with pharmacotherapy (as with antidepressants), it is important to look for signs of dry mouth and other adverse drug reactions in the orofacial region. Finally, patients with dementia can also benefit from dental care. But in many cases major dental procedures should not be undertaken in the advanced stages of Alzheimer's disease or other dementias. Sometimes the best intervention for these patients is maintenance and the alleviation of pain rather than major interceptive care. It is also important to consider the role of family caregivers for these patients and other elderly who are experiencing major physical and sensory losses.

## REFERENCES

1. Accardi FE, Gombos MM, and Gombos GM: Common causes of blindness: a pilot survey in Brooklyn, New York, Ann Ophthalmol 17:289, 1985.
2. Adams PF and Collings G: Measures of health among older persons living in the community. In Havlik RJ, Liu MG, and Kovar MG, editors: Health statistics on older persons, United States, 1986. Vital and Health Statistics, series 3, no 25, DHHS publ no PHS 87-1409, Washington, DC, 1987, US Government Printing Office.
3. American Psychiatric Association: Diagnostic and statistical manual of mental disorders, ed 3, Washington, DC, 1987, American Psychiatric Association.
4. Applegate WB, Miller JT, Elam JT, et al: Impact of cataract surgery with lens implantation on vision and physical function in elderly patients, JAMA 257:1064, 1987.
5. Arey L, Tremaine M, and Monzingo F: The numerical and topographical relations of taste buds to human circumvallate papillae throughout the life span, Anat Rec 64:9, 1935.
6. Arvidson K: Location and variation in number of taste buds in human fungiform papillae, Dent Res 87:435, 1979.
7. Atkinson JH and Schuckit MA: Alcoholism and over-the-counter and prescription drug misuse in the elderly. In Eisdorfer C, editor: Ann Rev Gerontol Geriatr 2:255, New York, 1981, Springer-Verlag, NY, Inc.
8. Bahrick HP, Bahrick PP, and Wittlinger RP: Fifty years of memory for names and faces: a cross-sectional approach, J Exp Psychol 104:54, 1975.
9. Barrett TR and Wright M: Age-related facilitation in recall following semantic processing, J Gerontol 2:194, 1981.
10. Bartoshuk LB, Riflein B, Marks LC, and Barns P: Taste and aging, J Gerontol 41:51, 1986.
11. Belsky JK: The psychology of aging: theory, research and practice, Monterey, Calif, 1984, Brooks/Cole Pub Co.
12. Blazer D: The epidemiology of mental illness in late life. In Busse E and Blazer D, editors: Handbook of geriatric psychiatry, New York, 1980, Van Nostrand Reinhold.
13. Blazer D: Depression in late life. St. Louis, 1982, The CV Mosby Co.
14. Blazer D, George L, and Landerman R: The phenomenology of late life depression. In Bebbington PE and Jacoby R, editors: Psychiatric disorders in the elderly, London, 1986, Mental Health Foundation.
15. Bollerup T: Prevalence of mental illness among 70-year-olds domiciled in nine Copenhagen suburbs, Acta Psychiatr Scand 51:327, 1975.
16. Borish JM: Clinical refraction, ed 3, Chicago, 1970, Professional Press.
17. Botwinick J: Aging and behavior, New York, 1978, Springer-Verlag, NY, Inc.
18. Botwinick J: Aging and behavior: a comprehensive integration of research findings, ed 3, New York, 1984, Springer-Verlag, NY, Inc.
19. Botwinick J and Storandt M: Memory related functions and age, Springfield, Ill, 1974, Charles C Thomas, Publisher.
20. Busse EW and Pfeiffer E: Behavior and adaptation in late life, Boston, 1975, Little, Brown & Co.
21. Butler RN: Psychiatry and the elderly: an overview, Am J Psychiatry 132:830, 1975.
22. Butler RN and Lewis M: Aging and mental health: positive psychosocial approaches, ed 3, St. Louis, 1982, The CV Mosby Co.
23. Canestrari RE: Paced and self-paced learning in young and elderly adults, J Gerontol 18:165, 1963.
24. Cavanaugh JC, Grady JG, and Perlmutter MP: Forgetting and use of memory aids in 20 and 70-year-olds' everyday life, Int J Aging Hum Dev 17:113, 1983.
25. Chien CP, Townsend EJ, and Townsend AR: Substance use and abuse among the community elderly: the medical aspect, Addictive Diseases: An International Journal 3:357, 1978.
26. Chiriboga DA and Cutler L: Stress and adaptation: life-span perspectives. In Poon LW, editor: Aging in the 1980's: psychological issues, Washington, DC, 1980, American Psychological Association.
27. Corso JF: Auditory perception and communication. In Birren JE and Schaie KW, editors: Handbook of the psychology of aging, New York, 1977, Van Nostrand Reinhold.
28. Cowart BJ: Relationships between taste and smell across the life span. In Murphy C, Cain WS, and Hegsted DM, editors: Nutrition and the chemical senses in aging: recent advances and current research needs, Ann NY Acad Sci 561:39, 1989.
29. Cummings JH, Sladen GE, James OFW, et al: Laxative-induced diarrhea: a continuing clinical problem, Br Med J 1:537, 1974.
30. Doty RL, Shaman P, Applebaum SL, et al: Smell identification ability: changes with age, Science 226:1441, 1984.
31. Eisdorfer C and Cohen D: The cognitively impaired elderly: differential diagnosis. In Storandt M, Siegler I, and Elias MF, editors: The clinical psychology of aging, New York, 1978, Plenum Pub Corp.
32. Eisdorfer C, Cohen D, and Veith R: The psychopathology of aging: current concepts, Kalamazoo, Mich, 1980, The Upjohn Co.
33. Eisdorfer C and Wilkie F: Stress, disease, aging, and behavior. In Birren JE and Shaie KW, editors: Handbook of the psychology of aging, New York, 1977, Van Nostrand Reinhold.
34. Erikson EH: Childhood and society, ed 2, New York, 1963, WW Norton & Co, Inc.
35. Evans DA, Funkenstein HH, Albert MS, et al: Prevalence of Alzheimer's disease in a community population of older persons, JAMA 262(18):2551, 1989.
36. Folkman S, Lazarus RS, Pimley S, and Novacek J: Age differences in stress and coping processes, Psychology and Aging 2:171, 1987.
37. Fozard JL: The time for remembering. In Poon LW, editor: Aging in the 1980's: psychological issues, Washington, DC, 1980, American Psychological Association.
38. Gaitz CM and Baer PE: Characteristics of elderly patients with alcoholism, Arch Gen Psychiatry 24:372, 1971.
39. Gerber I, Rusalem R, Hannon N, et al: Anticipatory grief and aged widows and widowers, J Gerontol 30:225, 1975.
40. Gerner R: Depression in the elderly. In Kaplan O, editor:

Psychopathology of aging, New York, 1979, Academic Press, Inc.

41. Gurland BJ and Cross PS: Epidemiology of psychopathology in old age, Psychiatr Clin North Am 5:11, 1982.
42. Gurland B, Dean L, Cross P, and Golden R: The epidemiology of depression and dementia in the elderly: the use of multiple indicators of these conditions. In Cole JO and Barrett JE, editors: Psychopathology in the aged, Englewood Cliffs, NJ, 1980, Prentice-Hall, Inc.
43. Gutmann DL: Alternatives to disengagement: aging among the highland Druze. In LeVine RA, editor: Culture and personality: contemporary readings, Chicago, 1974a, Aldine Pub Co.
44. Gutmann DL: The country of old men: cross-cultural studies in the psychology of later life. In LeVine RA, editor, Culture and personality: contemporary readings, Chicago, 1974b, Aldine Pub Co.
45. Gutmann DL: The cross-cultural perspective: notes toward a comparative psychology of aging. In Birren JE and Shaie KW, editors: Handbook of the psychology of aging, New York, 1977, Van Nostrand Reinhold.
46. Gutmann DL: Psychoanalysis of aging: a developmental view. In Greenspan SI and Pollock GH, editors: The course of life: psychoanalytic contributions toward understanding personality development, vol 3: Adulthood and the aging process, Washington, DC, 1980, US Government Printing Office.
47. Harkins SW and Warner MH: Age and pain. In Eisdorfer C, editor: Ann Rev Gerontol Geriatr 1:121, New York, 1980, Springer-Verlag, NY, Inc.
48. Holinger PC and Offer D: Prediction of adolescent suicide: a population model, Am J Psychiatry 139:302, 1982.
49. Hoyer WJ and Plude DJ: Attentional and perceptual processes in the study of cognitive aging. In Poon LW, editor: Aging in the 1980's: psychological issues, Washington, DC, 1980, American Psychological Association.
50. Hultsch DF and Dixon RA: Memory for text materials in adulthood. In Baltes PB and Brim OG, editors: Life-span development and behavior, vol 6, New York, 1984, Academic Press, Inc.
51. Hultsch DF and Plemons JK: Life events and life-span development. In Baltes PB and Brim OG, editors: Life-span development and behavior, vol 2, New York, 1979, Academic Press, Inc.
52. Inman VW and Parkinson SR: Differences in Brown-Peterson recall as a function of age and retention interval, J Gerontol 38:58, 1983.
53. Irion JC and Blanchard-Fields F: A cross-sectional comparison of adaptive coping in adulthood, J Gerontol 42:502, 1987.
54. Jung CG: Modern man in search of a soul, San Diego, 1933, Harcourt Brace & World.
55. Kay D: Schizophrenia and schizophrenia-like states in the elderly, Br J Hosp Med 8:369, 1972.
56. Kenshalo DR: Changes in the vestibular and somesthetic systems as a function of age. In Ordy JM and Brizzee KR, editors: Sensory systems and communication in the elderly, New York, 1979, Raven Press.
57. Kini MM, Leibowitz HM, Colton T, et al: Prevalence of senile cataract, diabetic retinopathy, senile macular degeneration and open-angle glaucoma in the Framingham Eye Study, Am J Ophthalmol 85:28, 1978.
58. Kisbourne M: Attentional dysfunctions in the elderly. In Poon LW, Fozard JL, Carmak LS, et al, editors: New directions in memory and aging, Proceedings of the George A. Talland Memorial Conference, Hillsdale, NJ, 1980, Lawrence Erlbaum Assocs, Inc, Pubs.
59. Kiyak HA, Beach BH, Worthington P, et al: The psychological impact of osseointegrated dental implants, Int J Oral Maxillofac Implants 5:61, 1990.
60. Koenig HG, George LK, and Siegler IC: The use of religion and other emotion-regulating coping strategies among older adults, The Gerontologist 28(3):303, 1988.
61. Kogan N and Wallach MA: Age changes in values and attitudes, J Gerontol 16:272, 1961.
62. Kornzweig AL: Visual loss in the elderly, Hosp Pract 12:51, 1977.
63. Kramer M: The increasing prevalence of mental disorders: a pandemic threat, Psychiatr Q 55:115, 1983.
64. Lawton MP: Schizophrenia forty-five years later, J Genet Psychol 121:133, 1972.
65. Lazarus RS and Cohen JB: The hassles scale, stress and coping project, Berkeley, 1977, University of California.
66. Lazarus RS and DeLongis A: Psychological stress and coping in aging, Am Psychol 38:245, 1983.
67. Lieberman MA: Adaptive processes in late life. In Datan N and Ginsberg LH, editors: Life-span developmental psychology: normative life crises, New York, 1975, Academic Press, Inc.
68. Leibowitz HM, Krueger DE, Maunder LR, et al: The Framingham Eye Study monograph, Surv Ophthalmol, suppl 24:335, 1980.
69. Lowenthal MF and Chiriboga D: Transition to the empty nest: crisis, challenge, or relief? Arch Gen Psychiatry 26:8, 1972.
70. Lowenthal MF, Thurnher M, and Chiriboga D: Four stages of life, San Francisco, 1975, Jossey-Bass, Inc, Pubs.
71. McCrae RR: Age differences in the use of coping mechanisms, J Gerontol 37:454, 1982.
72. McCrae RR: Age differences and changes in the use of coping mechanisms, J Gerontol 44:P161, 1989.
73. McIntire M and Angle C: The taxonomy of suicide and self-poisoning. In Wells C and Stuart J, editors: Self-destructive behavior in children and adolescents, New York, 1981, Van Nostrand Reinhold.
74. Meyer BJF and Rice GE: Learning and memory from text across the adult life span. In Fine J and Freedle RO, editors: Developmental studies in discourse, Norwood, NJ, 1983, Ablex Pub Corp.
75. Mignogna MJ: Integrity versus despair: the treatment of depression in the elderly, Clin Ther 8:248, 1986.
76. Miller IJ: Human taste bud density across adult age groups. J Gerontol 43:B26, 1988.
77. Miller M: Suicide after sixty: the final alternative, New York, 1979, Springer-Verlag, NY, Inc.
78. Mistretta CM: Aging effects on anatomy and neurophysiology of taste and smell, Gerodontology 3:131, 1984.
79. Moore NC: Is paranoid illness associated with sensory defects in the elderly? J Psychosom Res 25:69, 1981.
80. Moore RA: The prevalence of alcoholism in a community general hospital, Am J Psychiatry 128:638, 1971.
81. Morrant JCA: Medicine and mental illness in old age, Can Psychiatr Assoc J 20:309, 1975.

82. National Center for Health Statistics: Advance report of final mortality statistics: 1980, Monthly Vital Statistics Rep 32 (suppl), 1983.

83. Neugarten BL: Adaptation and the life cycle, J Geriatr Psychiatry 4:71, 1970.

84. Neugarten BL: Time, age and the life cycle, Am J Psychiatry 136:887, 1979.

85. Neugarten BL, Havighurst RJ, and Tobin SS: Personality and patterns of aging. In Neugarten BL, editor: Middle age and aging, Chicago, 1968, University of Chicago Press.

86. Niessen LC and Jones JA: Alzheimer's disease: a guide for dental professionals, Spec Care Dent 6(1):6, 1986.

87. Norris ML and Cunningham DR: Social impact of hearing loss in the aged, J Gerontol 36:727, 1981.

88. O'Hara MW, Hinrichs JW, Kohout FJ, et al: Memory complaint and memory performance in depressed elderly, Psychology and Aging 1:208, 1986.

89. Ordy JM, Brizzee DR, Beavers T, and Medart P: Age differences in the functional structural organization of the auditory system in man. In Ordy JM and Brizzee KR, editors: Sensory systems and communication in the elderly, New York, 1979, Raven Press.

90. Ordy JM and Brizzee KR, editors: Sensory systems and communication in the elderly, New York, 1979, Raven Press.

91. Palmore E, Cleveland WP, Nowlin JB, Ramm D, and Siegler IC: Stress and adaptation in late life, J Gerontol 34:841, 1979.

92. Pastalan LA: Designing housing environments for the elderly, J Architectural Educ 31:11, 1977.

93. Pastalan L et al: Age-related vision and hearing changes: an empathic approach, Slide tape program developed at the University of Michigan, Ann Arbor, 1976.

94. Pfeiffer E and Busse EW: Mental disorders in later life: affective disorders; paranoid, neurotic, and situational reactions. In Busse EW and Pfeiffer E, editors: Mental illness in later life, Washington, DC, 1973, American Psychiatric Association.

95. Poon LW: Differences in human memory with aging: nature, causes, and clinical implications. In Birren JE and Schaie KW, editors: Handbook of the psychology of aging, ed 2, New York, 1985, Van Nostrand Reinhold.

96. Post F: The functional psychoses. In Isaacs AD and Post F, editors: Studies in geriatric psychiatry, New York, 1978, John Wiley & Sons.

97. Powers JK and Powers EA: Hearing problems of elderly persons: social consequences and prevalence, J Am Speech Hearing Assoc (ASHA) 20:79, 1978.

98. Rice GE and Meyer BJF: Reading behavior and prose recall performance of young and older adults with high and average verbal ability, Educational Gerontol 11:57, 1985.

99. Rice GE and Meyer BJF: Prose recall: effects of aging, verbal ability, and reading behavior, J Gerontol 41:469, 1986.

100. Ringler RL: Aging perspective. In Miller NE and Cohen GD, editors: Clinical aspects of Alzheimer's disease and senile dementia, New York, 1981, Raven Press.

101. Rockstein M and Sussman M: Biology of aging, Belmont, Calif, 1979, Wadsworth Pub Co.

102. Rosin AJ and Glatt MM: Alcohol excess in the elderly, Q J Alcoholism 32:53, 1971.

103. Rosow I: Socialization to old age, Berkeley, 1974, University of California Press.

104. Ryan C and Butters N: Further evidence for a continuum of impairment encompassing male alcoholic Korsakoff patients and chronic alcoholic men, Alcoholism: Clin Exp Res 4:190, 1980.

105. Schiffman SS and Warwick ZS: Flavor enhancement of foods for the elderly can reverse anorexia, Neurobiol Aging 9:24, 1988.

106. Schmidt GL: Depression in the elderly, Wisc Med J 82:25, 1983.

107. Schonfield D and Stons MJ: Remembering and aging. In Kihlstrom JF and Evans FJ, editors: Functional disorders of memory, Hillsdale, NJ, 1979, Lawrence Erlbaum Assocs, Inc, Pubs.

108. Schuckit MA: Geriatric alcoholism and drug abuse, Gerontologist 17:168, 1977.

109. Schuckit MA and Miller PL: Alcoholism in elderly men: a survey of a general medical ward, Ann NY Acad Sci 273:558, 1976.

110. Schuckit MA, Miller PL, and Berman J: The three-year course of psychiatric problems in a geriatric population, J Clin Psychiatry 41:27, 1980.

111. Seeman M: Empirical alienation studies: an overview. In Geyer RF and Schweitzer DR, editors: Theories of alienation, Leiden, 1976, Martinus Nijhoff, Social Services Division.

112. Shamoian CA: Assessing depression in elderly patients, Hosp Community Psychiatry 36:338, 1985.

113. Shanan J: The Jerusalem study of mid-adulthood and aging, Isr J Gerontol 2:37, 1978.

114. Siassi I, Crocetti G, and Spiro HR: Drinking patterns and alcoholism in a blue-collar population, Q J Studies on Alcohol 34:917, 1973.

115. Small GW, Liston EH, and Jarvik LF: Diagnosis and treatment of dementia in the aged, West J Med 135:469, 1981.

116. Smith-DiJulio K, Heinemann ME, and Ogden L: Diagnosis and care of the alcoholic patient during acute episodes. In Estes NJ and Heinemann ME, editors: Alcoholism: development, consequences, and interventions, St. Louis, 1977, The CV Mosby Co.

117. Stenback A: Depression and suicidal behavior in old age. In Birren JE and Sloane RB, editors: Handbook of mental health and aging, Englewood Cliffs, NJ, 1980, Prentice-Hall Inc.

118. Stevens JC, Plantinga A, and Cain WS: Reduction of odor and nasal pungency associated with aging, Neurobiol Aging 3:125, 1982.

119. Stevens-Long J: Adult life, Palo Alto, Calif, 1979, Mayfield Pub Co.

120. Straatsma BR, Foos RX, and Horwitz J: Aging-related cataract: laboratory investigation and clinical management, Ann Intern Med 102:82, 1985.

121. Subby P: A community based program for the chemically dependent elderly, Presented at North American Congress on Alcohol and Drug Problems, San Francisco, 1975.

122. Terry RD and Wisniewski H: Structural aspects of aging of the brain. In Eisdorfer C and Friedal RO, editors:

Cognitive and emotional disturbance in the elderly, Chicago, 1977, Year Book Medical Publishers.
123. Thomae H: Personality and adjustment to aging. In Birren JE and Sloane B, editors: Handbook on mental health and aging, Englewood Cliffs, NJ, 1980, Prentice-Hall Inc.
124. Thomas PD, Hunt WC, Garry PJ, et al: Hearing acuity in a healthy elderly population: effects on emotional, cognitive and social status, J Gerontol 38:321, 1983.
125. Tylenda CA and Baum BJ: Oral physiology and the Baltimore Longitudinal Study of Aging, Gerodontology 7:5, 1988.
126. Verillo RT: Age-related changes in the sensitivity to vibration, J Gerontol 35:185, 1980.
127. Weale RA: Senile changes in visual acuity, Trans Ophthalmol Soc UK 95:36, 1975.
128. Weiffenbach JM, Baum BJ, and Burghouser R: Taste thresholds: quality specific variation with human aging, J Gerontol 37:372, 1982.
129. Wells CA: Pseudodementia, Am J Psychiatry 136:895, 1979.
130. Whanger AD and Wang HS: Clinical correlates of the vibratory sense in elderly psychiatric patients, J Gerontol 29:39, 1974.
131. Wilsnack RW, Wilsnack SC, and Klassen AD: Women's drinking and drinking problems: patterns for a 1981 national survey, Am J Public Health 74:1231, 1984.
132. Worchel P and Byrne D, editors: Personality change, New York, 1964, John Wiley & Sons.
133. Zimberg S: The elderly alcoholic, The Gerontologist 14:222, 1974.
134. Zung WWK: Depression in the normal aged, Psychosomatics 8:287, 1967.

# 3

# The Biology of Aging

*What is aging?*

S. Michal Jazwinski
Henry Rothschild

*Adapted by* **Sidney Epstein** *and* **Barnet M. Levy***

Human orofacial growth and development has been fairly well defined. Not so well understood is orofacial aging, which is obviously a component of the general aging process. In recent years, the field of the biology of aging has burgeoned, resulting in the enunciation of many "theories" of aging. Much of what we have learned has yet to be applied to the field of orofacial aging and geriatric dentistry. Some changes that occur with age—with time— are "natural." When they affect the orofacial areas, they affect the way we look; that is, we "look" young—we "look" old, based primarily on our orofacial appearance. Other changes that occur with age are a consequence of the imposition of disease, the effects of drugs, and the effects of society and culture on the aging person. Most important, aging itself is not a disease!

The oral diseases associated with aging can be understood only when examined in the light of known biologic changes. The so-called theories of aging are many and varied. All add something to our understanding of the orofacial changes that occur with age and therefore should be reviewed in that context. In later chapters, application of what we know of the biology of aging is directly applied to orodental problems of older persons.

## MANIFESTATIONS OF AGING

Individuals vary considerably in both the rate and the magnitude of age-related changes in cells, tissues, and organs. A common observation is that some people age rapidly, whereas others remain "well preserved." This observation, coupled to individual differences in longevity and the wide variations in performance by persons of the same chronologic age, have led to the concept of functional or physiologic aging as distinguished from chronologic aging. Those who age rapidly usually perform less well on age-related measures of function than those who age slowly.

The time of onset of age-dependent changes varies, as well as the patterns of change. Alterations in one system or structure do not always signal aging of the whole organism, but any deterioration in one organ system must influence changes in other organs. Some functions show predictable decline with age: vital capacity, cardiac output, renal

*From Jazwinski SM and Rothschild H: The biology of aging. In Rothschild H: Geriatrics for the internist, St. Louis, Mosby-Year Book, Inc. (In progress.)

plasma flow, glomerular filtration rate, swallowing, tongue function, taste acuity, grip strength, and reaction time are but a few. The rate of yearly loss seems to occur at about 0.8% to 0.9% of the functional capacity present at 30 years of age. Other functions, such as pH and electrolyte content of blood and verbal intelligence, show no age-associated changes.

The aging process may then be defined as the sum of all morphologic and functional alterations that occur in an organism and lead to function impairment, which decreases the ability to survive stress. Before the intrinsic properties of the aging process are dissected, however, it is necessary to separate processes and events that are only incidental to it.

## PATHOLOGIC PROCESSES

Superimposed on the basic biologic changes that occur with age is an increasing vulnerability to disease. Disease-related causes of death should therefore be separated from the "normal" physiologic processes that give rise to the manifestations of old age.

Delineating where the normal aging processes end and disease processes begin is difficult. Modern management of disease is reflected in the greatly increasing human life expectancy. This increase in life expectancy has been correlated with the control, elimination, or amelioration of pathologic processes by improved sanitation, nutrition, and drugs. By contrast, the maximum life span (which may be considered a measure of physiologic aging and independent of disease) has not changed.

## MORTALITY

The end point of the physiologic decrements that encompass aging is death. Disease may be viewed as the immediate cause of death in the elderly, but ultimately the biologic age changes that make disease more probable determine dying. Except for that caused by accident, death generally occurs when the body's capacity to withstand a specific challenge has been surpassed. Pneumonia, for example, is not an uncommon cause of death in the elderly. By contrast, in a young person, the same severity of lung infection caused by the same organism will usually be effectively resisted and overcome. The physiologic decrements that may

lead to pneumonia-caused death are the decrease in pulmonary function and reserve and reduced immune function. Thus pneumonia, a disease, is the proximate cause of death; however, the physiologic losses associated with aging are major determinants of the risk of dying. Furthermore, even though a given stress may not be sufficient to tax the body's tolerance, the functional impairments of old age may increase the frequency with which that stress is experienced.

Although aging may proceed linearly, the risk of mortality undergoes a sharp exponential increase with advancing years. For humans, the actuarial data, first analyzed by the English actuary Gompertz in the first quarter of the nineteenth century, show that mortality doubles every 7 years beyond 30 years of age, that is, after maturity, the rate and probability of dying increase exponentially with increasing age. In fact, the exponential increase in mortality is taken as a hallmark of "normal" aging and is characteristic of the aging process in most species (Fig. 3-1). Presenting aging as a linear process may be an oversimplification. To understand the aging process, one must strive to distinguish between physiologic decrements and superimposed pathologic processes. Such a distinction, however, is not *easily* apparent.

## FACTORS INFLUENCING AGING

Two alternative views on the nature of aging are prevalent: first, it is the result of *random damage*, and, second, it is the result of some *programed*, hence controlled, degeneration of the organism.

Aging, in essence, reflects a complex interaction of hereditary and epigenetic factors with environmental factors.

## GENETIC FACTORS

Evidence that genetic factors play a role in aging is substantial. The principal evidence that aging, as expressed by life span, is genetically determined derives from the following kinds of observations.

*Mutations.* Several mutations reduce the life span. However, in *Caenorhabditis elegans* a single mutation is known to increase it. It is unclear whether life-shortening mutations occur in specific longevity genes or the anomalies they produce are fundamentally inconsistent with maintenance of viability.

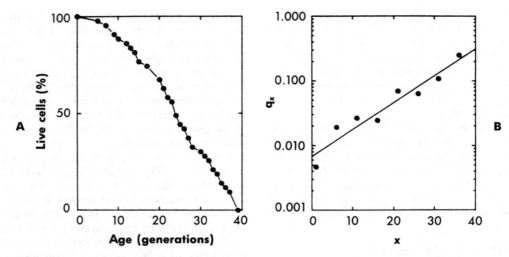

**Fig. 3-1** Survival characteristics of *Saccharomyces cerevisiae* X2180-1A. Life spans were determined for 43 individual cells. Buds were removed from mother cells at maturity by micromanipulation and deposited in isolated spots on an agar slab. These virgin cells, which had never budded before, were used to initiate the experiment. Every time the cell budded, the daughter was removed at maturity and the mother was scored one generation older. In **A,** the results are presented in the form of a survival curve. In **B,** the mortality $q_x$ (that is, $q_x = d_x h^{-1} L_x^{-1}$, where $d_x$ is the number of deaths in the interval $x + h$ [here 5 generations] at age $x$ and $L_x$ is the number living at age $x$) is plotted as a function of age, $x$, on a semilogarithmic scale. (From Jazwinski SM, Egilmez NK, and Chen JB: Exp Gerontol 24(5-6):423, 1989.)

***Species-specific life spans.*** Each species is characterized by its own pattern of aging and maximum (potential) life span (Table 3-1). Among mammals, the longevity ranges from that of humans, about 120 years, to that of small rodents, about 2 years. Differences in life spans of members of various animal groups argue strongly in favor of a species-specific genetic basis for longevity.

***Hybrid vigor.*** The effect of genetic constitution on longevity is perhaps best exemplified by those experiments in which hybrid vigor has been demonstrated. However, the increased longevity, seen in hybrids, does not exceed the maximum life-span characteristic of strains in the wild.

***Sex.*** In humans and most animals studied, the male is shorter lived than the female. For example, a white female born in the United States in 1974 can expect to outlive her male counterpart by 7.7 years. Leaving aside societal factors such as smoking, it has been hypothesized that if genes carried on the sex chromosomes indicate life span then genes on the X chromosome may decrease vulnerability to degenerative diseases. Contrariwise, genes on the Y chromosome may exert life-shortening effects that are incidental to their main function. Although the male is the shorter lived in most species, the opposite is true in some mouse, rat, and *Drosophila* strains.

***Parental age.*** Persons whose parents live to an older age have a greater life expectancy than persons whose parents died young. It has been shown that the summed age at death of the six immediate ancestors of centenarians and nonagenarians was significantly greater than those of persons in a control series. Persons older than 70 had at least one long-lived parent. Of nonagenarians, 48.5% had two such parents, and of centenarians, 53.4% had two long-lived parents. These figures are significantly higher than those found in the general population.

***Twin studies.*** The mean difference in life span for monozygotic twins has been found to be consistently less than that for dizygotic twins. As twins age, however, the differences decrease, attributable

**Table 3-1** Maximum life spans

| Organism | Maximum life span (in years) |
|---|---|
| Marion's tortoise | >152 |
| Man | 120 |
| Freshwater mussel | 100 |
| Sea anemone | 90 |
| Elephant | 70 |
| Eagle owl | 68 |
| Horse | 62 |
| Giant salamander | >52 |
| Chimpanzee | 45 |
| Domestic dog | 34 |
| Domestic cat | 28 |
| Mouse | 3.5 |

perhaps to the approaching maximum life span. Dizygotic twins show more variation in age at death than monozygotic twins do, but the difference was significant only in younger females. Thus individual genetic factors may shorten life expectation rather than increase it.

*Premature aging syndromes.* Single gene changes result in premature senescence in humans. Genetic diseases, such as progeria, are discussed later.

*Cells in culture.* A direct relationship exists between species longevity and replicative capacity of cells derived from the species. If one accepts the concept that cells in culture are an in vitro reflection of in vivo aging, the cell transformation that leads to immortality is difficult to explain, except through the abrogation of the genetic controls for limiting life span.

## ENVIRONMENTAL FACTORS

It has not been possible to convincingly document the action of any environmental factor or factors on the rate of aging. Nevertheless, it has been suggested that four categories of environmental factors influence the rate of aging in humans.

1. Physical and chemical components of the environment have been implicated as causing differential rates of aging. Some investigators have claimed that environmental pollutants, such as radiation, affect aging. Investigations of both laboratory animals and humans, how-

ever, do not support this contention. Comparisons of observed and expected numbers of deaths from all causes provide no evidence that occupational exposure to ionizing radiations leads to a detectable nonspecific shortening of the life expectation of radiologists. Hiroshima survivors, who have an increased incidence of leukemia, do not show symptoms of premature aging. In this population, no differences in age-related functions were determined by periodic measurement of blood pressure, vital capacity, heart size, gastric achlorhydria, hearing acuity, skin elasticity, and several immunologic tests. Only hand grip strength as a measure of neuromuscular function varied significantly between exposure groups and control subjects.

2. Biologic factors such as *nutrition* as a probable cause of differential aging in humans is discussed elsewhere in this volume. In fact, caloric restriction in laboratory rats, mice, and other animals is the only reliable method for lengthening their life span. It is not clear whether this treatment would extend the life span of humans.

3. Pathogens and parasites have been implicated in influencing the rate of human development and aging, particularly, in low-income groups and in tropical countries. Although they are important determinants of life expectancy (disease effect), there is no evidence that they influence the aging process.

4. Socioeconomic factors, such as bad housing, poor working conditions, or the stresses of life, are commonly believed to accelerate the aging process. This acceleration may, in fact, occur; however, it is difficult to confirm.

## MODELS FOR STUDYING SENESCENCE

Several systems, ranging from the analysis of cellular changes to clinical observations and testing in humans, each with its own inherent advantages and disadvantages, have been proposed as models for studying the aging process. The focal point in studies conducted with these models ranges from the molecular level to the intact organism.

## CULTURAL MODELS

For humans, the maximum life span is similar among geographically dispersed populations. Exaggerated claims of extreme longevity have been made for and by particular ethnic groups. For example, oft-quoted claims of longevity, with few debilitating diseases, have been made for three groups: one in the Andean village of Vilcabamba in Ecuador; the second in the Hunza state in the Karakoram Mountains of the Pakistani region of Kashmir; and the third in the Abkhazia and Ossetia regions in the Caucasus of the Georgian Republic of the Soviet Union. To appreciate the magnitude of those claims, one must realize that in other parts of the world the number of centenarians in the population is normally about two or three per 100,000, and the highest documented age attained has been about 120 years. Yet, in the three regions mentioned, not only have higher proportions of centenarians been claimed, but also many persons claim ages of 130 and even up to 160 years. Geographic, climatologic, dietary, genetic, and life-style situations were initially claimed as accounting for the increased life span and vigor of these populations. However, the claims of superlongevity have not been substantiated in any of these regions. Although many of the subjects in these areas are elderly, even centenarians, their exact age and their proportion in the total population have been questioned. Most records invariably involved recording errors and may have suffered from the tendency of extremely old persons to exaggerate their age. The best-studied situation, that in the Soviet Union, arose from a combination of social mores, politics, and fraud. Nevertheless, many of the older persons in those ethnic groups were more vigorous than similarly aged persons in other areas.

## HUMAN DISEASE ASSOCIATED WITH PREMATURE AGING

Human diseases, with accelerated aging phenotypes, have been used to study aging. The major limitation of this approach is the rarity of patients with these syndromes.

*Progeria.* Persons with progeria (Hutchinson-Gilford syndrome) show premature aging and bear uncanny resemblances to one another (Fig. 3-2). Invariably present in childhood, the condition has these characteristics: short stature (comparable to loss of height in the aged), decreased weight for height, diminished subcutaneous fat, craniofacial disproportion, micrognathia, prominent scalp veins, alopecia, prominent eyes, delayed dentition,

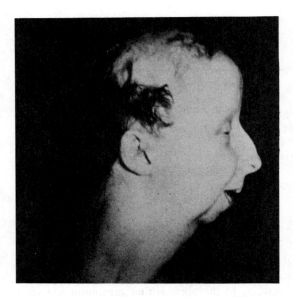

**Fig. 3-2** Patient with progeria (Hutchinson-Gilford syndrome). Age of this person at death was 16 years.

piriform thorax, a wide-based and shuffling gait, and stiff joints. Persons with this syndrome have normal intelligence. The median age at death is 12 years, with more than 80% of deaths attributed to cardiovascular disease. Widespread atherosclerosis and interstitial fibrosis of the heart are apparent at autopsy. Some features frequently associated with aging, such as diabetes, increased frequency of tumors, cataracts, or osteoporosis, are not found. The incidence is about one in 4 to 8 million live births. The low frequency of recurrence in families and the lack of consanguinity in those families, coupled to a paternal age effect, indicate that the source of progeria may be a dominant mutation. A reduced cumulative cell population doubling has frequently been found for cultured fibroblasts derived from patients with progeria.

*Cockayne's syndrome.* Cockayne's syndrome is a rare, autosomal recessive disease with some features of premature aging and some features that are not necessarily associated with senescence (Fig. 3-3). After apparently normal early development, the child in late infancy starts to show evidence of failure to grow, microcephaly, mental retardation, a peculiar facies and sunken eyes, prominent nose, prognathism, photosensitive der-

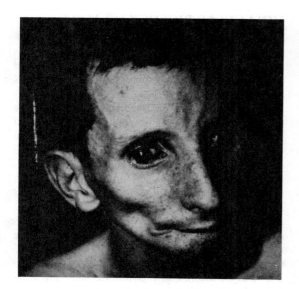

**Fig. 3-3** Person suffering from Cockayne's syndrome who died at 26 years of age.

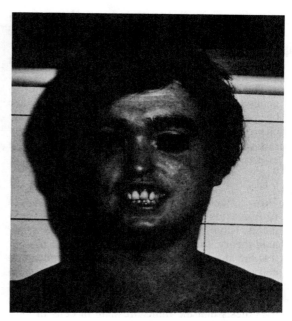

**Fig. 3-4** Person afflicted with Werner's syndrome who died at 29 years of age.

matitis, pigmentary retinal degeneration, partial deafness, and a progressive neurologic disorder characterized mainly by gait disturbance. Additional features include disproportionately long extremities with large hands and feet, limited joint movements, optic atrophy, cataracts, carious teeth, and thickened skull bones. Death usually occurs in late childhood or early adolescence.

*Werner's syndrome.* Werner's syndrome is a rare, autosomal recessive disease characterized by growth retardation during the teenage years, short stature, premature graying and hair loss, juvenile cataracts, thin skin, thick subcutaneous tissue, leg ulcers, loss of teeth, osteoporosis, soft-tissue calcification, insulin-dependent diabetes mellitus, and generalized atherosclerosis (Fig. 3-4). The mean age of survival is 47 years, and the incidence of neoplasms (carcinomas and sarcomas) is high (about 10%). Cultured fibroblasts from these patients have reduced life span with normal levels of ultraviolet and x-irradiation damage repair capacity.

None of the above syndromes can be considered simply as accelerated aging because each lacks some of the features of the normal aging process. Taken together, however, they do exhibit most of the major features of human aging. These syndromes illustrate the fact that simple genetic changes can profoundly alter the rates at which many of the processes of aging take place.

Inasmuch as the fibroblasts taken from patients with these syndromes display decreased life spans, it is hoped that an analysis of the cells grown in culture will lead to an understanding of aging at the molecular and genetic level.

## ANIMAL MODELS

Much information on physiologic aging derives from data obtained from wild, laboratory, and inbred vertebrates. The usefulness of mammalian model systems, from the molecular level to the whole organism, is proportional to their similarity to the human aging process. The advantage of some of these models is that the life spans of the animals are shorter than that of humans (Table 3-1); the disadvantage lies in the complexities of extrapolating from one species to another. It is usually accepted that genetically controlled animals should be used; however, no evidence has been presented that this stricture is valid. Inbred strains can pose difficulties of their own. Some strains of mice, for example, clearly display a propensity for the development of tumors that may confound certain kinds of aging studies.

The appropriateness of the model system depends on the question to be studied. Primates have been useful in studying the neuropathologic changes of aging. Laboratory rodents, particularly rats and mice, have been useful in studies on the effects of nutrition on longevity.

## CELLS IN CULTURE

Growing cells in culture has become a paradigm for the study of senescence. In his classic experiments, Hayflick found, in contrast to the previously held theory, that cells grown in culture are mortal, that the ability of normal fibroblasts to replicate in cell culture is finite, and that the number of population doublings is universally related to donor age and longevity of the species. He advanced the hypothesis that the finite life span of cells in vitro may be an expression of in vivo aging and therefore that such systems may be suitable models for the study of aging. Human fibroblasts can proceed through an average of about 50 population doublings before a sharp decline in proliferation occurs.

Other evidence to support the validity of this system as a model for aging includes the following:

1. Early-passage fibroblasts from old donors show a decreased population-doubling capacity similar in character to that of late-passage cells from embryos.
2. Cells from patients with progeria have curtailed life spans in vitro relative to cells from age-matched controls.

This model system lends itself to sophisticated manipulations and has led to the discovery of an inhibitory factor in old cells that can block replication of young cells and cells from many tumor cell lines. The study of cells as they age in culture has also permitted investigation of cellular events independent of the complexity of the whole organism. The conditions of cells in culture are not entirely physiologic, however, and allow study of only restricted classes of cells.

## MOLECULAR BIOLOGY OF AGING

The biochemical analysis of a variety of aging systems has revealed a wide assortment of changes associated with the aging process. Any variable subjected to analysis displays alterations as cells age. Overt manifestations of aging may be expected to have an even larger array of metabolic determinants. The most obvious manifestations of aging only scratch the surface. The problem with most of the biochemical studies is that they fail to establish causal relationships between the phenomena subjected to analysis and longevity. Frequently, even the efforts at establishing correlations are not altogether successful. The establishment of the biochemical phenomena underlying the aging process is of utmost importance as an initial step in the elucidation of the aging process. Such studies, as they become increasingly sophisticated, will undoubtedly continue to provide valuable information. However, there is need for new approaches to the problem.

The development of the powerful tools of recombinant DNA and their application to molecular genetics makes this new approach feasible. When coupled to the availability of classical genetics in an experimental system, this tool becomes exceptionally powerful. All these recent developments have given rise to a field that one may call the "molecular biology of aging." This term should not be understood to mean simply the biochemical analysis of macromolecules, but instead to include also the molecular study of the process of information storage and transfer during aging. Clearly, this brings the field into the realm of gene function and regulation. The methods of molecular biology have already found application in the study of gene expression during aging, and great potential exists for the analysis of control of proliferation in senescent cells, as mentioned above.

In metazoans, the interaction between various tissues and organs plays a predominant role in the maintenance of homeostasis. This is perhaps most clearly discerned in the neuroendocrine system. In keeping with this, adaptive failure at this hierarchical level of organization, rather than at the level of the individual cell, would be expected to have an overwhelming influence on aging. Consistent with this, the life span of any renewable cell type does not seem to be exhausted before the death of the organism. Many of the genes that are differentially expressed during the life span will probably play a role in aging at the cellular level. In an indirect way, they may influence aging of the organism. Even though a cell has not exhausted its own life span, incremental deficits in its function, which occur during aging, will undoubtedly play a role in senescence.

## BIOLOGIC THEORIES OF AGING

Numerous molecular models have been proposed to explain the mechanisms of aging. One is left with the impression that there is about one theory per investigator in the field with one theory not necessarily being an alternative to any of the others. The abundance of theories indicates the multitude of interpretations possible from the data on aging and the early stages of development of this field.

Many theories of aging presume that a single mechanism is responsible for all the characteristic changes seen with aging. Moreover, most focus only on the derangements that occur at some target molecule. In addition, most ignore the possibility that aging may be the result of several independent events involving genetically programed decay, random genetic changes, and environmental insults. If a unifying theory of such a complex process as aging is possible, it should account for aging in both replicative and postmitotic cells and should differentiate between programed senescence and that resulting from environmental damage to sensitive systems.

There is no simple way to catalog the various proposed theories. Those most often referred to are the following.

## GENETIC THEORIES

*Error theories.* The error theories of aging propose that senescence is related to the progressive accumulation of metabolic errors in macromolecules. In aging, DNA, RNA, and protein synthesis are now considered to be interconnected.

The possibility of a dramatic acceleration of error frequency was suggested by Orgel in 1963 in his "error catastrophe" theory. Because cellular metabolism, cellular and tissue interactions, and most life functions depend on the quality of proteins, the accumulation of errors in the production of these macromolecules would eventually become

great enough to impair function. The appeal of this theory was that it offered a simple translational explanation for aging and appeared testable.

The implications of this theory are particularly serious for cells that do not divide after they have differentiated, such as brain and muscle cells. If they function poorly, they die and are not replaced. The results are less serious for dividing cells, such as those of the liver or the lining of the gastrointestinal tract. Obviously, this statement is true only in situations in which the damage does not occur in stem cells.

The current data now argues preponderantly against the error catastrophe theory as well as against the idea of a less than catastrophic degree of errors occurring in proteins with age.

*Somatic mutations.* The basic assumption of the somatic mutations hypothesis is that just as spontaneous mutations occur in germ line cells, so also they may occur in somatic cells. Szilard postulated that random events called aging "hits" occur with a constant probability per unit of time throughout life. Because mutations cause some change in cell and tissue function, a sufficient number of cells carrying such mutations could affect tissue or organ function. More often than not, functional capacity declines. This theory is losing favor among the majority of scientists in the field of biologic aging.

*Redundancies.* Medvedev suggested that aging is attributable to the loss of unique, nonrepeated, genetic information from the genome. The repetitions of some genes, the bulk of which are repressed, are postulated as being not only an evolutionary reserve, but also a reserve to reduce the rate of aging. Medvedev believed that different species' life spans may be a function of the degree of repeated sequences.

Although many genes are present in multiple copies, these extra copies are frequently pseudogenes that cannot be expressed or variants that play specific roles during development or under certain conditions. Protein-coding sequences are largely absent from repetitive DNA. Thus this theory possesses historical interest only.

*Genetically programed senescence.* The theory of genetically programed senescence is the most general and the most comprehensive of the genetic theories. It is a deterministic theory, unlike the others that rely on randomly determined events. It is, however, consistent with the probabilistic nature of the aging process and can accommodate random components. The theory of programed senescence likens the aging process to the processes involved in development of the organism; in some renditions, aging is considered an extension of development. Development is a genetically determined process though epigenetic events play a crucial role. Thus, when we speak of programed aging, we talk about developmental (genetic) programs. This theory has seldom been explicitly enunciated; and, despite the fact that it makes strong predictions, it has never been subjected to experimental test. Instead, it has only been argued.

One of the most basic predictions of the theory is the genetic specification of life span. As mentioned earlier in this chapter, the genetic specification of life span is now widely accepted. Life span is clearly a polygenic trait. The acceptance of these views does not denote an acceptance of the existence of a genetic program that implies gene regulation. However, programed senescence need not mean that all manifestations of the aging process or age changes are part of a program. The existence of a program involving gene regulation becomes apparent only when such a program is altered to produce new and readily identifiable phenotypes. These phenotypes need not bear any relationship to what we normally consider age changes, such as the graying of hair. Thus not all the manifestations of the aging process must be programed.

*Disposable soma theory*. The disposable soma theory presents an attempt at a unifying theory for aging. It does not deal with mechanism directly. Rather, it is concerned with the ramifications of evolutionary or adaptive influences on the organism as they become manifested in senescence. In this theory, the function of the somatic cells of the organism, the soma (Greek 'body'), is to provide a vehicle for the germ line for assuring reproduction. A trade-off exists between devoting too few or too many resources to the soma. Too few resources will not allow the organism to survive for a time sufficient to guarantee a reasonable reproductive potential. Too many resources devoted to the soma will simply subtract from those devoted to the germ line, resulting in a lowered reproductive potential. It is the exhaustion of the resources avail-

able to the soma that results in aging and death. This disposable soma theory is applicable only to species that produce offspring repeatedly.

## NONGENETIC THEORIES

*Immunologic theories*. With aging, the immune system tends to be less able to distinguish normal molecules from abnormal ones, and so abnormal cells may proliferate and autoimmune reactions take place. As primarily advocated by Burnet, forbidden clones capable of a minor attack on tissues arise with greater frequency as age advances. Walford suggested that aging results from long-term, minor histoincompatibility reactions in the cell population. In humans, the frequency of autoantibodies in supposedly healthy older persons increases remarkably. In C3H mice and parabiotic hamsters, life has been shortened by an increase in low-grade histoincompatibility reactions. These features of the aging immune system, along with age-related decline in the ability to mount an immune response, might be called "immunosenescence."

More recently, Walford proposed that the major histocompatibility complex (MHC), though playing a role in the aging of the immune system itself, might also be one of a limited number of genes or gene complexes that actually play a regulatory role in aging, apart from their influence on certain specific aspects of the aging process. The MHC would be involved in the maintenance of "hierarchical homeostasis." In this form, the immunologic theory becomes a genetic theory. In any case, immunologic theories, though provocative, are not proved. The MHC, as compared to other chromosomal regions, does not appear to occupy a priviledged position in the aging process.

*Free-radical theory*. Free radicals are ubiquitous, short-lived, highly reactive chemicals produced during normal metabolic reactions. This theory postulates that free radicals combine with essential molecules, causing damage to DNA or other cellular structures. These reactions contribute to aging and age-associated diseases. Abnormal or uncontrolled free-radical reactions have been considered an important source of cellular damage in a variety of pathologic processes. Studies in mice have shown that administration of free-radical scavengers results in increased mean, but not maximum, life span. The free-radical theory, in its original version, is difficult to uphold. It has been modified to postulate that free radicals are implicated in processes that shorten life span below the maximum possible for a given organism. This effect is achieved by the involvement of free radicals, in certain chronic diseases, that are life limiting.

*Cross-linking theory*. Aging has been postulated to be caused by molecules becoming irreversibly immobilized as a result of strong cross-linking of substances having a profound effect on physiologic function. For example, cross-linking of collagen, which is 25% of total body protein, could affect the flow of nutrients and waste products from cells. These, in turn, are believed to produce changes that are, in effect, aging. Recently, another form of chemical modification of macromolecules has been proposed to play a fundamental role in aging. This is the nonenzymatic glycosylation of nucleic acids and especially proteins referred to as "glycation."

*Metabolic-rate or wear-and-tear theory*. It has been proposed that an increased metabolic rate, which presumably would result in greater wear-and-tear on the organism, results in a shorter life span. Thus Sacher has calculated that, among mammals, those species that have lower metabolic rates, defined as watts per gram of body weight, have longer life span. He also suggested that food (caloric) restriction lengthened life span by lowering the metabolic rate, which would seem to be intuitively obvious. Masoro's studies on food restriction in rats, however, do not support this concept.

## CONCLUSION AND PERSPECTIVES

We still have not answered "What is aging?" This difficulty in definition may arise from the varied causes of senescence, which may resemble cancer in this regard. The molecular basis for the multicausality of cancer seems to reside in the fact that the number of genes associated with it is large. These genes, the oncogenes, are derived from normal cellular homologs, the proto-oncogenes, whose expression or function has been altered by mutation or by genetic rearrangements. Evidence has been accumulating that the action of oncogenes can be suppressed by "anti-oncogenes." Anti-oncogenes may be considered normal components of signal-transduction pathways that function in the propagation of growth-inhibitory signals. Their presence manifests itself by preventing the expression of the transformed phenotype. The effects of these anti-oncogenes may be mediated at several levels, including gene transcription, that correspond to the various activities of oncogenes. Anti-oncogenes may perform hitherto unidentified cell cycle–regulatory functions.

Some of the genes involved in determining life span, seemingly, might easily fall into the category of anti-oncogenes. In this way, they would transmit signals that inhibit cell proliferation and ultimately lead to cell senescence.

How can we explain the physiologic aspects of aging by what we know at the basic level? This question translates directly into the question, "What is aging?" An important lesson learned from the study of cancer and cell cycle and growth control at the molecular level is that many crucial functions are analogous; and that the genes involved are homologous from lower eukaryotes to man. Only when we can describe how cell-cell interactions and the influences of the environment, that is, epigenetic factors, impinge on the mutual interactions of the "aging" genes, oncogenes, and anti-oncogenes will it be possible to arrive at the integration necessary to explain the key physiologic manifestations of the aging process. We are far from this goal. It is heartening, however, to know that a similar approach is bearing fruit in the analysis of the no-less-complex biologic processes of development and differentiation.

Old age is inevitable but need not be debilitating. Identifying and understanding the underlying cause or causes of senescence would be beneficial for intervening in and slowing the aging process, thus allowing for a longer period of well-being during a person's life, with a relatively quick denouement.

## SUMMARY

Geriatric dentistry is part of the health team that is responsible for intervening in and slowing the orofacial aging process or processes. The remaining chapters of this book build on the biologic concepts developed in this short review of the biology of aging.

## SELECTED READINGS

Cristofalo VJ, Adelman RC, and Roth GS, editors: CRC handbook of cell biology of aging, Boca Raton, Fla, 1985, CRC Press Inc.

Finch CE and Hayflick L, editors: Handbook of the biology of aging, New York, 1977, Van Nostrand Reinhold.

Finch CE and Schneider EL, editors: Handbook of the biology of aging, New York, 1985, Van Nostrand Reinhold.

Johnson TE and Mitchell DH, editors: Invertebrate models in aging research, Boca Raton, Fla, 1984, CRC Press Inc.

Rothstein M: Biochemical approaches to aging, New York, 1982, Academic Press Inc.

Rothstein M, editor: Review of biological research in aging, vol 1 to 3, New York, 1983, 1985, 1987 (respectively), Alan R Liss, Inc.

Sauer HW, editor: Cellular ageing, Basel, 1984, S Karger, AG.

Schneider EL, editor: The genetics of aging, New York, 1978, Plenum Press.

Warner HR, Butler RN, Sprott RL, and Schneider EL, editors: Modern biological theories of aging, New York, 1987, Raven Press.

Woodhead AD, Blackett AD, and Hollaender A, editors: Molecular biology of aging, New York, 1985, Plenum Press.

# 4

# The Effects of Aging on Drug Therapy

*Joseph M. Scavone*

The use of drugs in the elderly patient is an issue of social and medical concern. Problems associated with the proper selection of drugs, the patient's ability and desire to take medications as prescribed, the effects of aging on drug therapy, and the misunderstandings about the goal or goals of drug therapy have led to many discussions about the use of drugs in elderly patients. It is extremely important for dentists to be well informed about all drugs. Many elderly patients are taking several medications, which may interact with drugs prescribed by the dentist. Patients may also be taking over-the-counter drugs, which could affect a treatment plan. Thus, whenever a patient's clinical status is evaluated, both prescription and nonprescription drugs must be reviewed with the patient. Appropriate choice of drug therapy, dose selection, duration of therapy and potential interactions with a patient's coexistent disease states, other drug therapies, cigarette smoking, ethanol use, and life-style requirements must all be delicately balanced in an elderly patient.

Evaluating drug therapy in the elderly is difficult because both the frequency of drug therapy and the number of drugs taken progressively increases with age. It has been estimated that two thirds of all Americans over 65 years of age take at least one prescription drug. At hospital discharge, 25% of the aged patients receive prescriptions for six or more drugs. In nursing homes it is not uncommon for some patients to be receiving 12 to 15 drugs.

Almost 70% of aged people regularly use over-the-counter medications compared to about 10% of the general adult population. Approximately 55% of the over-the-counter drugs used by the aged are analgesics. It is estimated that the over-the-counter preparations account for at least 40% of all drugs used by the elderly. Since the incidence of adverse drug effects increases with age and number of medications used, the elderly may suffer adverse drug reactions one and a half to three times more than the younger and middle-aged adult population.[35]

Compliance with prescribed drug regimens by elderly patients is variable. It has been estimated that more than 60% are noncompliant to their prescription drug regimens. This is related to the frequency of administration and the number of drugs taken daily. Many patients either omit doses or take extra ones as dictated by their symptoms. Furthermore, it is not uncommon for the aged to self-medicate with nonprescription drugs or to take the wrong medication for a particular symptom.

The purpose of this chapter is to present information about the use of drugs by elderly patients and to describe the elements of drug therapy that are affected by the aging process. Therefore it is necessary to explain factors, such as physiologic changes, mechanisms of drug interactions, and adverse effects, that govern drug disposition and response. It is imperative that dentists have a working knowledge of these concepts so that they can better understand the effect of their treatments on the elderly patient.

## BASIC CONCEPTS OF DRUG THERAPY

Since the elderly react to medications differently from the way younger patients do, it is important to understand some basic concepts of body responses to drugs. The patient should receive the most appropriate drug for the disease in the right dosage, at a correct interval, and by an acceptable route of administration. When a certain drug is chosen for a patient, the pharmacologic action of the drug is always considered. The positive effect is referred to as its "therapeutic effect," and the unacceptable effects are known as "toxic, adverse, or side effects." Each drug has a certain mechanism of action that results in an acceptable and often coexistent unacceptable result or results. One has to weigh the positive and negative effects when selecting a certain drug therapy. Many drugs such as digoxin, theophylline, warfarin, phenytoin, lithium carbonate, antiarrhythmics, antibiotics, analgesics, and antianxiety agents have to be dosed so that the resultant drug concentration in the patient's serum or plasma lies within a defined "therapeutic range." Some drugs correlate very well to a range that will offer the most benefit with the least toxic effects. Thus drugs are categorized into two major groups: those with a "narrow" therapeutic range and those with a "wide" therapeutic range (see box and Fig. 4-1). A wide therapeutic range indicates that large fluctuations in serum or plasma drug concentration may occur without resulting in toxicity. Drugs with a narrow therapeutic range can cause the most problems in the aged patient when new therapies are added or changed, since pharmacologic and toxic effects closely parallel serum and plasma drug concentration.

## DRUG SENSITIVITY IN THE ELDERLY

It is well known that the elderly may exhibit an exaggerated response to medications. A therapeutic response may develop in aged patients at doses far below what is recommended for younger adults. Elderly patients may also experience drug toxicity

---

### THERAPEUTIC RANGES

**Examples of drugs with narrow therapeutic range**

Phenytoin
Theophylline
Digoxin
Gentamicin
Tobramycin
Kanamycin
Vancomycin
Lithium salts
Quinidine
Procainamide
Lidocaine

**Examples of drugs with wide therapeutic range**

Diazepam
Chlordiazepoxide
Lorazepam
Oxazepam
Temazepam
Propranolol
Atenolol
Ibuprofen
Imipramine
Amitriptyline
Buspirone

---

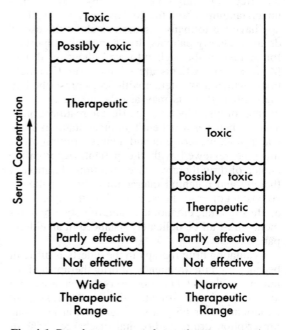

**Fig. 4-1** Based on serum or plasma drug concentrations, some drugs are associated with having wide or narrow therapeutic margins. Small fluctuations in plasma or serum drug concentration are unlikely to be clinically important for drugs with a wide therapeutic margin, but for drugs with a narrow therapeutic margin small fluctuations in concentration most likely will result in a change in clinical response.

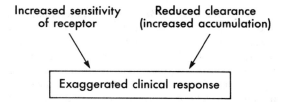

**Fig. 4-2** Drug sensitivity in the elderly resulting in alterations in clinical response can be explained by the complex interaction of pharmacokinetics and pharmacodynamics.

at doses that are within the usual therapeutic range.

Studies of drug response in the elderly have indicated that at least two types of phenomena may explain these changes in sensitivity (Fig. 4-2). The ability to biotransform (metabolize) and eliminate drugs from the body declines with age. If the total elimination (clearance) of drug is reduced, chronic therapy with any given dose will lead to higher steady-state (mean drug concentration after multiple dosage) blood concentrations, and the likelihood of toxicity is increased. The second explanation, a pharmacodynamic one, is that receptor site sensitivity to pharmacologic action of drugs may increase with age. Thus at any given drug concentration the presence of the drug at the receptor site may lead to a greater response. Such an increase in drug sensitivity may be evident clinically as a greater likelihood of excessive drug effect or effects or toxicity at what are usually regarded as safe therapeutic doses. Reduced drug sensitivity in the aged can also occur, but it has been described only in a few cases.

## PHARMACOKINETICS AND PHARMACODYNAMICS

When studying about the effects of drugs in the aged, one is quickly introduced to many terms that are used to describe the consequences of drug therapy. The term "pharmacokinetics" is often encountered and usually causes a fair amount of apprehension to those who are not familiar with the basic concepts. Pharmacokinetics is the mathematical analysis of the course of drug concentration in a body fluid or tissue. It describes the amount of drug in the body over time and includes factors that control the time course of drug absorption,

---

**FACTORS THAT CAN AFFECT THE PHARMACOKINETICS OF DRUGS**

**Patient variables**
Age
Gender
Body composition
Body weight
Drugs
Nutritional status
Ethanol use
Cigarette smoking

**Medical conditions**
Congestive heart failure
Kidney disease
Cirrhosis
Hepatitis
Fever
Sepsis
Burns (severe)
Anemia
Shock

---

distribution, biotransformation, and elimination, parameters collectively referred to as "drug disposition."

The pharmacokinetic profile of a drug is based on several interrelated factors that include the relationship of plasma or serum drug concentrations to the size and frequency of dose, the free or unbound drug concentration to the amount that is bound to proteins or other blood components, the equilibrium of ionized and unionized bound and unbound drug with receptors, and the dissipation of drug effects in relationship to the elimination of the drug from the receptor site.[33] Other factors that can influence the pharmacokinetics of drugs are listed in the box above.

It is important to realize that absorption, distribution, biotransformation (often referred to as metabolism), and elimination occur simultaneously at rates that change over time. The process is complex, but the essentials of pharmacokinetics should be understood by all persons involved in prescribing and monitoring the effects of pharmacologic agents. Since the goal of drug therapy is to treat a patient in such a way that medications provide a

| Blood | Receptor | Drug Action |
|---|---|---|

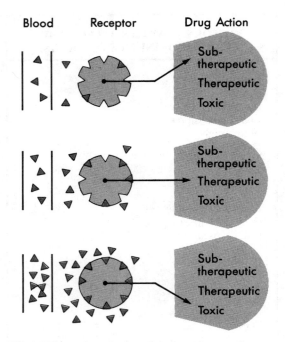

**Fig. 4-3** For many drugs a relationship between plasma or serum drug concentration and the availability of drugs at the receptor site translates to clinical effect.

therapeutic yet nontoxic way to manage various conditions, understanding and cautious application of pharmacokinetic principles can assist the dentist in making correct decisions when choosing or evaluating a patient's drug therapy.[17] It can also allow for more educated decisions about drug selection, dose, frequency of administration, route of administration, and monitoring therapeutic response, ineffectiveness, or toxicity. The application of the principles of pharmacokinetics are extremely important for safe and effective drug therapy, but it should never replace clinical judgment. Pharmacokinetics provides the framework for understanding drug behavior, but it oversimplifies the complicated physiologic events that govern drug disposition.

The other term that often appears in discussions about drug therapy in the aged is "pharmacodynamics." Pharmacodynamics refers to the interaction of the drug molecule with its target receptor site. The interaction of drug and receptor is analogous to an enzyme substrate or lock-and-key type of interaction (Fig. 4-3). To fully understand how and why a drug causes a particular effect or the mechanism of drug interactions, its pharmacodynamics must be defined. The effects of aging on receptor sensitivity, specificity, number, and affinity are now being studied. When the pharmacodynamic effects of aging are correlated with pharmacokinetic changes, it will enable the dentist to more accurately predict the effects of drugs in the aged patient.[8]

## ABSORPTION

The oral route is the safest, most convenient and economical delivery route for drugs intended to have a systemic effect. Orally administered drugs are absorbed from the gastrointestinal tract into systemic circulation and distributed to the site of action. Numerous factors govern the absorption process. In discussions of drug absorption three variables that describe the bioavailability (systemic availability in terms of rate and extent) of a drug should be identified: time of peak plasma drug concentration ($T_{max}$), peak plasma drug concentration ($C_{max}$), and the area under the plasma drug concentration–time curve (AUC). Knowledge of the bioavailability of a drug is important because it can be used as a guide when choosing between a brand name and a generic form of a drug, or when changing from one dosage form or product to another. For example, solutions are absorbed faster and often more completely than either suspensions, capsules, or tablets. Likewise suspensions are absorbed more quickly than capsules, which are absorbed quicker than tablets. Soft gelatin liquid-filled capsules are more quickly absorbed than the hard gelatin-dry powder-filled capsules. The intention of drug therapy is also an important factor. Drugs can be administered as a single dose for a specific time-limited situation or in multiple doses for chronic therapy. For example, if the patient is taking a medication as a single dose for the treatment of acute pain or as a sedative, it is important that the drug is absorbed quickly and that it produces a high enough blood level for a long enough time to be clinically effective. However, if a medication such as an antibiotic is needed for a long period of time, it is more important that the drug provides an average or steady state (constant) concentration in the blood.

After a tablet or capsule is swallowed, it must

disintegrate before the active drug can dissolve and become absorbed into the bloodstream. If a drug does not get absorbed from the stomach, it will pass into the small intestine where most drugs are actually absorbed. Factors that govern the absorption of drugs from the gut include the amount of fluid that is coingested with the dosage form, pharmaceutical aspects of the dosage form (such as tablet coatings, formulation, and hardness), the presence of other substances (other drugs, antacids, food, or ethanol) in the stomach, gastric emptying time, and intestinal transit time. All these variables influence the bioavailability profile of a drug. Other considerations include medications that can delay gastric emptying and gastrointestinal transit time (anticholinergics or opiates), drugs that accelerate gastric emptying (metoclopramide), and drugs that can bind other drugs (antihypercholesterolemic resins, Kaopectate, or psyllium type of laxatives).

Another concern is that some drugs such as nonsteroidal anti-inflammatory agents (including salicylates), potassium tablets and capsules, and iron supplements can be extremely irritating to the gut mucosa. Gastrointestinal bleeding, ulceration, and perforation have been reported with the aforementioned drugs. A simple way around this problem is to require the patient to take these drugs with food or milk or at least 4 to 6 ounces of fluid, which will buffer the effects of the drug on the gastrointestinal mucosa. Such a simple instruction is often forgotten.

The presence of food or milk usually causes a delay in drug absorption, but it should not be a clinically important problem if the drugs are taken as chronic therapy. If, however, the patient requires an immediate analgesic effect, the first dose should be taken on an empty stomach with one-half to one cup of water (Fig. 4-4). The risks of gastrointestinal ulcerations, bleeding, and perforation associated with nonsteroidal anti-inflammatory drug therapy, especially in aged and debilitated patients, are so important that the U.S. Food and Drug Administration requires the manufacturers of these drugs to include a highlighted warning about the occurrence of these problems in the package information inserts and in the *Physicians' Desk Reference (PDR)*.

Enteric coated tablets are specially coated to dissolve in the higher pH of the small intestine. This type of tablet is especially useful in preventing ir-

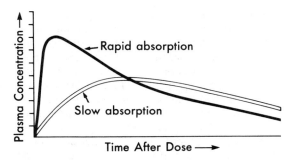

**Fig. 4-4** The rate of absorption is an important determinant of the onset of clinical activity (such as analgesics, sedatives, hypnotics). Shown here is an example of a drug administered in the fasting state (rapid absorption) and the same drug coadministered with food (slow absorption).

ritation by the drug to the gastric lining. Since the tablet is designed to dissolve in a higher pH, drugs that increase gastric pH such as antacids and histamine$_2$ antagonists (that is, cimetidine, ranitidine, nizatidine, famotidine) may cause the tablet to dissolve in the stomach. Therefore these drugs should be taken separately or coadministered with meals. This dosage form of aspirin is best used for chronic therapy rather than for the management of acute pain because of erratic absorption patterns. Sustained-release tablets, which provide a slow release of medication either by dissolution over varying ranges of pH, by ion exchange, or by leaching of the drug slowly out of a special matrix, may also be affected by changes in gastrointestinal pH transit time.

Other routes of administration that involve drug absorption include the oral route in which a drug can be used sublingually, buccally, or as a perioral spray, the intramuscular route, the subcutaneous route (including injection and implantation), the intranasal route, the ophthalmic route, and the transdermal route. There is not much information about the effects of aging on the absorption of drugs from these other routes. It is assumed that aging does not significantly affect the absorption of drugs from these routes either. Anecdotal information indicates that if an aging person has diminished salivary production and if he or she is taking an anticholinergic drug such as an antihistamine, tricyclic antidepressant, or antipsychotic medication, these may sufficiently dry the mouth so that it takes longer for the tablet to dissolve. Although this has not yet been studied in a controlled fashion, it may explain why some aged patients have difficulty with sublingual dosage forms. The sublingual route of drug administration is becoming more popular because in some patients oral administration may be undesirable because of nausea, vomiting, or other situations when the use of the gastrointestinal tract needs to be avoided. Drugs such as triazolam, alprazolam, captopril, opiate analgesics, antiarrhythmics, nitroglycerin, and other drugs are administered by this route.[38-39]

The coingestion of food and other drugs can significantly affect the bioavailability of a drug. Certain drugs such as propranolol and griseofulvin actually have an increased bioavailability when taken with food, whereas the coingestion of food can delay absorption of analgesics, hypnotics, and other drugs so dramatically that the desired clinical effect after a single dose will not occur.

When drugs are given in multiple doses as chronic therapy, the amount of drug absorbed (AUC) is more important than either $T_{max}$ or $C_{max}$. Since the object of drug therapy is to maintain an average blood level of the drug, the course of absorption is less important than the actual amount of drug that replaces what has been cleared by the body.

Numerous studies performed on the effects of aging on the gastrointestinal tract indicate the possibility of altered drug absorption in the aged gut.[21.34] Reasons for this include increased gastric pH because of a reduction in gastric parietal-cell function resulting in decreased gastric acid output,[13] decreased splanchnic blood flow resulting from a decrease in cardiac output,[41] a reduction in gastric emptying time, and a decrease in gastrointestinal motility.[10] In addition, altered active-transport processes of some nutrients in the aged have led to the belief that drug absorption may be similarly impaired.[29] However, for most drugs used in clinical practice, the rate and extent of absorption are determined by passive diffusion during contact with the surface of the proximal small intestine.[21] Despite speculation to the contrary, there is essentially no evidence that drug absorption is impaired in the aged.[26.31-32] Any changes, if they actually do occur, are often small and unlikely to be of any clinical importance, especially during chronic therapy.[6.18] In summary, changes in drug absorption

appear to be the least important of the age-related pharmacokinetic changes. Knowledge of how drug absorption affects the onset and duration of clinical effects for drugs that are given as single doses can assist the dentist in targeting the desired therapeutic effects of a drug for a specific situation.

## DISTRIBUTION

Once in the body a drug will be distributed to various body fluids and tissues. Fat-soluble drugs such as digoxin, diazepam, and imipramine are distributed readily and have relatively large distribution volumes, whereas water-soluble drugs such as cephalosporins, penicillins, and aminoglycosides are considered to have small volumes of distribution. Understanding drug distribution is sometimes difficult because the distribution volumes or compartments are actually derived from mathematics rather than anatomy and physiology. Thus pharmacokinetic compartments are imaginary mathematical spaces and do not correspond to actual anatomic entities, even though the compartments are assigned numeric dimensions of volume (milliliters, liters).[17]

After a drug reaches systemic circulation, its passage into body tissue and fluids depends on the drug's molecular size, degree of ionization, solubility, and ability to cross biologic membranes. The goal is to have the drug reach the receptor at the intended site of activity and to cause the desired effect. If too much reaches the receptor site, toxicity could result, and if not enough drug reaches the target, a subtherapeutic response can result. Furthermore, if the drug is available to reach other sites, adverse effects may occur. For example, an antihistamine may be prescribed for the treatment of an allergy, coughs, or colds, but in addition to alleviating the symptoms, it can act in the central nervous system to cause drowsiness and confusion, in the eyes to cause a mydriasis and a blurring of vision, in the gastrointestinal tract to cause a decrease in gut motility resulting in constipation, and in many other areas to cause urinary retention, diminished salivary flow, and various other effects.

If the drug is able to penetrate many areas in the body, the range of adverse effects can be dramatic. Certain drugs are specifically designed to have different lipid- and water-solubility characteristics so that the intended action is more predictable based on its distribution profile. Since many drugs need to be present at the site of activity at a certain minimum effective concentration, a drug's distribution profile can be used clinically so that one may actually plan a desirable duration of effect. For example, benzodiazepines such as midazolam and diazepam are administered intravenously as a pre–anesthetic/induction agent for surgery or orally (diazepam, alprazolam) for conscious sedation or as anxiolytics.[42] They are extremely fat-soluble substances that are readily distributed throughout the body after the administration of the dose. Because of their extensive distribution, the central nervous system concentrations diminish to a level where the drug is not active any longer. Thus the termination of clinical effect is governed by the distribution of the drug throughout the body, causing a dilution of the amount available to the brain and not by the biotransformation or excretion of drug from the body. If a lipid-soluble drug with a large volume of distribution is given chronically, as is often the case with diazepam, the compartments will sequester drug and the result will be the accumulation of drug in various tissues. This can lead to residual effects secondary to increased total body levels of drug. Benzodiazepines, which are relatively more hydrophilic, will exhibit longer durations of clinical effect than their more lipophilic counterparts after single doses but will accumulate to a lesser extent after chronic dosing (Fig. 4-5). The level of response to a medication may increase over time independent of an increase in dose to the patient. Although this concept is extremely important, many dentists and physicians forget that drug accumulation can occur. Some reasons for this include the ability of the body to maintain homeostasis through adaptive mechanisms at the receptor site. It is a rather complicated process, but the message is that, despite the protective mechanisms, the body's homeostatic mechanisms can be overridden after a period of time because of changes in reserve capacity.

Several factors such as decreased cardiac output, increased peripheral vascular resistance, decreased blood flow to the liver and kidney blood flow, and increased fraction of cardiac output to cerebral, coronary, and skeletal muscle circulations affect the distribution of drugs in the aged person.[3,34] In addition age-related changes in body habitus (composition) can affect drug distribution. The aged generally experience a decrease in body water, ex-

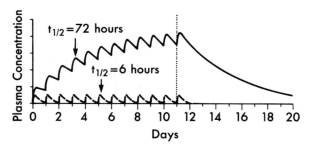

**Fig. 4-5** Accumulation of a drug with a long elimination half-life versus no accumulation of a drug with a short elimination half-life after the administration of multiple doses.

tracellular fluid, muscle, and lean body mass and a relative doubling in the proportion of adipose tissue (Fig. 4-6). For example, the fat content in the body of young adult males is approximately 18% and can increase to approximately 36% in aged males. The percentage of fat in young adult females is approximately 33% and can increase to approximately 48% in aged females.[21] These changes in body habitus can affect the volume of drug distribution, depending on the drug's fat and water solubility. Thus it appears that there is a gender-related difference in the aged regarding the volume of distribution of drugs. Women will have a larger distribution of fat-soluble drugs[2,19-20] and a smaller distribution volume for relatively water-soluble drugs.[7,22] Various fat-soluble drugs such as diazepam and lidocaine are more extensively distributed in the aged, whereas various relatively water-soluble drugs (less lipid soluble) such as ethanol, antipyrine, and acetaminophen have a decreased volume of distribution in aged persons.[21,25,30,45]

After drugs enter the systemic circulation, they become bound to circulating plasma proteins. Albumin and alpha$_1$ acid glycoprotein (AAG), an acute-phase reactant, are the two most important proteins to which drugs can bind. The attachment of drugs to a protein involves a reversible bonding of the ionic, hydrogen, or van der Waal's type, which is relatively weak and loose.[36] Acidic drugs preferentially bind to albumin (such as nonsteroidal anti-inflammatory agents, salicylates, benzodiazepines, warfarin, and phenytoin) whereas basic drugs (tricyclic antidepressants, beta-adrenergic receptor antagonists, lidocaine, and other drugs) bind

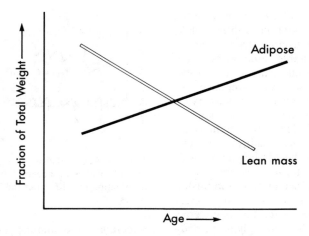

**Fig. 4-6** Changes in body habitus as a function of age are shown here. As one ages, there tends to be a reduction in lean body mass and total body water and an increase in adipose tissue.

to alpha$_1$ acid glycoprotein. Not all drugs are equally bound, and the actual binding of drugs is a dynamic process. In any given situation there is an equilibrium that is established between the amount of drug that is bound and the amount of drug that is unbound or free. The percentage of free drug is known as the free fraction and represents a ratio between the free drug concentration and the total (free plus bound) drug concentration. The distribution of drug to plasma proteins contributes to the actual volume of distribution because only the unbound drug is available to leave the systemic circulation and travel to the receptor site. Additionally, it is the free drug that is available for elimination from the body and to other body tissues and fluids. Although some controversy exists, an age-related reduction in plasma albumin concentrations and age-related increases in alpha$_1$ acid glycoprotein have been consistently reported.[9,15] Aged patients who are undernourished, are severely debilitated, or have advanced disease especially have a substantial decrease in plasma albumin concentrations.[27] Healthy, well-nourished aged persons have lower albumin concentrations than young persons have even though they may not fall below the usual normal range.[21] The degree of drug binding to plasma proteins may be reduced in the aged because of the decrease in the amount of albumin and because of suspected alterations in the affinity of albumin for drugs.[34,36]

The clinical implications of protein binding have often been overestimated. Plasma protein binding, or changes in binding that may occur as a result of drug interactions or disease, seldom have any direct clinical importance. It is neither a benefit nor disadvantage for a drug to be extensively bound to plasma protein because the free drug concentration is that which is available for pharmacologic activity, distribution, and clearance. The free concentration depends only on the drug dosing rate and the clearance of free drug, not on the actual extent of protein binding.[16] Drugs that are considered highly protein bound are generally greater than 80% bound (see box, next page). Changes in free fraction could be important for drugs that are 80% to 90% bound but much more important for those that are greater than 90%. When the free fraction is small, slight variations can have important consequences. Drugs that are less than 80% bound generally imply that the consequences of protein binding are relatively unimportant.[17]

Although protein binding interactions do not directly influence clinical activity, alterations in binding can have an enormous effect on the interpretation of total serum or plasma drug concentrations. When drug levels in the serum, plasma, or whole blood are monitored, the laboratory reports the total (free plus bound) amount of drug even though it is only the free drug that is available to cross cell membranes and interact with the receptor. Luckily

## EXAMPLES OF PROTEIN-BOUND DRUGS

**Greater than 90% bound**

Warfarin
Ibuprofen
Phenylbutazone
Indomethacin
Diazepam
Chlordiazepoxide
Temazepam
Oxazepam
Furosemide
Thiazide diuretics
Oral hypoglycemics (first generation)
Propranolol*
Chlorpromazine*

**80% to 90% bound**

Lorazepam
Sulfisoxazole
Salicylates
Phenytoin
Oxazepam
Clofibrate
Haloperidol*
Methadone*
Quinidine*
Tricyclic antidepressants*

*Bound to alpha$_1$ acid glycoprotein; drugs without an asterisk are bound to albumin.

the free concentration remains stable over the course of a patient's therapy, and the variability between and within patients is relatively small.[12]

When more than one highly protein-bound drug is given to a patient, drug binding to serum protein may be substantially altered. A "new" drug added to a therapeutic regimen can displace the present drug or drugs from their protein binding site or sites resulting in a reduction in binding accompanied by an increase in free fraction.[24,40] Such interactions have been misinterpreted. In reality these interactions are unlikely to be clinically important because the transient increase in free concentrations will equilibrate rapidly and will be available for clearance.[21,24,28,40] The total drug concentration will be reduced as a result of redistribution and may result in a lowering of the therapeutic and toxic ranges for the total serum or plasma drug level.[12]

For example, if a patient who was taking phenytoin (Dilantin) for the treatment of a seizure disorder and routinely had steady-state plasma concentrations averaging about 15 μg/ml and was well controlled (seizure and side effect free) received a prescription for aspirin, a drug interaction will most likely occur because of the displacement of phenytoin from protein binding sites by the salicylate. However, this drug interaction would unlikely be of clinical importance, since only the total blood level of phenytoin would decrease.[11] Protein binding interactions are complex, yet transient, and the net result is usually harmless to the patient. The misinterpretation of what actually occurs is the main problem and could result in an inappropriate and potentially hazardous intervention. Since the elderly take more medications, the frequency as well as the confusion of such interactions is much greater than in younger patients.

In summary, a change in drug binding to plasma proteins does not itself alter clinical drug effects. However, alterations in binding may influence the interpretation of plasma or serum drug concentrations (blood levels) used to monitor therapy.[21] For highly protein-bound drugs whose binding is decreased and resulting free fraction is increased, dentists should anticipate lower ranges of both toxic and therapeutic plasma or serum concentrations of total (free plus bound) drug. Regarding drug distribution, altered drug distribution itself in the aged will not alter steady-state plasma concentrations during chronic drug administration because the maintenance of steady-state plasma concentrations depends only on the dosing rate and the total clearance of the drug.

## CLEARANCE

In order to understand how the body eliminates drugs, it is important to be familiar with terms such as "clearance" and "elimination half-life."

The concept of total clearance is extremely important when evaluating the pharmacokinetic properties of all drugs. Clearance is expressed in units of volume divided by time (such as milliliters per minute (ml/min), or liters per hour (L/hr) and is the single most reliable index of an organism's capacity to biotransform (metabolize) or excrete a given drug.[16] Most clinicians are familiar with the concept of clearance in the context of renal function, for which the clearance of creatinine is used as an index of kidney function. Creatinine clearance schematically represents the total volume of blood from which creatinine is completely removed per unit of time. The clearance of drugs is conceptually similar. Most drugs are primarily cleared by either the liver or the kidney. A given drug's clearance numerically describes the capacity of a given person to remove that drug from the body. A drug's clearance cannot exceed the rate of drug delivery or blood flow to the clearing organ.

Clearance is important in clinical practice because it is a major determinant of steady-state plasma or serum concentration during multiple dosage. In fact, the total clearance of a drug will influence a patient's therapeutic outcome. When a medication has been administered as a multiple dose long enough for steady state to occur, the general equation describing the steady-state concentration in blood, plasma, or serum ($C_{ss}$) is as follows:

$$C_{ss} = \frac{\text{Dosing rate}}{\text{Clearance}}$$

It is important for dentists and physicians to appreciate this equation because dosing rate is the variable over which they have control; it is the rate of drug administration, expressed in units of amount of drug divided by time (such as milligrams per hour (mg/hr), or grams per day (g/d). By varying the size of each dose or the interval between doses (dosage schedule), the dentist or physician can directly control the dosing rate and ultimately the steady-state concentration. Clearance appears in the denominator of this equation as the biologic variable describing the person's capacity to remove the drug from the body. However, in a medically stable patient the clearance of a drug is assumed to be constant. Changes in hepatic or renal status secondary to aging or disease or the addition or deletion of drugs that affect the function of the liver, such as the chemicals in cigarette smoke, ethanol, and drugs that are hepatic microsomal enzyme inducers or inhibitors, and the function of the kidney, such as drugs that compete for renal tubular absorption or secretion, may dramatically change a person's clearance rate. Thus, at any given dose rate, $C_{ss}$ will increase as clearance decreases.[21] If aging is associated with the reduction in total clearance of a given drug, $C_{ss}$ will increase accordingly, and the clinician can either extend the dosing interval or give a lower maintenance dose to the aged patient for a desired steady-state concentration.

Knowledge of a drug's pathway of biotransformation and of factors that could influence its clearance can help dentists to anticipate how patient characteristics, drug interactions, or disease states might alter clearance. Many drugs yield active metabolites upon biotransformation that contribute to the therapeutic or toxic effect of the parent compound. The ultimate goal of multiple-dose drug administration is to achieve a steady-state plasma concentration that lies within a "therapeutic" range and to avoid toxic or clinically ineffective blood levels.[16]

## ELIMINATION HALF-LIFE

Elimination half-life is probably the most commonly discussed and most misinterpreted pharmacokinetic variable for drugs used in clinical practice. Most drugs are eliminated by a characteristic kinetic behavior known as "first-order process." For a drug to fit this first-order model, the rate of change of drug concentrations over time must vary continuously in relation to the concentration.[17] Drug concentration in body fluids usually declines with time; when the concentrations are high (that is, after drug administration), the rate of decline is also high, and when concentrations are low the rate of decline is smaller. Since the rate of drug disappearance varies continuously as a function of time as the concentration changes, an exponential function is used to describe this behavior. Luckily, first-order exponential processes can be described by use of the concept of half-life. The elimination half-life of a drug is the time necessary for the drug concentration in blood, serum, plasma, or any other body fluid or tissue to fall by one half, or 50%. Each time an interval equal to a half-life elapses, the concentration falls to one half the value at the beginning of that interval. The amount of drug that has been eliminated from the system decreases with the passing of each half-life, but the percentage or ratio of change (50%) is always constant. The important facts[17] to remember about the clinical use of half-lives is that:

1. All first-order processes are more than 90% complete after four half-life intervals have elapsed.

2. First-order processes are never 100% complete no matter how much time elapses.
3. It takes approximately four to five half-lives to elapse before a drug is considered to be in the steady-state condition.
4. It takes approximately four to five half-lives to elapse before a drug is considered to be virtually eliminated from the system even though first-order processes are considered to be essentially complete after approximately eight half-life intervals.

It is also important that dentists understand that the elimination half-life is a dependent biologic variable related to a drug's volume of distribution ($V_d$) and inversely related to its total clearance as follows:

$$\text{Elimination half-life} = \frac{0.693 \times V_d}{\text{Clearance}}$$

If the volume of distribution is relatively constant, the elimination half-life will be inversely related to total clearance. Therefore, when clearance is low, half-life is long, and conversely, when clearance is high, half-life is short. However, when the volume of distribution is not constant, changes in the volume of distribution may influence the elimination half-life without a change in clearance.[1] The potential pitfalls of elimination half-life must always be recognized.

Elimination half-life is a clinically important variable because it is related to the rate and extent of drug accumulation during multiple dosage. When a drug is administered at dosing intervals that are shorter than its elimination half-life, a large fraction of each prior dose will remain in the body when the next dose is administered. This leads to drug accumulation, which continues until the steady-state condition is reached, at which point there is no further accumulation. Likewise the time necessary to reach steady state after the start of multiple-dose therapy is also related to the drug's elimination half-life. This concept is used clinically in situations where a loading dose is administered to a patient in order to quickly initiate a therapeutic response.

Many categories of drugs contain representatives in their class that vary widely in their elimination half-life. This raises questions about which type of drug is more appropriate for a particular patient. There are benefits as well as disadvantages for both long half-life and short half-life compounds. Drugs with relatively short values of elimination half-life (such as ibuprofen, triazolam, temazepam, lorazepam, and alprazolam) are usually termed "nonaccumulating." For these drugs, the steady-state condition is reached rapidly after the start of therapy. This may provide some therapeutic benefit in terms of ease of dosage titration because little delay occurs between initiation of treatment and the attainment of steady state. Short half-life compounds also have some potential disadvantages, since multiple daily doses are usually required to maintain adequate plasma levels throughout the day. Furthermore when treatment is discontinued, or if doses are inadvertently or deliberately missed, serum concentrations will fall rapidly, and such change may lead to rapid recurrence of symptoms, withdrawal, or rebound effects. For long half-life compounds (such as piroxicam, digoxin, diazepam, chlordiazepoxide, and desmethyldiazepam), a theoretic disadvantage is that attainment of steady state may be delayed. There is also a delay in the achievement of a new steady-state condition if the dosage must be increased or decreased. There is also a long elimination (washout) phase upon discontinuation of the drug, and it must be accounted for when a patient's treatment response is reevaluated after a different drug therapy is started. On the other hand, a potential advantage is that the number of doses that the patient takes per day is decreased, and such reduction could possibly translate into enhanced patient compliance. Furthermore, when treatment is discontinued, or when doses are missed, plasma levels will not fall promptly, thereby minimizing the likelihood of a rapid recurrence of symptoms.

## BIOTRANSFORMATION

Biotransformation, commonly referred to as "drug metabolism," is a considerably complex process that primarily occurs in the liver. Liver cells carry out many biotransformation reactions that contribute to the removal of drugs from the body. Oxidation and conjugation are the two most important subdivisions of hepatic clearance. These reactions can be categorized into either phase I, also referred to as "preparative reactions," or phase II, also

## EXAMPLES OF DRUGS THAT ARE BIOTRANSFORMED

**By phase I (preparative) reactions**

Alprazolam
Amitriptyline
Antipyrine
Barbiturates
Carbamazepine
Chloramphenicol
Chlorpromazine
Clonazepam
Codeine
Desipramine
Desmethyldiazepam
Diazepam
Dimenhydrinate
Doxylamine
Flurazepam
Glutethimide
Ibuprofen
Imipramine
Lidocaine
Meperidine
Methamphetamine
Nortriptyline
Midazolam
Phenacetin
Phenylbutazone
Phenytoin
Prazepam
Quinidine
Trazodone
Triazolam
Warfarin

**By phase II (synthetic) reactions**

Acetaminophen
Acetylsalicylic acid (aspirin)
Clonazepam
Hydralazine
Lorazepam
Nitrazepam
Oxazepam
Phenelzine
Procainamide
Sulfanilamide
Temazepam

known as "synthetic reactions." Phase I biotransformation includes the oxidation reactions such as hydroxylation, dealkylation, sulfoxidation, nitroreduction, and hydrolysis. These reactions generally constitute minor molecular modifications usually resulting in a more water-soluble (polar) metabolite. The products of these reactions also retain part or all of the pharmacologic activity of the parent compound.[21] Examples of drugs that undergo phase I biotransformation reactions that yield active metabolites include (parent drug to active metabolite): diazepam to desmethyldiazepam, flurazepam to desalkylflurazepam, imipramine to desipramine, and amitriptyline to nortriptyline. Hepatic microsomal oxidation is often termed a "susceptible" metabolic pathway, in that its activity can be impaired by numerous factors such as old age, hepatitis, cirrhosis, severe debilitation, or the coadministration of many agents known to impair oxidizing capacity.[14,47] The hepatic microsomal enzymes responsible for phase I reactions appear to be significantly impaired in the aged. The result is a reduction in total drug clearance, higher steady-state plasma drug concentrations during multiple dosage, and an increase in elimination half-life. Phase II reactions involve the attachment or conjugation of the drug molecule to a glucuronide, sulfate, or acetate moiety. The resulting conjugates are generally pharmacologically inactive (except for some acetylated metabolites), are much more polar than the parent molecule, and are usually excreted in the urine.[21] Hepatic conjugation is considered to be a "nonsusceptible" pathway and is relatively not influenced by old age, disease states, or drug interactions.[16,20] Thus a prior knowledge of a drug's major metabolic pathway (oxidation versus conjugation) may be of help to the dentist in predicting whether clearance is susceptible to change in a specific clinical situation (see the box and Fig. 4-7). In addition, it can be helpful in drug selection for the aged patient. For example, the benzodiazepines diazepam, chlordiazepoxide, desalkylflurazepam, and desmethyldiazepam are all subject to oxidation reactions during the clearance from body. The clearance of many drugs is reduced in aged patients, and the likelihood for increased accumulation is a concern in this patient population. Since the metabolism of the parent drug yields metabolites that are also clinically active, there is

**Biotransformation**

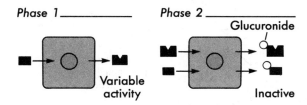

**Fig. 4-7** Phase I (oxidation) versus phase II (conjugation) biotransformation pathways are shown. Phase I reactions may yield the formation of active metabolites, whereas phase II reactions result in the inactivation of a drug.

a concern about the accumulation of not only the parent drug, but the active metabolites as well. The accumulation of metabolites could theoretically contribute to the development of adverse or increased effects. On the other hand, the benzodiazepines oxazepam, temazepam, and lorazepam undergo conjugation reactions, have no active metabolites, and are relatively unaffected by aging. Thus drug selection for the aged patient can essentially make more sense if the prescribing dentist considers the drug's metabolic fate.

Hepatic blood flow can be more important for some drugs than microsomal enzyme activity as a major determinant of total drug clearance.[46] Partially as a result of an age-related reduction in cardiac output, liver blood flow declines an estimated 40% to 45% in aged persons as compared to young adults.[13] Hepatic size, both in absolute terms and as a percentage of total body weight, decreases with age. One would expect that the clearance of liver blood flow–dependent drugs would be uniformly affected, but the data are conflicting. For example, a reduction in the total clearance occurs for propranolol but not for lidocaine.[4,30,44] Theoretically the bioavailability of drugs that have a high first-pass hepatic extraction (after drug absorption from the gastrointestinal tract before reaching the general systemic circulation) may also be affected by aging, but there is no conclusive evidence available at this time.

It is difficult to predict the influence of age on biotransformation, since hepatic drug-metabolizing capacity may not be uniformly affected. Changes in total clearance of hepatic microsomal enzyme–mediated drug-oxidation reactions can be impaired in an aged person even though the patient has normal liver function tests. Thus normal values on liver function tests do not imply normal drug metabolism. In addition, the effect of age on hepatic drug clearance depends on the metabolic pathway of the drug in addition to the influence of liver blood flow, size, and other coingested substances and drugs.

## ELIMINATION (RENAL CLEARANCE)

The effect of age on renal drug clearance is more straightforward and predictable. Glomerular filtration rate decreases by about 35% over a person's lifetime, and so drugs excreted mainly by the kidney can be expected to have reduced total clearance.[21,34,37,43] To adequately predict the effect of the aging kidney on total drug clearance, one needs to know the status of a patient's level of renal function. This is usually accomplished by evaluation of a serum creatinine level of estimation of a glomerular filtration rate (GFR) using creatinine clearance as an indicator. Serum creatinine concentration depends on endogenous creatinine production as well as renal creatinine clearance. Evaluating renal function based on serum creatinine is often misleading because the age-related decrease in lean body (muscle) mass results in a decrease in daily endogenous creatinine production. As a result, in the aged creatinine clearance must fall to a greater extent than in a younger person before the serum creatinine increases.[37] Thus the use of serum creatinine concentration as the only indicator of renal function may actually overestimate renal function (Fig. 4-8). In an aged patient, serum creatinine may be in the normal range while renal function

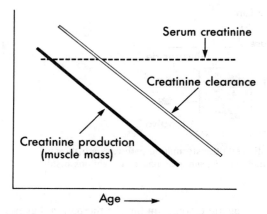

**Fig. 4-8** Serum creatinine values may result in an over-estimation of renal function in the elderly. With less muscle mass, less creatinine is formed and is presented to a kidney with reduced function. Normal serum creatinine values usually result even when there is a significant decline in renal function.

is substantially reduced.[21,34] Ideally, creatinine clearance determinations based on 24-hour urinary excretion should be used along with serum creatinine to evaluate renal function. In reality this is not always feasible, and so clinicians must rely only on serum creatinine concentrations. However, there are various nomograms and formulas available to estimate creatinine clearance from serum creatinine. One formula[5] that is considered useful is the following:

Creatinine clearance in males
$$= \frac{(140 - \text{Age}) \times \text{Body weight (kg)}}{72 \times \text{Serum creatinine level}}$$

Creatinine clearance in females
$$= 0.85 \times \text{(Above value)}$$

where creatinine clearance is in milliliters per minute (ml/min), serum creatinine is in milligrams per deciliter (mg/dl), age is in years, and weight is in kilograms (kg).

In general, the dosage of a drug that is excreted principally by the kidney must be reduced to prevent excessive accumulation of the drug (see box). After reduction in the initial doses of drugs excreted by the kidney, the clinical status of the patient can be reviewed and dosage adjustments can be made.

| EXAMPLES OF DRUGS THAT ARE EXCRETED BY THE KIDNEY |
| --- |
| Amantadine |
| Amikacin |
| Cephalosporins |
| Cimetidine |
| Digoxin |
| Erythromycin |
| Furosemide |
| Gentamicin |
| Lithium salts |
| Mefenamic acid |
| Nitrofurantoin |
| Penicillins |
| Phenobarbital |
| Procainamide |
| Quinidine |
| Sulfonamides |
| Tetracycline |
| Tobramycin |
| Vancomycin |

## APPLICATIONS TO PATIENT CARE

The information presented in this chapter offers a comprehensive review of clinical pharmacology and the effects of aging on drug therapy. Absorption processes do not appear to be affected by the aging process, but distribution, metabolism (biotransformation), and renal elimination may be altered so that clinically significant effects result. When one is choosing dosages for elderly patients, a smaller dose should be tried initially, and depending upon the desired clinical response, subsequent doses should be titrated upward or downward. For actual drug selection, the dentist should choose drugs that will not interact with a patient's preexisting drug therapies. In pharmacokinetic terms, drugs that alter gut motility could affect the absorption or toxicity profile of other agents. Drugs that may compete for protein binding should especially be noted in case potential drug interactions occur. In this type of situation the patient's other health care providers may have to be consulted, especially if the patient is receiving warfarin or anticonvulsants.

Accumulation can also occur depending on a

drug's route of clearance or metabolite profile. Care should be taken in noting which drugs the patient is currently using that could alter the metabolism of the drug being selected, or if the new therapy could affect the clearance of a patient's coexisting drug therapy. If drugs that are excreted intact by the kidney are selected, care must be used by the dentist so that the appropriate dose is selected. When antibiotics are used, if the dose is too low, the patient's infection will not be treated effectively; however, if the dose is too high, the risk of toxicity may be unacceptable.

A complete review of a patient's medications is extremely important. This review should include a listing of all current medications, both over the counter and prescription. A review could also help to reveal the source of a patient's dental problem. Drugs with anticholinergic activity can dramatically diminish salivary production and flow.[23,48] These drugs include $H_2$-receptor blockers, antihistamines, antidepressants, antiparkinsonians, diuretics, antipsychotics, and muscle relaxants. Some over-the-counter drugs with anticholinergic effects include sleeping pills, appetite suppressants, antispasmodics, antidiarrheals, calmatives, and cough and cold preparations. Special attention should be given to the possibility of patients taking numerous anticholinergic agents in which there exist additive effects. A complete drug history should also include questions about prior drug sensitivities, adverse drug reactions, and allergies.

Whenever a prescription is written, it should be properly explained to the patient. Information should be provided as to what the generic and brand names are, what the drug is for, how it should be taken, what the patient should expect in terms of therapeutic effects and side effects, and what the patient should do if he or she experiences any problems. This information should all be provided by the prescribing dentist and should be explained in sufficient detail so that the patient understands the medications that are being prescribed. This may also positively influence compliance, since a patient is more likely to trust his or her drug therapy if it is understood. The dentist should also try to choose drugs that can be taken in a dosing pattern similar to that of the rest of the patient's medications. This will help to ensure that the patient takes the drug on schedule.

In summary, there are many factors that govern appropriate drug therapy in the aged patient. With the number of new drugs introduced each year, the increasing numbers of elderly patients, and the sophistication of medical care, choosing drugs for a patient can be extremely difficult. Often a patient's clinical condition is delicately balanced and care must be taken not to upset homeostatic compensatory mechanisms. Knowledge of clinical pharmacology, pharmacokinetics, pharmacodynamics, and the effects of aging on all these parameters will help the dentist to provide the most appropriate care for his or her patients.

## REFERENCES

1. Abernethy DR et al: Alterations in drug distribution and clearance due to obesity, J Pharmacol Exp Ther 217:681, 1981.
2. Allen MD et al: Desmethyldiazepam kinetics in the elderly after oral prazepam, Clin Pharmacol Ther 28:196, 1980.
3. Bender AD: The effect of increasing age on the disturbances of peripheral blood flow in man, J Am Geriatr Soc 13:192, 1965.
4. Casteleden CM and George CF: The effect of age on the hepatic clearance of propranolol, Br J Clin Pharmacol 7:49, 1979.
5. Cockroft DW and Gault MH: Prediction of creatinine clearance from serum creatinine, Nephron 16:31, 1976.
6. Divoll M et al: Age does not alter acetaminophen absorption, J Am Geriatr Soc 30:240, 1982a.
7. Divoll M et al: Acetaminophen kinetics in the elderly, Clin Pharmacol Ther 31:151, 1982b.
8. Dorris RL and Taylor SE: Significant adverse interactions of drugs in dentistry, Dent Clin North Am 28:555, 1984.
9. Dybkaer R et al: Relative reference values for clinical chemical and haematological quantities in 'healthy' elderly people, Acta Med Scand 209:1, 1981.
10. Evans MA et al: Gastric emptying rate in the elderly: implications for drug therapy, J Am Geriatr Soc 29:201, 1981.
11. Fraser DG et al: Displacement of phenytoin from plasma binding sites by salicylate, Clin Pharmacol Ther 27:165, 1980.
12. Friedman H and Greenblatt DJ: Rational therapeutic drug monitoring, JAMA 256:2227, 1986.
13. Geokas MC and Haverback BJ: The aging gastrointestinal tract, Am J Surg 117:881, 1969.
14. Gibaldi M and Perrier D: Clinical pharmacokinetics, N Engl J Med 293:702, 964, 1975.
15. Greenblatt DJ: Reduced serum albumin concentration in the elderly: a report from the Boston Collaborative Drug Surveillance Program, J Am Geriatr Soc 27:20, 1979.
16. Greenblatt DJ and Scavone JM: Pharmacokinetics of oxaprozin and other nonsteroidal antiinflammatory agents, Sem Arthritis Rheum 15(suppl 2):18, 1986.
17. Greenblatt DJ and Shader RI: Pharmacokinetics in clinical practice, Philadelphia, 1985, WB Saunders Co.

18. Greenblatt DJ et al: Pharmacokinetics and bioavailability of intravenous, intramuscular, and oral lorazepam in humans, J Pharm Sci 68:57, 1979.
19. Greenblatt DJ et al: Diazepam disposition determinants, Clin Pharmacol Ther 27:301, 1980.
20. Greenblatt DJ et al: Clobazam kinetics in the elderly, Br J Clin Pharmacol 12:631, 1981.
21. Greenblatt DJ et al: Drug disposition in old age, N Engl J Med 306:1081, 1982.
22. Greenblatt DJ et al: Antipyrine kinetics in the elderly: prediction of age-related changes in benzodiazepine oxidizing capacity, J Pharmacol Exp Ther 220:120, 1982.
23. Handelman SL et al: Hyposalivatory drug use, whole stimulated salivary flow, and mouth dryness in older, longterm care residents, Special Care Dent, Jan-Feb:12,1989.
24. Koch-Weser J and Sellers EM: Binding of drugs to serum albumin, N Engl J Med 294:311, 526, 1976.
25. Klotz U et al: The effects of age and liver disease on the disposition and elimination of diazepam in adult man, J Clin Invest 55:347, 1975.
26. Kramer PA et al: Tetracycline absorption in elderly patients with achlorhydria, Clin Pharmacol Ther 23:467, 1978.
27. MacLennan WJ et al: Protein intake and serum albumin levels in the elderly, Gerontology 23:360, 1977.
28. McElnay JC and D'Arcy PF: Protein binding displacement interactions and their clinical importance, Drugs 25:495, 1983.
29. Montgomery R et al: The ageing gut: a study of intestinal absorption in relation to nutrition in the elderly, Q J Med 47:197, 1978.
30. Nation RL et al: Lignocaine kinetics in cardiac patients and aged subjects, Br J Clin Pharmacol 4:439, 1977.
31. Ochs HR et al: Effect of age and Billroth gastrectomy on absorption of desmethyldiazepam from clorazepate, Clin Pharmacol Ther 26:449, 1979.
32. Ochs HR et al: Diazepam absorption: effects of age, sex, and Billroth gastrectomy, Dig Dis Sci 27:225, 1982.
33. Ogilvie RI: An introduction to pharmacokinetics, J Chron Dis 36:121, 1983.
34. Ouslander JG: Drug therapy in the elderly, Ann Intern Med 95:711, 1981.
35. Picozzi A and Neidle EA: Geriatric pharmacology for the dentist: an overview, Dent Clin North Am 28:581, 1984.
36. Richey DP and Bender AD: Pharmacokinetic consequences of aging, Annu Rev Pharmacol Toxicol 17:49, 1977.
37. Rowe JW et al: The effect of age on creatinine clearance in man: a cross-sectional and longitudinal study, J Gerontol 31;155, 1976.
38. Scavone JM et al: Enhanced bioavailability of triazolam following sublingual versus oral administration, J Clin Pharmacol 26:208, 1986.
39. Scavone JM et al: Alprazolam kinetics following sublingual and oral administration, J Clin Psychopharmacol 7:332, 1987.
40. Sellers EM: Plasma protein displacement interactions are rarely of clinical significance, Pharmacology 18:225, 1979.
41. Stevenson IH: Drugs for the elderly. In Lemberger L and Reideberg MM: Proc Second World Conference on Clinical Pharmacology, Washington, DC, American Society of Pharmacology and Experimental Therapy, Bethesda, Md, pp 64-73, 1984.
42. Terezhalmy GT et al: Pharmacotherapeutics in urgent dental care, Dent Clin North Am 30:399, 1986.
43. Vestal RE: Drug use in the elderly, Clin Pharmacokinet 1:280, 1978.
44. Vestal R et al: Reduced beta-adrenoceptor sensitivity in the elderly, Clin Pharmacol Ther 26:181, 1979.
45. Vestal RE et al: Aging and ethanol metabolism, Clin Pharmacol Ther 21:343, 1977.
46. Wilkinson GR and Shand DG: A physiological approach to hepatic drug clearance, Clin Pharmacol Ther 18:377, 1975.
47. Williams RL: Drug administration in hepatic disease, N Engl J Med 309:1616, 1983.
48. Wright JM: Oral manifestations of drug reactions, Dent Clin North Am 28:529, 1984.

# 5

# Oral Physiology

*Bruce J. Baum*
*Anthony J. Caruso*
*Jonathan A. Ship*
*Andy Wolff*

It is the purpose of this chapter to provide the reader with a general overview of oral physiology and aging. We have chosen to focus our discussion on key functions of the oral cavity that are fundamental to human physiology. From our perspective, the oral cavity has two essential roles: (1) to initiate alimentation and (2) to permit communication (speech). All the tissues and structures in the mouth have developed to subserve these functions. We cannot survive as a species in a complex society without the successful routine accomplishment of these functions. In addition, the oral cavity has another responsibility and that is to protect itself. The mouth is exposed to the outside world with a limitless number of insults available to affect local tissues and functions as well as to put the host at systemic risk. Accordingly, specialized protective mechanisms (saliva, a mucosal barrier, the commensal flora) have evolved to allow the two key oral physiologic processes to occur. We are potentially quite vulnerable to considerable morbidity and even at some fatal risk if our oral defenses are significantly compromised.

Specifically in this chapter we address salivary gland secretion, the oral mucosal barrier, and motor/sensory performance. For each topic, we first provide a current understanding of the general physiologic mechanism involved in the accomplishment of the function. This ranges from being quite detailed for salivary secretion and some sensory tasks to being less specific for mucosal barrier

function; a circumstance that reflects true limitations in our knowledge of these subjects. Secondly, we try to convey what is known about the performance of these physiologic tasks in the aging person.

One should understand that we know relatively little about aging and oral physiology. There are not many groups of investigators at work in this area, and there are not much available data describing true physiologic status with age. It is important to emphasize here that aging and disease are different. To describe normal human physiology one must measure functions in essentially healthy persons, regardless of their age. Many literature reports on the effects of aging are based on the evaluation of patients with diseases and who are using various pharmaceuticals. We cannot be sure that such effects truly reflect age-related alterations. Furthermore, even in studies conducted with healthy persons, most reported findings are of a cross-sectional nature. Cross-sectional aging studies compare different persons of two or more age groupings, such as those 20 to 40 years old with others 60 to 80 years old. Although such studies are useful, interpretation of the results must be made with considerable caution because different people, with different experiences, are involved. True aging data, based on longitudinal evaluations of oral physiologic functions in the same persons over time, are indeed sparse. Thus, in reading this chapter, you should proceed with care.

## SALIVARY GLANDS

There are three major pairs of salivary glands (parotid, submandibular, sublingual) and several minor glands (such as labial, palatal, buccal) whose primary function is the exocrine production of saliva. Saliva plays a critical role maintaining and preserving oral health. Each gland type makes an unique secretion derived from either mucous cells or serous cells, forming the fluid in the mouth termed "whole saliva." In addition to the secretions from the major and minor salivary glands, whole saliva contains many other constituents that are not salivary in origin (such as desquamated mucosal epithelial cells, food debris, bacteria and their products, and serum factors). In the evaluation of salivary gland function, therefore, it is more appropriate to evaluate individual gland secretion and not whole saliva.

It is generally believed that two steps are involved in the formation of saliva.[90] Initially, salivary gland acini secrete an isotonic fluid (such as 140 mEq/L NaCl) called "primary saliva," which contains most (approx. 85%) of the exocrine salivary proteins. These proteins are derived from the exocytotic release of secretory granule contents into the forming saliva.[18] This primary saliva is then modified as it passes through the ductal system before being secreted into the oral cavity.[56] This represents the second step in the secretory process and principally involves the reabsorption of NaCl. The second stage results in a final gland saliva entering the mouth which is considerably hypotonic (such as 20 mEq/L NaCl). Ductal cells also contribute the remaining 15% of salivary proteins.[102]

The principal control of salivary secretion is the autonomic nervous system by means of parasympathetic and sympathetic innervation.[11] Stimulation of neurotransmitter receptors located on the basolateral membrane surface of salivary gland acini activates intracellular events that lead to fluid production and protein release. Much less is known about neural control of ductal cell functions, but it is believed that stimulation of neurotransmitter receptors on ductal cells will influence the ion fluxes by reabsorption and secretion of electrolytes in the ducts, and such events lead to the final hypotonic saliva. It is likely that salivary gland dysfunction exists when neurotransmitter receptors are altered, or when neural signals to the salivary gland receptors are impaired.

---

### MAJOR ROLES OF SALIVA IN THE MAINTENANCE OF ORAL HEALTH

Preparation and translocation of the food bolus
Lubrication of oral mucosa
Preservation of microbial ecologic balance
Mechanical cleansing
Antibacterial and antifungal activities
Maintenance of oral pH
Remineralization of dentition
Mediation of taste acuity

---

As noted above, saliva is critical for the maintenance of oral health.[54] The presence of saliva protects the oral cavity, the upper airway, and the digestive tract and facilitates numerous sensorimotor phenomena. The absence of saliva, not surprisingly, has many deleterious consequences to the host. The specific functions of saliva are multiple and are listed in the box.

Saliva contributes to the digestion of food by assisting in food bolus formation and translocation. Salivary fluid (water) and lubricatory proteins thus facilitate deglutition. The lubricatory glycoproteins found in saliva also help maintain the integrity of oral mucous membranes. The microbial ecologic balance of the oral cavity is carefully preserved, and most oral flora do not pose a severe threat to the host. Saliva possesses antibacterial and antifungal components, which are essential in maintaining the balance of the oral flora. In addition, saliva buffers intraoral pH and directly protects the dentition. Saliva is supersaturated with calcium and phosphate salts, which help to remineralize incipient caries. There are several salivary proteins (such as anionic proline-rich proteins) that also assist in the remineralization of the dentition. Finally, taste-sensory phenomena partially depend on the presence of saliva to dissolve tastants and bring them into contact with oropharyngeal taste buds.

The salivary glands are known to undergo quantitative and qualitative histologic changes with increased age. Morphometric studies on submandibular and parotid gland samples obtained from essentially healthy persons show that the proportion of gland parenchyma occupied by acinar cells is reduced 25% to 30% over the adult life span.[73-74]

With advancing age there is an atrophy of acinar tissue, a proliferation of ductal elements, and some degenerative changes in the major salivary glands. These alterations tend to occur linearly with increasing age and can even be detected in early adult life. Minor salivary glands also undergo similar degenerative changes with advancing age. Therefore there appears to be a normal, uniform decrease in the acinar content of salivary gland tissue accompanying the aging process.

Salivary secretion has long been believed to be reduced with increased age. Recent functional studies have not, however, supported this general stereotype. It is now generally accepted that parotid saliva output is stable across all ages in healthy persons.[10] There is no uniform agreement on submandibular saliva production. One study reported that submandibular salivary flow rates were significantly diminished in an older group of healthy persons when compared to younger subjects,[65] whereas another recent study indicated no significant age-related trends in a population of healthy adults.[92] At present, there is only one report of minor salivary gland fluid output in different aged persons. In this study significant reductions in stimulated labial gland saliva flow rates were found in healthy older persons compared to younger subjects.[31] Therefore it is difficult to make a general conclusion about the age-related status of fluid output from all the salivary glands. It appears, however, that decreased saliva flow does not uniformly accompany aging in healthy persons. A few studies have evaluated salivary composition in different aged persons and generally show similar constituent levels with increased age.[13,19,30]

These functional observations contrast with the morphologic changes seen in aging salivary glands mentioned above. Since it is known that acinar components are primarily responsible for the secretion of saliva,[102] it is not understood why, in the presence of a significant reduction in the gland acinar volume, total fluid production does not similarly diminish with increasing age. One explanation that has been hypothesized to account for these apparently inconsistent results is that salivary glands possess a functional reserve capacity,[73,92] enabling the glands to maintain a constant fluid output throughout the human adult life span.

In distinction to these normal physiologic phenomena, morphologic and functional changes in salivary glands have been associated with certain systemic diseases and their pharmacologic treatment.[53,55] The elderly are most susceptible to systemic disease. Eighty percent of the senior population have one or more chronic illnesses or ailments necessitating treatment.[1] Greater than two thirds of all adults over 65 years of age are taking prescription medications,[21] and many of these drugs are suggested to alter salivary gland performance.[83] The single most common disease affecting salivary glands is Sjögren's syndrome, an autoimmune exocrinopathy predominantly occurring in postmenopausal women. It has been conservatively estimated that there are one million such patients in the United States. Common forms of oncologic therapy, such as radiation for head and neck neoplasms and cytotoxic chemotherapy, can have direct and dramatic deleterious effects on salivary glands. Older persons thus are at considerable risk to suffering reductions in saliva secretion as a result of systemic disease or its treatment.

Regardless of the cause of a salivary dysfunction, any of the major physiologic roles of saliva (see box on facing page) may be adversely affected. In such circumstances, rampant dental caries may occur, leading to discomfort and possible tooth loss. The oral mucosa can become desiccated, painful, and cracked and leave the host susceptible to microbial infection. Food bolus formation and translocation will become more difficult, resulting in dysphagia, and food enjoyment may be significantly diminished. Finally, these changes can contribute to alterations in the nutritional intake pattern of geriatric patients and may result in nutritional deficiencies.[63] All these oral and systemic sequelae of salivary gland dysfunction may increase morbidity and reduce the quality of life experienced by the elderly person.

In summary, the secretion of saliva is essential for normal oral health and function. Despite the appearance of age-related morphometric changes in salivary glands, functional output and composition do not appear to be consistently altered in older, essentially healthy persons. The geriatric populations at greatest risk for developing salivary gland dysfunction and related oral morbidities are those with systemic disease and taking medications.

## ORAL MUCOSAL BARRIER

The oral mucosa performs essential protective functions that profoundly affect the general health and well-being of the host. These protective functions are of two broad types. The oral mucosal barrier (covered in this section) limits the access of innumerable environmental insults (microbes, chemicals) to the systemic circulation and provides a first line of active defense. Specialized mucosal sensory detectors serve to warn us of many potentially harmful situations such as spoiled foodstuffs, temperature extremes, and sharp objects (covered in the next section). It is therefore obviously important to understand whether any changes occur in these functions of the oral mucosa with increasing age. The protective-barrier functions of the oral mucosa are accomplished by both nonimmunologic and immunologic mechanisms. Clearly, a decline in the protective-barrier function of the oral mucosa could expose the aging host to myriads of pathogens and chemicals that enter the oral cavity during daily activities.

Both histologic layers of the oral mucosa, the epithelium and the connective tissue, have important defensive functions. A stratified epithelium, containing closely apposed, attached cells, constitutes a physical barrier that interferes with the entry of microorganisms and toxic substances. Mucosal epithelial cells also synthesize several substances that are critical for the maintenance of the mucosal surface, such as keratin and laminin. Keratin is found only on specific sites in the oral cavity, that is, the masticatory mucosa (defined topographically by the attached gingiva and the hard palate) and the specialized mucosa covering the tongue.[51] It provides a superficial defense layer against abrasive insults from stiff food particles, which strike those areas frequently. Laminin plays a role in cellular attachment to the basement membrane and therefore may be essential to preserve the epithelial structural integrity or to restore it in wound healing.[35] Oral mucosal surfaces also possess a protective self-cleansing mechanism provided by the natural turnover of epithelial cells. The rate of mitotic activity in these cells is believed to be dictated by functional requirements to replace abraded cells and expel superficial cell-colonizing microorganisms.[51] The main cell type of the connective tissue is the fibroblast, which produces and secretes most components of the intercellular matrix, including collagen, elastic fibers, fibronectin, and proteoglycans. This tissue layer provides both mechanical stability and elasticity to the mucosa.[82]

The existing literature on the structural integrity of the oral mucosa during aging is quite ambiguous. Although many authors report the occurrence of age-related histologic changes in the oral mucosa, very few base their assertions on studies performed with specimens taken from healthy, nonmedicated persons and none relate their histologic findings to any subjective complaints. Furthermore, in patient studies it has been difficult to appreciate the effects of disease and medication on the integrity of mucosal tissues. A brief review of this existing literature follows. However, please be aware that the cause of the changes that have been reported is not necessarily normal aging (that is, separate from disease).

There are numerous differences in reports between authors describing the histology of the aging oral mucosa. For example, advanced aging was found to be accompanied by thinning of the oral epithelium,[44] or by no changes in epithelial volume.[50] Similarly, the degree of oral mucosal keratinization has been reported to be decreased,[104] unchanged,[60] or increased.[44] Studies performed with healthy subjects report either an age-related increase in the mitotic index of the oral epithelium,[3,32] or no such variation.[52] Furthermore, controversy still exists as to whether menopause is associated with alterations in oral epithelial maturation and subjective complaints in women. Epithelial maturation has been shown to be increased in some such cases,[14] but also the opposite has been suggested, unless women were maintained on estrogen therapy.[23]

An additional complication in evaluating oral mucosal status in older persons is the use of prosthetic appliances by this population. Removable prostheses are in frequent use by elderly persons. These prostheses have considerable potential to alter mucosal integrity.[93]

In summary, the literature does not supply a clear picture of the histologic status of the oral mucosa with normal aging. It appears that if any histologic alterations of oral mucosal membranes occur because of normal aging they are mild and their clinical significance is questionable.

It is not the aim of this chapter to review the status of indigenous oral flora. Indeed, the scientific literature contains negligible information regarding the existence of oral microbial population shifts in different aged healthy adults. General reviews concerning oral microbial ecology are available.[70,86] The mucosal protective functions of saliva have been mentioned earlier. At present, mucins and epidermal growth factor are the salivary constituents most directly linked to protection of the oral soft tissues.[72,88] A mucous glycoprotein layer on the mucosal surface is crucial for lubrication, maintaining hydration and providing protection against abrupt osmotic changes.[57] This mucous layer grants immediate defense to the host when challenged for the first time with a pathogen, probably by competing as a receptor site for microbial adhesion with the epithelial cell surfaces.[20] Many salivary antimicrobial components (such as lysozyme, lactoferrin, lactoperoxidase, and secretory IgA) can associate synergistically with the mucous layer to provide additional protection to the oral mucosa.[57] Finally, another molecule found in saliva, fibronectin (a cell-surface attachment glycoprotein), has been shown to participate in the modulation of the flora colonizing the oral cavity by decreasing binding of gram-negative organisms to epithelial cells.[41] As noted earlier, there is no evidence to suggest that any biologically significant changes occur in salivary protective factors with increasing age.[30]

It should be clearly recognized that the exact mechanisms by which oral defense occurs are not yet understood. The most specific mucosal defense mechanisms that have been suggested to exist are related to salivary secretions (such as secretory IgA and lactoferrin). Only a few mechanisms appear inherent to the oral mucosa itself, and these are quite general in nature (mentioned above). In a recent study, however, we reported that substantial oral mucosal integrity was preserved, even in patients without normal major salivary gland secretion.[101] This preservation indicates the presence of important endogenous protective factors in the mucosa, and we proposed the existence of other factors in the oral cavity, unrelated to already-described salivary proteins. In particular, we hypothesized that oral mucosal cells may produce novel antimicrobial peptides similar to the magainins, recently described in frog skin.[103] Indeed, preliminary findings support this suggestion.[99] Considerable further study of intrinsic mucosal protective factors, including their relation to aging, is obviously needed.

Despite the multiple nonimmunologic mechanisms that protect the mucosa, the mucosal membranes are not impenetrable. An additional mechanism (immunologic) is therefore needed. The existence of a minor salivary gland duct–associated lymphoid tissue, similar to the gut- and bronchial-associated lymphoid tissues (GALT and BALT), has been suggested to be capable of evoking an immune response to antigens approaching it by retrograde passage through the excretory ducts.[62] In addition, within the oral mucosa, several types of immunocompetent cells (such as Langerhans, B and T cells) are present.[69] The best known immune component of the oral cavity is salivary IgA.[22] The functions of this immunoglobulin are varied and include inhibition of bacterial adherence to mucosal surfaces and neutralization of viruses and toxins.[57]

The human immune system undergoes significant alterations during the aging process. According to Hausman and Weksler,[42] "not only does aging affect immune competence but also immune competence may affect aging." Aging individuals display an increased heterogeneity in immune reactivity, compared to younger persons, and impairments in cell-mediated and humoral immune responses to foreign antigens are well documented in many species.[42] Studies in mice, however, have demonstrated that there is no age-associated deterioration in the mucosa-associated lymph nodes.[87] In human specimens no age-related changes either in the number of mononuclear cells residing in the oral mucosa[48] or in the concentration of salivary IgA[2,28,30] were observed. Mucosal immunity, in fact, may play a fundamental role in the protection of healthy elderly persons from infections, despite a decline in general immune competence. This too is a subject that requires much more study.

Many clinical reports indicate that changes exist in the appearance of the oral mucosa in older persons. However, these reports lack adequate documentation and are based primarily on "clinical impressions." There are only a few systematic studies on the appearance of the oral mucsoa during aging. In none of these, however, did investigators compare older with younger persons or attempt to separate aging from other confounding factors (such as disease, pharmaceuticals). The frequency of reported oral mucosal changes ranges from 60% among institutionalized persons[25] to less than 10% in a rural American elderly population.[38] Recently we conducted a prospective survey of the clinical oral mucosal condition of 182 healthy, nonmedicated persons between 20 and 95 years of age. The oral mucosae were found to remain essentially intact, regardless of age and sex.[100]

Conceivably, aging itself has no substantial effect on the oral mucosa or on its protective defense mechanisms, provided that the individual is in reasonably good health. It is likely that reported age-associated oral mucosal disorders are rather related to disease, malnutrition, drug usage, or wearing of ill-fitting dentures among elderly persons. These conditions, however, certainly need special attention because of their common occurrence in geriatric populations.

## ORAL MOTOR PERFORMANCE

Some of the most intricate, complex, and sophisticated of all human movements are those performed by the oral motor mechanism. The oral motor apparatus is a robust mechanism involved in three critical human functions: chewing, swallowing, and speech. Specifically, the upper lip, lower lip, jaw, and tongue are involved in several tasks requiring various motions with movement characteristics (such as position, velocity, timing, and force) that are often strikingly different. That is, their performance is function specific.[29,39,84-85] For example, several aspects of tongue activity (such as tongue shape and timing of tongue movements) can vary considerably for chewing, swallowing, and speech.[45, 84-85] In other words, although the same oral structures are involved in chewing, swallowing, and speech, the neuromotor control mechanisms underlying the movements of those oral structures are task specific. The importance of this concept cannot be underestimated, since it may explain, in part, why normal (nonpathologic) aging appears to differentially affect oral movements for chewing, swallowing, and speech. In addition, it should be recalled that there exists a considerable literature that demonstrates that significant age-related change occurs in the morphologic appearance and biochemical function of neural and muscle tissues.[37,67] Such changes also may partially account for certain oral motor performance events more than others. Unfortunately, although strides have been made in basic scientific investigations of oral structures involved in chewing,[39] speaking,[33] and swallowing,[58] parallel advances in objective and quantifiable clinical indices of oral motor performance have not developed at the same pace. The development of such clinical measures is critical to the practicing clinician who must discern if changes in oral motor performance are associated with the normal aging process or pharmacologic side effects or is indicative of a pathologic condition.

Although some age-related changes in oral motor performance for chewing, swallowing, and speech can be expected,[12,27,78,81] the normal aging process does not uniformly impinge on the three critical functions of the oral mechanisms. Perhaps the most frequently reported oral motor disturbance in the elderly is related to mastication. Ironically, mastication is the oral motor function that has been least rigorously studied. Clinical studies of chewing historically have suffered from (1) inadequate (such as capturing of movement of only one orofacial structure in only one or two dimensions) or inappropriate (such as use of x rays) instrumentation to study chewing motions; (2) a lack of objective, quantifiable indices to measure movements of oral or orofacial structures; (3) failure to control for size and shape of food particles that subjects were asked to chew (though most studies have controlled for food texture); and (4) failure to provide detailed information regarding the instructions to the subjects under investigation (such as "chew as you normally would," "chew on your left side," "chew on your right side," and "chew on your preferred side"). Recently there have been reported some well-designed clinical studies that discuss chewing in elderly patients. Feldman et al.[27] used an objective method of measuring food-particle size and found that even fully dentate older persons were less able to adequately prepare food for swallowing as compared to younger subjects and, as a result, tended to swallow larger-sized food particles than their younger counterparts did. Similar findings are reported by Heath.[43] It is not unlikely that these negative age-related changes in chewing are even further exacerbated in persons with compromised dentition.

Swallowing behavior may also be greatly affected by the normal aging process.[26,76,81] As stated earlier, compromised dentition in the elderly person may be related to a reduced ability to prepare food to a swallow-ready consistency. Several aspects of the oropharyngeal phase of swallow, even in persons with good dental status, have been specifically shown to differ between different aged persons, including the duration of the swallow and the presence of unusual or unnecessary structural movement.[79] Sonies and Caruso[79] speculated that the normal aging process has a pervasive effect on swallowing because the swallowing mechanism, unlike the speech mechanism, appears to have limited capability to successfully compensate for other age-related changes. Importantly, pathologic situations (such as disease or various pharmaceuticals) that affect an already diminished (aged) oropharyngeal mechanism may serve to all but eliminate the largely reflexive activity involved in swallowing. Such a circumstance would place the older person, who is medically compromised, at increased risk of choking or aspirations.

Speech production is the function of the oral mechanism that appears most resistant to aging. This does not mean that there are no age-related changes in speech. In fact, there have been reports from several different laboratories indicating differences in specific characteristics of speech production in old versus young adults.[46,49,78,98] Interestingly, however, there are little data to indicate that the normal (nonpathologic) aging process actually affects movements of the oral speech articulators (lips, tongue, and jaw) in any appreciable manner. Although it has been reported that listeners can perceive differences in young versus old talkers,[40,71] these age-related differences may be associated with laryngeal rather than oral events.[59] Moreover, we are aware of no published reports to indicate that listeners incorrectly perceive normal elderly speakers as disordered speakers. In essence, normal elderly persons are quite capable of producing normal-sounding speech.[80] Unlike swallowing, the robust neuromotor control processes underlying speech may provide the elderly talker with the ability to make "on-line" articulatory adjustments that compensate for any normal age-related physiologic changes in the oral mechanism.

One widely used clinical measure to assess oral articulatory movement is diadochokinetic syllable rates (DSRs). DSRs are measured as one instructs the speaker to produce syllables (such as /pa/, /ta/, /ka/) as rapidly as possible and comparing them to published reports of syllable rate (usually number of syllables per second) for different age groups.[8] Results of such studies with elderly subjects have not consistently demonstrated a reduction in oral movement abilities for speech. Whereas it was first reported that DSRs were somewhat slower for persons over 65 years versus those under 40 years,[68] subsequent studies have found DSRs to be equivalent or even slightly faster for older versus younger talkers.[47,75]

Much of what is known regarding oral speech movements in the elderly has often been derived from *indirect* measures (such as listeners' perceptions or analysis of the acoustic [speech] signal) rather than *direct* ones (such as position of the lips, tongue, or jaw). Although such studies have provided numerous insights regarding aging speech, indirect measurements of speech production may not be sufficient for studies of oral movements because (1) some of these indirect measures may not accurately and precisely reflect actual oral movement events,[16] (2) different patterns of oral movements can produce the same acoustic (speech) result,[7] and (3) some measures exclusively focus on performance extremes (such as the maximum number of times a syllable can be repeated in a second) rather than at different levels of oral motor performance.[46]

We are currently involved with the development of objective, clinical indices of oral motor performance that would be applicable for dynamic measures of speaking, chewing, and the oral phase of swallowing.[17] It is now possible to develop direct measures of oral motor performance during chewing, speaking, and swallowing that should be extremely sensitive to the normal aging process. For example, Fig. 5-1 displays actual speech movement data for the upper lip (UL), lower lip (LL), and jaw (J) in the anteroposterior (AP), mediolateral (ML), and superoinferior (SI) dimensions for a normal 75-year-old woman's production of the word /sapapple/. This figure shows five pro-

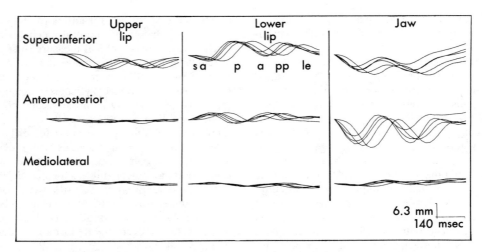

**Fig. 5-1** Upper lip, lower lip, and jaw movement traces in the anteroposterior (A-P), superoinferior (S-I), and mediolateral (M-L) dimensions during five productions of "sapapple" by a normal 75-year-old woman. On the graphs, traces moving toward the top of the page show structural movement in the S, A, and M (subject's right) dimensions. Likewise, traces moving toward the bottom of the page show structural movement in the I, P, and L (subject's left) dimensions.

ductions of the test word that have been overlaid on one another. As shown, these five utterances by this elderly speaker indicate that the UL, LL, and J movement patterns are quite variable in both timing and positioning across utterances, a finding similar to that reported for young adults.[34] Objective clinical measures such as these should ultimately be beneficial in understanding more specifically how the aging process affects oral motor performance. Moreover, such clinical indices of oral motor performance could have wide application in quantifying outcome of various orthodontic, prosthetic, and surgical treatments.

In conclusion, it should be recognized that there needs to be considerably more study of oral motor performance during aging. The current level of understanding is relatively minimal. Our present interpretation of the existing data is that the aging process does not uniformly alter the three critical functions of the oral motor mechanism. More specifically, the impact of aging on oral motor performance cannot be characterized as a simple, gradual diminution as we grow older, since the older motor mechanism has varying abilities across functions to make compensatory adjustments to age-related changes.

## ORAL SENSORY SYSTEMS

The sensory basis for our appreciation of foods is generally considered to result from the chemosensory systems of the mouth and nose. However, other oral stimuli, which are not chemosensory (such as tactile, thermal, textural), always accompany chemosensory stimulants. In concert, this battery of sensory detection systems allows us to savor the pleasures of eating and drinking and, importantly, serves to protect us from ingesting spoiled or harmful (and thus potentially dangerous) substances. Physiologically, the basic events that underlie olfaction and gustation are best understood. Only limited study has been directed at other oral sensory processes (except for pain, which is not addressed here).

Taste buds are equivalent to gustatory receptors. They are neuroepithelial cells and exist on many oral and contiguous structures including the tongue, soft palate, pharynx, larynx, and epiglottis. Taste buds recognize (bind) chemicals (tastants) from food that are dissolved in saliva and convert this initial binding event into a neural signal. The mechanisms by which this signal transduction process takes place is not established. Recently it has been suggested that gustatory receptors may transduce their stimuli by a receptor–second messenger (calcium ions, cyclic AMP) mechanism.[5,89] The role of second messenger mechanisms in transducing sensory stimuli is better established for olfaction (see below).

Most interest in gustation has focused on the tongue. Fungiform, foliate, and circumvallate papillae all have taste buds. Branches of cranial nerves V, VII, and IX provide the sensory innervation to the tongue. Taste bud cell turnover is quite frequent, showing a half-life of about 10 to 14 days. Earlier studies (before 1940) reported that the number of taste buds in humans diminishes with increased age.[4] Several recent reports (such as Arvidson's[6]), however, demonstrate that there is no significant reduction in taste bud number with age in humans, nonhuman primates, and rodents.

There are four basic taste qualities (sweet, sour, salty, and bitter). Taste cells do not respond uniquely to only one quality class of tastant. Objective measurements of clinical gustatory function are typically made at two levels: threshold and suprathreshold. Threshold values are most commonly employed. These represent a "molecular level" event reflecting either the lowest concentration of a tastant that a person can determine as being different from water (a detection threshold) or assign a quality recognition (a recognition threshold). Suprathreshold values allow measurement of the ability to taste the intensity of substances at daily-life, functional concentrations, such as the amount of sugar needed to sweeten coffee. Additionally, the hedonic component (degree of pleasantness) can be measured.

Many earlier assessments of gustatory function during aging have been complicated by methodologic limitations (see commentary in Weiffenbach[94]), including use of patients versus healthy subjects. Recent studies, however, have benefited from progress in measurement procedures using pure taste stimuli and by evaluation of different aged, generally healthy persons. Detection threshold studies have examined all four taste qualities. There was no general pattern of functional change observed with increased age.[36,95] Reduced performance (increased thresholds) was quality specific (salty—sodium chloride; bitter—quinine sulfate) and modest. No age-related decrements in sweet (sucrose) and sour (citric acid) detection thresholds were observed. Studies of suprathreshold gusta-

tory function have produced similar conclusions, that is, the absence of any general deterioration in the ability of older persons to judge taste intensity.[9,96]

Olfactory receptor cells recognize volatile chemicals as stimuli. They are bipolar, sensory neurons that are found, along with supporting and basal cells, in the olfactory epithelium lining the nasal septum. The dendritic part of the olfactory receptor cell possesses cilia and extends into the nasal cavity, and the axonal portions form the first cranial nerve. In the last few years there has been remarkable progress in identifying the mechanisms by which olfactory signals are transduced.[64,77] Pevsner et al.[66] have isolated and characterized an odorant binding protein from bovine and rat nasal mucosae. The protein contains two similar subunits, each about 20,000 daltons in size, and binds certain radiolabeled odorants (e.g. [$^3$H]-2-isobutyl-3-methoxypyrazine) in a specific and saturable manner. Odorants are capable of activating adenylate cyclase to form cyclic AMP in preparations of olfactory epithelium. Odorants appear to elicit the cyclic AMP signal through a transducing, specific GTP-binding protein (G protein) in a manner analogous to the signaling mechanism operative for many neurotransmitter and peptide hormone receptors. Indeed, there has been a report that patients with type Ia pseudohypoparathyroidism suffer an olfactory deficit because of a deficiency in a GTP-binding stimulatory protein.[97]

We are aware of no published studies examining the status of olfactory receptor cells with aging in humans. There are, however, several reports that evaluate olfactory function in different aged persons. Olfactory, like gustatory, function can be measured at both threshold and suprathreshold levels as well as by examination of odor recognition. Generally, most data support the view that olfactory performance declines with increased age.[24,94] We and others have employed a commercially available odor-recognition test (40 odorants encapsulated in a scratch-and-sniff, multiple-choice format) to demonstrate that most older persons have a reduced ability to identify correctly a broad range of presented odors; that is, older persons generally appear to be hyposmic.

It is important to recognize that in the course of daily living we do not taste a single tastant or react to a single olfactory cue. The situation in the clinic or laboratory, testing subjects with simple stimuli to assess chemosensory performance, is important but does not address the complex tasks required to detect and identify the chemosensory mixtures that exist in foods. Several studies have examined the more difficult problems associated with flavor perception, food recognition, and food preference in the elderly. In one study[61] using blended foods, younger persons were significantly better at recognizing stimuli than elders. If, however, younger subjects repeated the test with occluded airways, their level of performance fell to that of elderly persons. It thus appears that among generally healthy older persons diminished olfactory performance may be the cause of complaints associated with lessened food enjoyment.

As noted earlier, there has been little physiologic study of other oral sensory systems (such as tactile, thermal, and textural)[15] and virtually none as a function of age. Flavor, which results from the interactions of chemosensory systems, does not define the entire pleasurable sensory experience associated with eating and drinking. We, for example, are careful to prepare food to the correct temperature and texture. We have recently begun to assess what might be termed nontaste sensory contributions to the oral alimentary experience in different aged persons.[91] We have used a similar methodologic approach to one used in gustatory and olfactory studies—assessment of intensity perception of suprathreshold stimuli for local discrete pressure, viscosity, and temperature. Initial results indicate that older persons may use a smaller response range to judge pressure and viscosity and are not as reliable in making intensity judgments of pressure.

In general, it should be recognized that there needs to be considerably more study of oral sensory systems during aging. Our current level of understanding is minimal. However, existing data support a cautious conclusion that the effect of age on oral sensitivity is heterogeneous across modalities and cannot be characterized as a simple dulling of sensation as we grow old.

## REFERENCES

1. Aging America: trends and projections, edition 1985-1986, Washington, DC, 1986, American Association of Retired Persons.
2. Aguirre A et al: Immunochemical quantitation of α-amylase and secretory IgA in parotid saliva from people of various ages, Arch Oral Biol 32:297, 1987.
3. Ahuja SS: Effect of age on mitotic index of buccal mucous membrane, J Indian Dent Assoc 47:117, 1975.
4. Arey LB, Tremaine MJ, and Mozingo FL: The numerical and topographical relations of taste buds to human circumvallate papillae throughout the life span, Anat Rec 64:9, 1935.
5. Arkabas MH, Dodd J, and Al-Awqati Q: A bitter substance induces a rise in intracellular calcium in a subpopulation of taste cells, Science 242:1047, 1988.
6. Arvidson K: Location and variation in number of taste buds in human fungiform papillae, Scand J Dent Res 87:435, 1979.
7. Atal BS et al: Inversion of articulatory-to-acoustic transformation in the vocal tract by a computer-sorting technique, J Acoust Soc Am 63:1535, 1978.
8. Baken RJ: Clinical measurement of speech and voice, Boston, 1987, College-Hill Press.
9. Bartoshuk L et al: Taste and aging, J Gerontol 41:51, 1986.
10. Baum BJ: Salivary gland function during aging, Gerodontics 2:61, 1986.
11. Baum BJ: Neurotransmitter control of secretion, J Dent Res 66:628, 1987.
12. Baum BJ and Bodner L: Aging and oral motor function: evidence for altered performance among older persons, J Dent Res 62:2, 1983.
13. Baum BJ, Kousvelari EE, and Oppenheim FG: Exocrine protein secretion from human parotid glands during aging: stable release of the acidic proline-rich proteins, J Gerontol 37:392, 1982.
14. Bercovici B, Gron S, and Pisanty S: Vaginal and oral cytology of the menopause: a comparative study, Acta Cytol 29:805, 1985.
15. Bradley RM: Basic oral physiology, Chicago, 1981, Year Book Medical Publishers.
16. Caruso AJ and Burton EK: Temporal acoustic measures of dysarthria, J Speech Hear Res 30:80, 1987.
17. Caruso AJ et al: Three-dimensional analysis of multiarticulate speech movements: a new technique, ASHA 30:167, 1988.
18. Castle JD, Arvan P and Cameron R: Protein production and secretion in exocrine cells, J Dent Res 66:633, 1987.
19. Chauncey HH et al: Parotid fluid composition in healthy aging males, Adv Physiol Sci 28:323, 1981.
20. Clamp JR: The relationship between the immune system and mucus in the protection of mucous membranes, Biochem Soc Trans 12:754, 1984.
21. Cottone JA and Kafrawy AH: Medications and health histories: a survey of 4,365 dental patients, J Am Dent Assoc 98:713, 1979.
22. Crawford JM, Taubman MA, and Smith DJ: Minor salivary glands as a major source of secretory immunoglobulin A in the human oral cavity, Science 190:1206, 1975.
23. Croley TE and Miers C: Epithelial changes in the oral mucosa resulting from a variation in hormone stimulus, J Oral Med 33:86, 1978.
24. Doty RL, Shaman P, and Dann M: Development of the

University of Pennsylvania smell identification test, a standardized microencapsulated test of olfactory function, Physiol Behav 32:489, 1984.

25. Ekelund R: Oral mucosal disorders in institutionalized elderly people, Age Ageing 17:193,1988.
26. Elliott JL: Swallowing disorders in the elderly: a guide to diagnosis and treatment, Geriatrics 43:95, 1988.
27. Feldman RS et al: Aging and mastication: changes in performance and in the swallowing threshold with natural dentition, J Am Geriatr Soc 28:97, 1980.
28. Finkelstein MS, Tanner M, and Freedman ML: Salivary and serum IgA levels in a geriatric outpatient population, J Clin Immunol 4:85, 1984.
29. Folkins J and Abbs J: Lip and jaw motor control during speech: responses to resistive loading of the jaw, J Speech Hear Res 18:207, 1975.
30. Fox PC et al: Secretion of antimicrobial proteins from the parotid glands of different aged healthy persons, J Gerontol 42:466, 1987.
31. Gandara BK et al: Age-related salivary flow rate changes in controls and patients with oral lichen planus, J Dent Res 64:1149, 1985.
32. Gargiulo AW, Wentz FM, and Orban B: Mitotic activity of human oral epithelium exposed to 30 per cent hydrogen peroxide, Oral Surg Oral Med Oral Pathol 14:474, 1961.
33. Gracco V and Abbs J: Programming and execution processes of speech movement control: potential neural correlates. In Keller E and Gopnik M, editors: Motor and sensory processes in language, Hillsdale, NJ, 1987, Lawrence Erlbaum Associates, Inc.
34. Gracco V and Abbs J: Variant and invariant characteristics of speech movements, Exp Brain Res 65:156, 1987.
35. Grotendorst GR et al: Role of attachment factors in mediating the attachment, distribution, and differentiation of cells, Cold Spring Harbor Conferences on Cell Proliferation 9:403, 1982.
36. Grzegorczyk PB, Jones SW, and Mistretta CM: Age-related differences in salt taste acuity, J Gerontol 34:834, 1979.
37. Gutman E: Muscle. In Finch CE and Hayflick CE, editors: The biology of aging, New York, 1977, Van Nostrand Reinhold.
38. Hand JS and Whitehill JM: The prevalence of oral mucosal lesions in an elderly population, J Am Dent Assoc 112:73, 1986.
39. Hannam A; Mastication in man. In Bryant P, Gale E, and Rugh J, editors: Oral motor behavior: impact on oral conditions and dental treatment, Bethesda, Md, 1979, National Institutes of Health.
40. Hartman DE and Danhauer JL: Perceptual features of speech for males in four perceived age decades, J Acoust Soc Am 59:713, 1979.
41. Hasty DL and Simpson WA: Effects of fibronectin and other salivary macromolecules on the adherence of *Escherichia coli* to buccal epithelial cells, Infect Immun 55:2103, 1987.
42. Hausman PB and Weksler ME: Changes in the immune response with age. In Finch CE and Schneider EL, editors: Handbook of the biology of aging, ed 2, New York, 1985, Van Nostrand Reinhold.

43. Heath MR: The effect of maximum biting force and bone loss upon masticatory function and dietary selection of the elderly, Int Dent J 32:345, 1982.
44. Kaminsky AR et al: Envejecimiento de la mucosa bucal, Rev Circ Argent Odont 33:17, 1970.
45. Keller E: Factors underlying tongue articulators in speech, J Speech Hear Res 30:223, 1987.
46. Kent RD and Burkhard R: Changes in the acoustic correlates in speech production. In Beasley DS and Davis GA, editors: Aging: communication processes and disorders, New York, 1981, Grune & Stratton.
47. Kruel E: Neuromuscular control examination (NMC) for parkinsonism: vowel prolongations and diadochokinetic and reading rates, J Speech Hear Res 15:72, 1972.
48. Lebendiger M and Lehner T: Characterization of mononuclear cells in the human oral mucosa, Arch Oral Biol 26:1041, 1981.
49. Linville SE: Acoustic-perceptual studies of aging voice in women, J Voice 1:44, 1987.
50. Löe H and Karring T: The three-dimensional morphology of the epithelium-connective tissue interface of the gingiva as related to age and sex, Scand J Dent Res 79:315, 1971.
51. Mackenzie IC and Binnie WH: Recent advances in oral mucosal research, J Oral Pathol 12:389, 1983.
52. Maidhof R and Hornstein OP: Autoradiographic study on some proliferative properties of human buccal mucosa, Arch Dermatol Res 265:165, 1979.
53. Mandel ID: Sialochemistry in diseases and clinical situations affecting salivary glands, CRC Crit Rev Clin Lab Sci 12:321, 1980.
54. Mandel ID: The functions of saliva, J Dent Res 66:628, 1987.
55. Mandel ID and Wotman S: The salivary secretions in health and disease, Oral Science Rev 8:25, 1976.
56. Martinez JR: Ion transport and water movement, J Dent Res 66:638, 1987.
57. McNabb PC and Tomasi TB: Host defense mechanism at mucosal surfaces, Ann Rev Microbiol 35:477, 1981.
58. Miller AJ: Deglutition, Physiol Rev 62:129, 1982.
59. Morris RJ and Brown WS, Jr: Age-related voice measures among adult women, J Voice 1:38, 1987.
60. Mosadomi A et al: Effects of tobacco smoking and age on the keratinization of palatal mucosa: a cytologic study, Oral Surg 46:413, 1978.
61. Murphy C: Taste and smell in the elderly. In Meiselman HL and Rivlin RS, editors: Clinical measurement of taste and smell, New York, 1986, MacMillan Co.
62. Nair PNR and Schroeder HE: Duct-associated lymphoid tissue (DALT) of minor salivary glands and mucosal immunity, Immunology 57:171, 1986.
63. Navazesh M: Xerostomia in the aged, Dent Clin North Am 33;75, 1989.
64. Pace U and Lancet D: Olfactory GTP-binding protein: signal-transducing polypeptide of vertebrate chemosensory neurons, Proc Natl Acad Sci USA 83:4947, 1986.
65. Pedersen W et al: Age-dependent decreases in human submandibular gland flow rates as measured under resting and post-stimulation conditions, J Dent Res 64:822, 1985.
66. Pevsner J, Sklar PB, and Snyder SH: Isolation and characterization of an odorant-binding protein, Ann NY Acad Sci 510:547, 1987.

67. Pradham SN: Central neurotransmitters and aging, Life Sciences 26:1643, 1980.
68. Ptacek PH et al: Phonatory and related changes with advanced age, J Speech Hear Res 9:353, 1966.
69. Reibel J et al: Pattern of distribution of T lymphocytes, Langerhans cells and HLA-DR bearing cells in normal human oral mucosa, Scand J Dent Res 93:513, 1985.
70. Russell C and Melville TH: Bacteria in the human mouth: a review, J Appl Bacteriol 44:163, 1978.
71. Ryan W and Burk K: Perceptual and acoustic correlates of aging in the speech of males, Commun Disorders 7:181, 1974.
72. Sarosiek J et al: Role of salivary epidermal growth factor in the maintenance of physicochemical characteristics of oral and gastric mucosal mucus coat, Biochem Biophys Res Commun 152:1421, 1988.
73. Scott J: Structure and function in aging human salivary glands, Gerodontology 5:149, 1986.
74. Scott J: Structural age changes in salivary glands. In Ferguson DB, editor: Frontiers of oral physiology, Basel, 1987, S Karger, AG.
75. Shanks S: Effects of aging upon rapid syllable repetition. Percept Motor Skills 30:687, 1970.
76. Sheth N and Diner WC: Swallowing problems in the elderly, Dysphagia 2:209, 1987.
77. Sklar PB, Anholt RRH, and Snyder SH: The odorant-sensitive adenylate cyclase of olfactory receptor cells, Ann NY Acad Sci 510:623, 1987.
78. Smith B et al: Temporal characteristics of the speech of normal elderly adults, J Speech Hear Res 25:129, 1987.
79. Sonies BC and Caruso AJ: The aging process and its potential impact on measures of oral sensorimotor function, American Speech-Language-Hearing Association Rep 19:114, 1990.
80. Sonies BC: Tongue motion in elderly adults: initial in situ observations. J Gerontol 39:279, 1984.
81. Sonies BC et al: Durational aspect of the oral-pharyngeal phase of swallow in normal adults Dysphagia 3:1, 1988.
82. Squier CA, Johnson NW, and Hopps RM: Human oral mucosa, Oxford, 1976, Blackwell Scientific Publications.
83. Sreebny LM and Schwartz SS: A reference guide to drugs and dry mouth, Gerodontology 5:75, 1986.
84. Stone M and Shawker T: An ultrasound examination of tongue movement during swallowing, Dysphagia 1:78, 1986.
85. Stone M et al: Cross-sectional tongue shape during the production of vowels, J Acoust Soc Am 83:1586, 1988.
86. Sutter VL: Anaerobes as normal oral flora, Rev Infect Dis 6:S62, 1984.

87. Szewczuk MR and Wade AW: Aging and the mucosal-associated lymphoid system, Ann NY Acad Sci 404:333, 1983.
88. Tabak LA et al: Role of salivary mucins in the protection of the oral cavity, J Oral Pathol 11:1, 1982.
89. Teeter J and Gold GH: A taste of things to come, Nature 331:298, 1988.
90. Thaysen JH, Thorn NA, and Schwartz IL: Excretion of sodium, potassium chloride and carbon dioxide in human parotid saliva, Am J Physiol 178:155, 1954.
91. Tylenda CA and Baum BJ: Oral physiology and the Baltimore longitudinal study of aging, Gerodontology 7:5, 1988.
92. Tylenda CA et al: Evaluation of submandibular salivary flow rate in different age groups, J Dent Res 67:1225, 1988.
93. Watson IB and MacDonald DG: Oral mucosa and complete dentures, J Prosthet Dent 47:133, 1982.
94. Weiffenbach JM: Taste and smell perception in aging, Gerodontology 3:137, 1984.
95. Weiffenbach JM, Baum BJ, and Burghauser R: Taste thresholds: quality specific variation with human aging, J Gerontol 37:372, 1982.
96. Weiffenbach JM, Cowart BJ, and Baum BJ: Taste intensity perception in aging, J Gerontol 41:460, 1986.
97. Weinstock RS et al: Olfactory dysfunction in humans with deficient guanine nucleotide–binding protein, Nature 322:635, 1986.
98. Wilcox KA and Horii Y: Age and changes in vocal jitter, J Gerontol 35:194, 1980.
99. Wolff A et al: Magainin-like immunoreactivity in human submandibular and labial salivary glands, J Histochem Cytochem 38:1531, 1990.
100. Wolff A et al: Oral mucosal status in healthy, different aged adults, Oral Surg Oral Med Oral Pathol. (In press.)
101. Wolff A et al: Oral mucosal status and major salivary gland function, Oral Surg Oral Med Oral Pathol 70:49, 1990.
102. Young JA et al: Secretion by the major salivary glands. In Johnson LR, editor: Physiology of the gastrointestinal tract, New York, 1987, Raven Press.
103. Zasloff M: Magainins, a class of antimicrobial peptides from Xenopus skin: isolation, characterization of two active forms, and partial cDNA sequence of a precursor, Proc Natl Acad Sci USA 84:5449, 1987.
104. Zimmermann ER and Zimmermann AL: Effects of race, age, smoking habits, oral and systemic disease on oral exfoliative cytology, J Dent Res 44:627, 1965.

# 6

## Disease-Related Changes in Older Adults

*Barnet M. Levy*

Time passes! Everything ages. All living and even nonliving things get older and older, minute by minute, day by day, year by year. Aging is a natural phenomenon that has long been of great concern to religious and philosophic scholars. In the past few decades, along with the science information explosion, considerable knowledge about biologic aging has accumulated.[19,73,111] However, as Oota[73] points out, this knowledge seems almost random, arising from many disciplines and covering everything from molecules to societies. Only recently have we realized that aging itself is not a disease.

In this chapter, I attempt to distinguish between how normal aging processes affect oral diseases and how disease processes accentuate or accelerate normal orofacial aging.

Data on the gradual and often subtle changes in the aging oral tissues have for the most part been gathered from cross-sectional studies. Cross-sectional studies (gathering information from many individuals in specific age groups of a given population) have long been utilized in aging research in animals other than man, and so the application of this type of research to humans should come as no surprise. On the other hand, longitudinal studies (following the same person throughout his lifetime or at least from middle age onwards) are now developing, the most exciting of which is the ongoing Baltimore Longitudinal Study of the National Institute of Aging. Such studies may provide the needed data on the oral physiology of aging that will ultimately lead to a better understanding of the oral pathology of the aged. However, with nearly 30 million people in the United States over 65 years

of age there is a pressing need to understand the oral pathology associated with human aging. It is dentistry's most urgent priority.

Some of the theories of aging—of the biologic changes that accompany aging—are briefly reviewed. The oral diseases associated with the elderly then can be explored in the light of known underlying biologic changes. It is important to remember, however, that all orofacial diseases associated with the elderly can and frequently do occur in "middle age" or earlier. No oral disease occurs exclusively in the elderly.

What then differentiates the older person from the younger one? How or why do oral changes occur with age? Why are certain oral diseases associated with aging?

### OROFACIAL AGING

Orofacial aging, the way someone "looks," is a fairly good index of the rate at which that person has aged. We recognize our friends, relatives, and patients by their facial features, which do change with age. Facial skin (and skin from other exposed parts of the body, such as hands or neck) reflects the long time exposure to the physical environment—the wear and tear caused by the elements—as well as by diet, emotions, and physical activity (Fig. 6-1). Thus the way a person's genetic *constitution* responds to external and internal environmental forces helps determine the apparent effects of time on the skin of the face. In addition, there are intrinsic age changes that occur in the skin that are thought by many to be genetically controlled.

Skin thickness declines sharply at about 60 years of age.[29] Although the epidermis generally thins, it may greatly thicken in focal areas. The dermis becomes relatively dehydrated, has a diminished vascularity, and loses both strength and elasticity. In addition, subcutaneous fat is lost, and the melanocytes appear to lose the ability to spread their melanin granules evenly throughout the epidermis.[102]

These basic biologic changes may explain some of the skin changes associated with aging. Gilchrest[26] points out the histologic features of aging (Table 6-1) and the skin functions that decline with age (Table 6-2). All or part of these changes help to explain the clinical appearance of the "old" face. Although the loss of subcutaneous fat exaggerates the dermal changes to give a folded, lined, wrinkled, and lax appearance to the face,[5] the loss of elastin fibers also contributes to the wrinkled appearance of the old face[70] and old skin (Fig. 6-2). Despite the interest in wrinkles by the lay public, the plastic surgeon, and the dermatologist, the histogenesis of wrinkling is still unknown.

Studies of the histologic changes associated with aging human oral mucosa indicate a loss of submucosal elastin and fat similar to that found in skin, but wrinkling of the oral mucosa has not been reported.

The prominent loss of skin vascularity, especially of the vertical capillary loops, is believed by Gilchrest[26] and others[52] to underlie the gradual atrophy and fibrosis of the eccrine, apocrine, and sebaceous glands in the skin. Whether such vascular changes occur in the oral mucosa is still unknown. If they do, it may explain some of the atrophic and fibrotic changes seen in the mucosal minor salivary glands.

Although the above-mentioned skin changes may give rise to some of the changes responsible for the appearance of facial skin, sun damage is really responsible for the majority of clinically evident age-associated skin changes.[26] The interaction of sun damage with intrinsic age changes has not been well investigated, though many researchers suggest additive effects.

Age changes in the oral mucosa have not been as well documented. When several studies of the same type of tissue have been reported, they are frequently contradictory. One of the problems may lie in interpreting the results obtained by studying such disparate animals as rodents (mice, rats) and primates, including man. Another might be the criteria used to select a human study population. The literature of the past 15 to 20 years on the effects of aging is too large to review here. However, Table

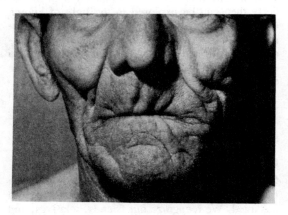

**Fig. 6-1** Face of old person with typical age changes.

**Table 6-1** Histologic features of aging human skin

| Epidermis | Dermis | Appendages |
| --- | --- | --- |
| Flattened dermo-epidermal junction | Atrophy (loss of dermal volume) | Depigmented hair |
| Variable thickness | Fewer fibroblasts | Loss of hair |
| Variable cell size and shape | Fewer mast cells | Conversion of terminal |
| Occasional nuclear atypia | Fewer blood vessels | to vellus hair |
| Fewer melanocytes | Shortened capillary loops | Abnormal nailplates |
| Fewer Langerhans cells | Abnormal nerve endings | Fewer glands |

From Gilchrest BA: Skin and aging processes, Boca Raton, Fla, 1984, CRC Press, Inc.

6-3 is an attempt to indicate the changes in the oral tissues that accompany age and to provide a reference source for the student interested in pursuing this problem. It also indicates the current level of

**Table 6-2** Functions of human skin that decline with age

| | |
|---|---|
| Cell replacement | Immune responsiveness |
| Injury response | Vascular responsiveness |
| Barrier function | Thermoregulation |
| Chemical clearance | Sweat production |
| Sensory perception | Sebum production |
| Vitamin D production | |

From Gilchrest BA: Skin and aging processes, Boca Raton, Fla, 1984, CRC Press, Inc.

knowledge (confusion) in oral gerobiology.

In summary, the local changes that might affect oral disease in the elderly are primarily changes in the connective tissues. There is a decrease in the ability of fibroblasts to synthesize new collagen. At the same time, there is an increase in the cross linking of collagen. Microscopically, the connective tissues become denser and coarser, giving the tissues a fibrotic look.

Changes in the rate of epithelial cell renewal with age have not been well established, though there seems to be some evidence that the epithelium of the oral mucosa appears clinically thinner in the aged.[62]

The so-called theories of aging have been numerous, probably because of the difficulty in dif-

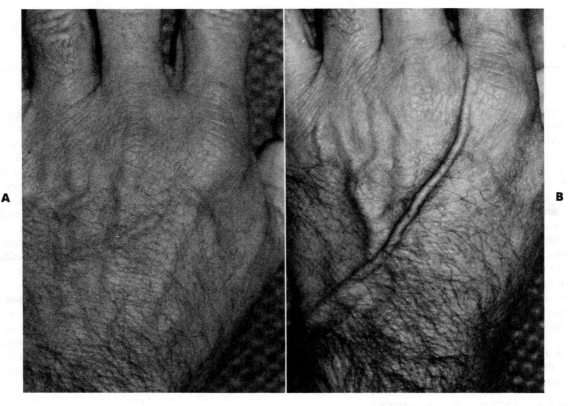

**Fig. 6-2** Skin of hand of 72-year-old man. Loss of elasticity is evident after pinching of the skin. **A,** Before pinching of skin. **B,** Thirty seconds after pinching of skin.

**Table 6-3** Changes in oral tissues with age

| Tissue | Measured | Reported structural change | Reference number |
|---|---|---|---|
| Epithelium | | | |
| | Width | Thinned | 82, 85, 90 |
| | Keratinization | Decreased | 75, 116 |
| | | Unchanged | 79 |
| | Rete pegs | Heightened | 60, 112 |
| | | Constant | 64 |
| | | Shortened | 90 |
| | Mitotic activity | Increased | 23, 68, 96, 101, 105 |
| | | Constant | 64, 84 |
| | | Decreased | 48, 57, 88, 104 |
| Connective tissue | | | |
| | Cellular elements | Decreased | 53, 84, 112 |
| | Fibers | Decreased | 22, 58, 86 |
| | Mitotic activity | Decreased | 96 |
| | Collagen synthesis | Decreased | 11, 97 |
| | Acid mucopolysaccharides | Decreased | 58, 67 |
| | Width of periodontal | Increased | 45, 51 |
| | ligament | Decreased | 12, 27, 30, 100-114 |
| | Gingival recession | Increased | 89, 100 |
| | | Stable | 4, 28, 114 |

ferentiating cause from effect. Given the number and diversity of changes that occur in cells, organs, and systems, the possibilities for theorizing and hypothesizing seem almost limitless. If we believe, as we must, that any deteriorative event in one organ influences changes in other organs in a kind of cascade effect, the theories of senescence become infinite. On the other hand, predicting such cascade effects may eventually lead to a few theories or even a unified theory of the mechanism or mechanisms of aging. The numerous theories that are an attempt at explaining the nature of biologic aging through an understanding of the mechanisms of aging can, however, provide a framework for discussion of those oral diseases associated with the aging patient.

Most of the current theories of the mechanisms of aging involve either "wear and tear" or genetically programed (clock) theories. Can we apply them to gerodontic pathology?

## WEAR-AND-TEAR THEORIES

The oldest theory on the mechanisms of aging posits that aging results from the accumulation of harmful by-products of essential, "normal" biochemical and physiologic processes. This simple wear-and-tear hypothesis[76,77] states that aging may result from the accumulation of damage at the cellular or intracellular levels, leading to cell loss and dysfunction.[54] In other words, aging and death result simply from the wear and tear of daily use, as happens sooner or later with any machine. But machines do not have the ability to self-repair, to heal. And so the analogy loses some of its value. As we will see, the inability to repair the results of wear and tear may be a sign of the aging process.

Probably the only area where wear and tear occurs in man is on his teeth—leading to the abnormality (disease?) that we know as "attrition." Although most tissues have a turnover rate, some do not. Nerve cells do not. Enamel and dentin do not, and that is what makes attrition possible. Attrition, the wearing away of the teeth as a result of tooth-to-tooth contact, occurs only on the occlusal, incisal, and proximal surfaces. It is associated with aging. In the human, modern diets vary greatly in consistency and abrasiveness, and so the correlation between attrition and age is not so great as it

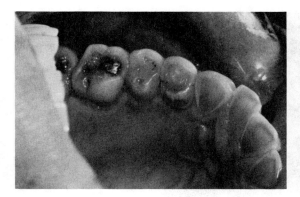

**Fig. 6-3** Attrition of the occlusal surfaces of teeth in a 78-year-old man.

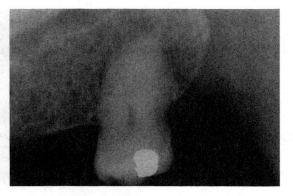

**Fig. 6-4** Radiograph of molar teeth of a 62-year-old man. The pulp chamber and root canals are almost obliterated by secondary dentin. (Courtesy Dr. Rahmat Barkhordar, San Francisco, Calif.)

it is in the horse, where age can be fairly well determined by examination of its teeth.

Attrition begins when the teeth first make occlusal contact. Early clinical signs are the appearance of small polished facets on cusps or ridges. There may also be flattening of the incisal edges of the anterior teeth. With age, there is a gradual reduction in cusp height with a consequent flattening of the occlusal plane. The process usually proceeds faster in men than in women, believed to be attributable to the greater masticatory force in men (Fig. 6-3). In addition to attrition, the enamel becomes less permeable but more brittle with age. The perikymata and imbrication lines are lost.[69] This loss alters the light reflection of enamel and results in tooth color changes. The changes in the thickness and type of dentin (secondary) with age also results in the yellowing and loss of translucency commonly seen in the teeth of aged persons.

The exposure of the dentin stimulates the pulp to lay down "secondary," or adventitious, dentin. The rate of this adventitious secondary dentin deposition is usually sufficient to prevent pulpal exposure through attrition, though thin tendrils of pulp horn may remain and become exposed to the oral cavity.

There are two other apparent changes in dentin associated with the aging process—physiologic secondary dentin formation and dentinal sclerosis.

*Secondary dentin* (irregular dentin) is formed after the deposition of primary dentin has been completed. It is characterized by its irregular mor-

phology. Secondary dentin may be considered a physiologic phenomenon associated with normal aging. As with almost all abnormal or pathologic aging processes, the change may not always be age related. Secondary dentin may form as a response to dental caries, attrition, and cavity preparation at any age.

Extensive secondary dentin formation partially explains the age-associated decrease in tooth sensitivity. Anterior teeth become less sensitive than molar teeth, since they have been shown to have a higher incidence of secondary dentin than molars in the same person.[6]

Radiographically the decreased size of the pulp chamber and root canals because of secondary dentin is apparent (Fig. 6-4). Histologically, the physiologic secondary dentin, though well demarcated from primary dentin, has somewhat fewer tubules but is otherwise similar to normal dentin. On the other hand, adventitious secondary dentin is usually quite irregular in appearance with few tubules, and those that are present are quite tortuous.

## PULP

Pulpal changes associated with age do not fit any of the wear-and-tear theories, or any of the other theories of aging. They are discussed here as a matter of convenience.

Histologically the pulp from the teeth of the el-

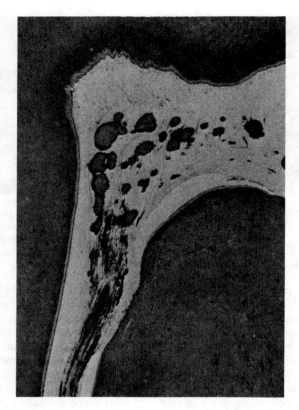

**Fig. 6-5** Photomicrograph of a tooth from a 68-year-old woman showing secondary dentin, fibrotic pulp, diffuse calcification, and false denticles.

derly is fibrotic and less cellular than that found in young persons. The blood supply, including the rich plexus of capillary loops in the subodontogenic region, is greatly reduced[5] (Fig. 6-5).

## Pulp calcifications

Although various forms of pulp calcifications are formed at almost every age, they apparently increase in frequency, number, and size during the aging process. Hill[41] found calcifications in 66% of all teeth examined in young people between 10 and 20 years of age but in 90% of all teeth examined in people 50 to 70 years of age.

There are two chief morphologic forms of pulp calcification: discrete pulp stones (pulp nodules, denticles) and diffuse calcification (Fig. 6-5). Pulp denticles, which have a tubular structure and re-

semble dentin, are called "true denticles." They are more frequently found in the pulp chamber than in the root canal. They may be continuous with the dentinal wall as "attached denticles" or may be lying completely within the pulp tissue as "free denticles."

*False denticles* are localized masses of calcified material that appear to be laid down in concentric layers around a central nidus (Fig. 6-5).

*Diffuse calcification* is most commonly seen in the root canals of teeth. It resembles diffuse calcifications seen in other parts of the body after fibrous degeneration or "calcific degeneration." Histologically, it appears as unorganized linear strands of amorphous deeply hematoxylin-staining material paralleling the blood vessels of the pulp (Fig. 6-5).

In summary then, the pulp diminishes in volume, probably because of continuous secondary dentin formation, which mechanically reduces its space. By age 75, the pulp space may be completely obliterated.[50] The changes in the blood and nerve supply reduce the perfusion and sensitivity of the aging pulp. Pulp stones and areas of diffuse calcification associated with dehydration of ground substance and fibrosis is a frequent finding; the incidence of all types of pulp calcifications increases with age.

## CEMENTUM

Cementum apparently continues to be laid down throughout life, but the rate of formation diminishes with age.[50] Under some circumstances, excessive amounts of cementum may be formed (hypercementosis) associated with accelerated elongation of an unopposed tooth or to an inflammatory stimulus.

The cementum may contain one of the very few real biologic markers of age. Countable, microscopically clear anular cemental rings have been found in all animals examined, including man.[49,98,99] Although this phenomenon has not been extensively explored in humans, it has great potential as a biologic tool for the forensic pathologist.

## OTHER WEAR-AND-TEAR THEORIES
### Waste accumulation

The theory of waste accumulation is based on the idea that old cells and postmitotic cells, which do not replicate or turn over, have a hard time disposing of their waste products of metabolism. This "garbage," some of which is a fatty, fluorescent, yellow-pigmented, granular substance, is called "lipofuscin."[95] It is one of the most ubiquitous, age-related changes in the cytoplasm of postmitotic, slowly dividing cells. It may occupy 30% to 75% of the available cytoplasmic space of heart muscle and nerve cells. The age-related increase of lipofuscin is inversely correlated with RNA content. Thus lipofuscin may interfere with the normal metabolic activity of cells. Currently, lipofuscin is believed to arise through a variety of processes, such as autophagocytosis, oxidation of lipids, and co-polymerization of organic molecules.[49] Many gerontologists viewed this phenomenon as a result rather than a "cause" of aging. Evidence now is accumulating to indicate that lipofuscin accumulation may be a by-product of reactions that do play a causal role in the aging process.[94]

As of now, the presence of "wear-and-tear" pigments have not been described and studied in oral tissues, an indication of a need for research in this area.

### Free radicals

Free radicals are small, highly charged pieces of interacting molecules containing an unpaired electron. These highly reactive molecules, which commonly have a short half-life, normally occur in metabolic reactions, especially those involving chains of enzymes.[21,33]

Harmon[35-37,39] postulates that free radicals are the central agents that cause the changes seen in aging tissues and cells. Although free-radical reactions are commonplace in all living things, it seems probable that the sum of *deleterious* free-radical reactions, which continuously go on in all cells and tissues, is indeed the aging process or one of them. The free radicals produced during normal cell metabolism form part of a structured system and therefore cannot diffuse within the cell. It is the diffusible free radicals that produce deleterious effects such as impaired information transfer in the cell (caused by lipid peroxidation with malonaldehyde production, leading to release of free bases from nucleotides, especially DNA), cross-linking (typical of aging collagen and elastin), and reorganization of mucopolysaccharides of connective tissue ground substance, among others.[50] It is the possible role of oxidative DNA damage in the aging process as well as in the diseases of the aged that remains an uncertainty in the free-radical theory of aging. On the other hand, antioxidants do not influence *maximum life span* because they cannot reset the internal clock. This does not negate the concept that there is free-radical involvement in many chronic diseases that are *life limiting*.[81] Free-radical reactions are implicated in the two major causes of death in the elderly—cancer and atherosclerosis. It is interesting to note that although antioxidants cannot increase maximum life span they can increase life expectancy in many animal species.

Although *atherosclerosis* may not be *directly* involved in oral pathologic conditions, it certainly is an important disease for the dentist to understand.

There are few clinical oral changes associated with atherosclerosis. It occurs in the tongue at a very early age (22 days) and increases in incidence and severity with increasing age. However, the structures supplied by the atheromatous vessels are not detectably disturbed by the vascular lesions, no matter the degree of atherosclerotic severity.[15]

*Oral cancer,* on the other hand, is an important oral disease of the elderly. Just how the free-radical theory might influence oral malignant disease should be discussed here. Other theories of aging that may influence the development of oral cancer are discussed later.

There is now evidence to support the idea that radicals are involved in cancerogenesis. Oberly and Oberly[72] theorize that carcinogenesis is a two-step process. Step 1 is the attainment of immortality (not to be confused with initiation), and step 2 is the loss of cell division (not to be confused with promotion). They believe that both steps are caused by free radicals, which play a great part in the final type of tumor. They beleive that the target cell in carcinogenesis is the stem or transit cell of the cell type that will eventually become malignant. They hypothesize that "cancer arises because the initiator causes a halt in differentiation by damaging the regulatory genes for MnSOD and/or CAT.* This damage opens the way for promotion and selection of a phenotype resistant to oxygen radicals. . . . We propose that the initial sites of damage are different in cancer from those in aging. We propose that the initial site of damage in cancer is the nuclear genes that regulate MnSOD and/or CAT. In contrast, we propose that the initial site of damage in aging is the mitochondrial DNA, not the nuclear DNA."[72]

Additional evidence for a role of oxygen free

radicals in carcinogenesis is proliferating. For example, there is an extensive literature on the oxidation of polynuclear aromatic hydrocarbons (PAH) to carcinogenic compounds by radicals, based on the finding that oxidation of PAH's can be catalyzed by the prostaglandin endoperoxide synthetase system (PGS).[81]

Tumor *promotion* also involves radicals.[16,40,65,93] For example, tetradecanoyl phorbol acetate (TPA), a well-known tumor promotor in experimental carcinogenesis, binds to membrane receptors and causes the release of superoxide from cells. In addition, the finding that antioxidants frequently act as anticarcinogenic compounds lends additional support to the idea of free-radical involvement in carcinogenesis.[106,115]

Whether free radicals play a role in oral tobacco carcinogenesis in long-time users (Fig. 6-8) or in early lip lesions associated with tobacco use (Fig. 6-9) or sun exposure (Fig. 6-10) remains to be seen. This is another important area for exploratory research, both clinical and experimental.

In any event, in Harmon's words,[38] "The aging process, beyond reasonable doubt, is the sum of the deleterious free radical reactions going on continuously throughout the cells and tissues. . . . The relationship between aging and diseases involving free radical reactions seems to be a direct one. . . . The number of diseases in which free radical reactions are recognized to be involved is increasing and includes the two major causes of death, cancer and atherosclerosis."

But don't be discouraged. He goes on to say, "It is reasonable to expect on the basis of present data that the healthy life span can be increased by 5-10 or more years through the judicious selection of diets and antioxidant supplements." (For an update on current experimental and theoretical information on the formation of oxygen radicals and their relation to tissue injury, see Halliwell.[32])

But that really does not settle the matter. There are still several well thought-out theories of aging; the most important for an understanding of oral pathology in the elderly is the immunologic theory. This theory postulates that the decline in immune function and the active destruction of vital organs by the immune system "causes" aging.[109,110]

Anatomists and anatomical pathologists from the time of Galen have known that the thymus reaches

---

*The discovery of the enzyme superoxide dismutase (SOD) by McCord and Fridovich[67] provided scientists with a sensitive and specific probe for superoxide radicals. It also suggested that oxygen free radicals were produced during normal cell metabolism. It paved the way for the conceptualization of antioxidant defense systems within cells and for the considerable research on the effects of antioxidants (vitamin E) on aging. The enzymatic system consisted of a copper and zinc–containing superoxide dismutase (Cu-ZnSOD) in the cytoplasm of a cell and a manganese-containing superoxide dismutase (MnSOD) in the mitochondria of cells. In addition, catalases (CAT) and peroxidases (glutathione peroxidase, GPX) are commonly found in mammalian cells.

its maximum size in childhood and rapidly involutes during puberty. All lymphoid tissues undergo involutional changes with advancing age,[1] a finding that explains some of the age-associated immune deficits. In fact, Burnet described the thymus as the pacemaker or "aging clock," its shrinkage being responsible for the falloff in immune capacity and the increase in autoantibodies, which characterize aging.[10] However, the evidence for the role of the immune system in aging is more convincing for the diseases of old age than for the process or processes of aging itself.[55]

On would assume that the student brings a background in basic immunology to the study of orofacial geropathology. Therefore only a brief review to remind the student of the interplay between subsets of lymphocytes needs be provided. (References have been selected to include literature reviews for the interested student.)

You may remember that stem cells arise during embryogenesis. Before birth, some of the hematopoietic stem cells differentiate into lymphoid precursor cells, some of which colonize the thymus, others the spleen, lymph nodes, and tonsils, and still others the bone marrow. Depending on the microenvironment, these cells differentiate and mature into at least two functionally different species of immunocompetent lymphocytes. Those under thymic influence become T-cells; those under bone marrow influence become B-cells. The T-cells populate the thymus-dependent areas of lymph nodes and spleen. Functionally, the T-cells are responsible for delayed-type or cell-mediated immunity, which involves direct contact of lymphocytes for destruction of foreign cells of all types. Such immunity has been termed "cell-mediated or cellular immunity" because it can be transferred from animal to animal only by transfer of lymphocytes, not cell-free serum. In addition, T-lymphocytes produce lymphokines (interleukin-1, interleukin-2, and so on), which are responsible for graft rejection, and "natural killer" cells (NK cells). They act as "helpers" to or suppressors of B-cell activity, as restrictors of cytotoxic effector cells, and as regulators of the level of humoral antibody response.

The B-cells interact with T-cells (and other accessory cells, such as macrophages) in the presence of antigen to multiply and subsequently differen-

tiate into plasma cells, which secrete specific antibody.

The decline in immune function is one of the most striking correlates with age. It has long been known that the cortex of the thymus begins to atrophy at sexual maturity. By 40 years of age the entire thymus has involuted to the extent that almost 90% of it is connective tissue and fat, with only about 6% of the cortex and 4% of the medulla remaining.[7] The thymic hormone thymosin decreases with age. Other lymphoid tissues also reach their maximum size at or immediately after puberty but undergo much more gradual atrophy with age.

In the B-cell arm of the immune system, the response to an antigen (such as bacteria) it is encountering for the first time (primary immune response) also has an age-related decline. This is especially so in those responses requiring a T-cell interaction with a B-cell.

Of even greater importance is the finding that secondary immune responses (those seen after a second, or "booster," encounter with an antigen) show no age-associated decline. This finding may explain why childhood diseases are not commonly seen in adults.

It is interesting that the number of circulating B-cells (and in the spleen and lymph nodes of mice) remain relatively constant.[14] However, subpopulations of B-cells may fluctuate because the level of serum IgG and IgA tends to increase with age whereas that of IgM decreases.[8] The total numbers of T- and B-cells remain constant, but their ability to respond to mitogenic stimulus is depressed in older people.[31]

Almost all studies indicate that the decline in immune function with age may be attributable to changes in the T-cell population of lymphocytes.[44] There is, for example, an age-related decrease in delayed hypersensitivity to skin test antigens to which a person has not been previously sensitized.[61] On the other hand, the skin reaction (delayed hypersensitivity) to tuberculin appears to be adequate in old age.[15]

Aging is also associated with a decrease in the magnitude of the immune response. Although conventional theory indicates that the loss of immune vigor is directly responsible for an increase in infections and perhaps tumors, Siskind[92] suggests the alternative view ". . . that despite the marked decrease in immune responsiveness, elderly ambulant persons remain remarkably free of infection. Certainly their susceptibility to infection is far less than that of patients with classical immune deficiency syndromes." He also points out that, except for reactivation of tuberculosis and herpes zoster (probably a chicken pox reactivation, not uncommon in the elderly), many infectious diseases such as pneumonias and renal infections occur in people "confined to bed or restricted in mobility, suggesting that mechanical factors, rather than immunologic ones, may be responsible for their increased susceptibility to infection." What he suggests is that the elderly produced antibodies to a wide range of pathogens in their early or youthful years and are thus provided with protection despite their reduced response to a *new* antigen.

In summary, there is an apparent age-related immunodeficiency, but the relations of age-diminished immune function to susceptibility to infection and to malignant disease has not been established. The thymic arm of the immune system loses vigor, especially the helper, effector, and suppressor T-cells, but the B-cells still produce antibodies when stimulated. In addition, there is an increased prevalence of autoantibodies of various types.

It is important to point out that chronologic aging itself may not be the only non–drug related immunodepressant for the elderly. Psychological stress factors alter the immune system and increase susceptibility to infections and neoplasias.[66] Severe depression, which is frequently found in older people, reduces helper T-cells and lowers NK cell activity. The stress-immune connections have been well reviewed by Hall et al.[30] and by Osterweis et al.[74]

Of the many theories of aging, that is, wear and tear, cross-linking of macromolecules, biologic clocks, finite replicative potential, free-oxygen radicals, and decreasing immunologic vigor, the diminution in immune vigor is the one that lends itself best to the study of the genetic control of aging. This is not the place for an in depth analysis of the genetics of immunology. Suffice it to say that genes of the major histocompatibility gene complex (MHC) are implicated in the control of the immune system and have been associated with diseases of the aged such as autoimmune diseases, rheumatoid arthritis, and cancer. Numerous MHC-regulated functions have been identified, a few of which may

be important in understanding oral geropathology. Among those are the regulation of helper and suppressor T-cells, immune response to T-dependent antigens, level of humoral antibody response, regulation of T-B cell interaction, control of cytotoxic effector cells and natural killer cells, T/B lymphocyte ratios, and maturation of immune function.[80]

An understanding of immunology is necessary if we are to examine and study the oral diseases of the aged, since most oral diseases are, after all, reactions to injury. Sometimes the injurious agents are known; frequently they are not. As indicated before, we can react to an injurious agent only within our genetic capabilities.

## ORAL INFECTIOUS DISEASES
### Herpes zoster

Herpes zoster (shingles) is an extremely painful and frequently incapacitating disease. It is characterized by inflammation of the dorsal root ganglia or extramedullary cranial nerve ganglia and by vesicular eruptions of the skin or mucous membranes in areas supplied by the affected sensory nerves. Evidence indicates that the signs and symptoms are caused by a reactivation of the latent V-2 (varicella, or chicken pox) virus acquired during a previous attack of chicken pox.

The disease is most common in adults, causing fever, general malaise, and pain and tenderness along the course of the involved sensory nerves. The trunk is often involved (Figs. 6-6 and 6-7). Within a few days, there is a linear papular or vesicular eruption of the skin or mucosa supplied by the affected nerves.

The triggering factors initiating the onset of herpes zoster include trauma and immunosuppressive therapy. When neither of the above factors are evident, the disease is often attributed to the loss of immune vigor because of age.

### Candidiasis

Candidiasis (candidosis, moniliasis, thrush) is a disease caused by a yeastlike fungus, *Candida albicans*, though other species such as *C. tropicalis*, *C. parapsilosis*, and *C. krusei* may be involved. The *Candida* species is one of the most opportunistic organisms we know. Although it is a relatively common organism of the mouth, gastrointestinal tract, and vagina, it apparently does not produce

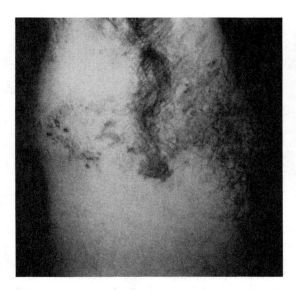

**Fig. 6-6** Herpes zoster involving T3 and T4 nerves. (Courtesy Dr. Samuel Dreizen, Houston, Texas.)

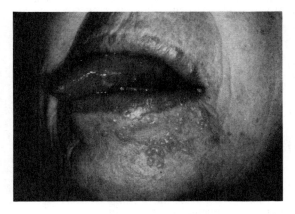

**Fig. 6-7** Herpes zoster involving the third division of the trigeminal nerve. (Courtesy Dr. Deborah Greenspan, San Francisco, Calif.)

disease until it actually penetrates the tissues. The incidence of candidiasis has increased remarkably since the widespread use of antibiotics, which upset the normal oral environment and destroy bacteria that apparently inhibit the growth of *C. albicans*. The disease is also common in patients who use immunosuppressive drugs, as in patients under treatment for leukemia or other malignant disease,

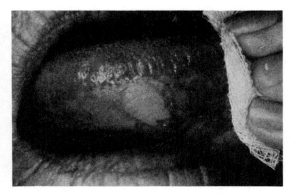

**Fig. 6-8** Acute pseudomembranous candidiasis in a 72-year-old woman.

transplant patients, and others using large doses of corticosteroids.

*Chronic mucocutaneous candidiasis* is characterized by chronic involvement of the skin, scalp, nails, and mucous membranes. These patients have some immunoabnormality—impaired cell-mediated immunity, isolated IgA deficiency, reduced serum candidacidal activity—and many are frail elderly. It is a relatively rare disease.

*Acute pseudomembranous candidiasis,* on the other hand, is a more common form of the disease. Although it too may occur at any age, the debilitated, chronically ill, or frail elderly are especially at risk. Oral lesions are characterized by the appearance of soft, white, slightly raised plaques on the buccal mucosa and tongue (Fig. 6-8). The palate, gingiva, or floor of the mouth may also be involved.

*Chronic atrophic candidiasis* is now considered to be synonymous with "denture sore mouth," a diffuse inflammation of denture-bearing areas. Although there is no absolute age correlation with this form of atrophic candidiasis, most of the patients with this lesion are over 55 years of age.[9] Contributing factors, in addition to age, are denture trauma, continual denture wearing, poor oral hygiene habits, poor denture cleanliness, and possibly diet.

## DENTAL CARIES

**Myth** Dental caries is a disease of the young; destructive periodontitis is a disease of the old.

Dental caries is an infectious disease of the teeth

characterized by demineralization of its inorganic portion and destruction of its organic portion. The cause and pathogenesis of dental caries in the elderly is similar to or identical with those disease processes in younger people. It is assumed that the student is already familiar with clinical and microscopic carious lesions, and so a reiteration of these basic phenomena need not be repeated. There are, however, special considerations for understanding and treating dental caries in the elderly.

As mentioned earlier, enamel changes with age. It is less translucent, and so enamel caries in the elderly may have a different clinical appearance from that seen in young people. In addition, proximal caries, especially where an adjacent tooth is missing, are frequently arrested and show a dark brown to black discoloration. Microscopic examination of these arrested carious lesions in the elderly show demineralized areas intermingled with areas of dense mineralization.

All teeth in which an enamel lesion extends to the dentin show dentinal and pulpal changes.[18] When attrition occurs after a carious lesion is established, the lesion may be seen in the exposed dentin. These findings are of importance in the treatment of caries in the elderly and are discussed in more detail in Chapter 9.

With increasing age, the gingiva gradually recedes, and such recession exposes the root surfaces to the oral environment. Depending on the amount and composition of saliva, the amount and composition of microbial plaque, and the amount and composition of dietary carbohydrates, the exposed root surfaces are at risk for dental caries. Unfortunately, little is known about root caries.[71] The literature on the epidemiology and histopathology is reviewed in Chapter 9 and by Fejerskof and Nyvad.[17]

## PERIODONTAL DISEASE

Both the cellular and humoral arms of the immune system are implicated in the destructive aspects of periodontal inflammation. There has been good correlation between clinical severity of periodontitis and plaque-induced peripheral lymphocyte mitogenesis.[42,43,63] In addition, patients with primary immunodeficiency syndromes, though always very young, without exception have less gingivitis than immunocompetent, age-, and plaque-matched controls.[83] Immunosuppressed adult patients were also

found to have little or no gingivitis, even in the presence of large accumulations of plaque.[47,103] In other words, destructive periodontal inflammatory reactions to injury can occur only in people able to mount an immunologic response to dental plaque. The various immunological deficits and the gradual loss of immune vigor, especially in the T-cell arm of the immune system, complicate the clinical response to plaque in the elderly. If the "old old" cannot mount a T-cell response to plaque organisms, the massive destructive aspects of periodontitis, so well illustrated by Levy et al.[59] in nonhuman primates as a response to tuberculin in sensitized animals, will not occur.

When one realizes that there are defects in osteoblastic activity in the elderly[2] and that wound healing in the elderly is or may be greatly reduced, the problems of periodontal therapy in the aged are understandably complex. These problems are discussed in Chapter 11. Suffice it to say here, current evidence does not support the concept that periodontal disease is predominantly a disease of the old, though it may occur in the older population. When it does, all the biologic factors previously mentioned interact with the bacterial dental plaque to produce a clinical change in the periodontal tissues, about which very little is known.

## OROFACIAL TUMORS

As indicated earlier, there are no tumors or other oral or orofacial lesions that are limited exclusively to the elderly. On the other hand, many tumors are found predominantly in the elderly.

### Benign tumors

Keratoacanthoma is a benign epithelial lesion that closely resembles epidermoid carcinoma. It occurs twice as frequently in men as in women, with the majority of cases occurring between 50 and 70 years of age.[24] About 90% of these tumors occur on the exposed skin, most often on the cheeks, nose, and dorsum of the hands. The lesion occurs on the lips in about 8% of the cases. Intraoral lesions are rare.[20,91] The lesion usually first appears as a 5 to 8 mm, firm elevated umbilicated or crateriform nodule with a depressed central keratin core. It may reach 1 to 1.5 cm in diameter within 4 to 8 weeks, persist for 4 to 8 weeks, expel the keratin core, and regress over the next 6 to 8 weeks. Some lesions have been reported to persist for as

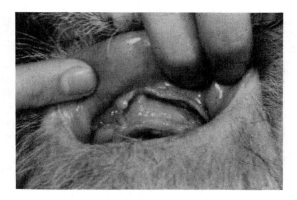

**Fig. 6-9** Fibrous hyperplasia in the labial fold of an 83-year-old man with ill-fitting dentures for about 10 years.

long as 2 years. Since spontaneous regression does not occur in every case, surgical excision is the usual treatment.[34]

*Fibrous hyperplasia* (inflammatory fibrous hyperplasia, epulis fissuratum, redundant tissue), though not a tumor in the usual sense of the word, is one of the most common tissue reactions to ill-fitting dentures. It usually occurs along the denture borders but may be seen on the gingiva, buccal mucosa, or angle of the mouth, wherever chronic irritation of any type exists.

This lesion is characterized by the development of elongated rolls of tissue in the mucolabial or mucobuccal fold into which a denture flange fits (Fig. 6-9). The lesion is firm and fibrous feeling on palpation and may or may not be ulcerated at its base. It is important to recognize the mass for what it is and treat it accordingly.

### Premalignant lesions

*Leukoplakia* is a white plaque on the mucosa (which cannot be identified as a diagnosable entity, such as lichen planus, white sponge nevus, candidiasis, or chemical burns) and carries no histologic connotation. The WHO (World Health Organization) Collaborating Center for Oral Precancerous Lesions was established in 1967 to characterize oral lesions that should be considered precancerous and uses a similar definition. An extensive review of oral leukoplakia was published by Waldron and Shafer[107] almost 30 years ago and not much new knowledge has been added since then. The report of the WHO Collaborating Center

for Oral Precancerous Lesions, published some 20 years ago, presents an excellent critical review of the lesion.[113]

Of importance here is the fact that oral leukoplakia is a disease that occurs primarily in the 50 to 80 year old group. Certain sites of predilection have been identified. Although the site as well as the prevalence and incidence varies throughout the world, the findings by Waldron and Shafer,[108] based on a review of over 3250 cases in the United States, found that the greatest number of cases of leukoplakia occurred on the mandibular alveolar ridge, gingiva, or mucobuccal fold (25%). The next most common site was the buccal mucosa (22%). In men, the lower lip was the site of leukoplakia in 16% of those examined, but the lip lesion was found in only 4% of the women. The tongue and floor of the mouth were not frequent sites for leukoplakia in their study. For a more universal discussion of the incidence and site of predilection of oral leukoplakias, the student is referred to the excellent review by Pindborg.[78]

Clinically, patches of leukoplakia vary from a nonpalpable, faintly translucent white area to thick, fissured, papillomatous, indurated lesions. The surface may be wrinkled and feel rough to palpation. The lesions are white, gray, or yellowish white. In heavy tobacco users, especially smokeless-tobacco users, the lesion may be brownish yellow. Some leukoplakia lesions undergo malignant transformation to epidermoid carcinoma. However, there is no correlation between the clinical appearance of leukoplakia and its histologic configuration. Some large, "ugly-looking" leukoplakias show no histologic atypia, whereas small "mild-looking" leukoplakias are invasive carcinoma. Biopsy is mandatory for definitive diagnoses (Figs. 6-10 and 6-11).

*Actinic elastosis* (solar elastosis, senile elastosis) of the orofacial areas is a dermatologic disease of elderly men who have spent a good deal of time outdoors, such as farmers and fishermen. Although it does not occur on the oral mucous membranes, it frequently involves the lower lip.

Clinically, the affected skin is wrinkled, dry, atrophic, and flaccid. The sharp demarcation between the vermilion and the skin disappears (Fig. 6-12). There may be a mild keratosis on the lip.

Cancer of the vermilion border is often preceded by actinic elastosis.[78]

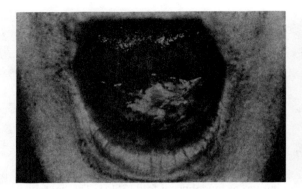

**Fig. 6-10** Leukoplakia in floor of mouth. (Courtesy Drs. Sidney Epstein, San Francisco, and Paul Jacobs, Palo Alto, Calif.)

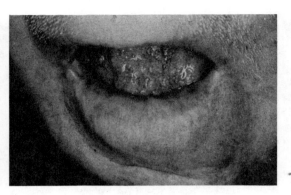

**Fig. 6-12** Actinic elastoses of lip. The vermilion border is obliterated in this 73-year-old fisherman.

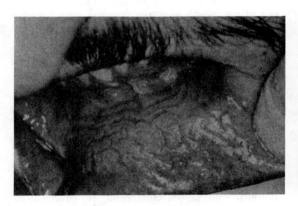

**Fig. 6-11** Leukoplakia, lower lip mucosa in a 64-year-old smokeless tobacco user of 45 years. (Courtesy Drs. Sidney Epstein, San Francisco, and Paul Jacobs, Palo Alto, Calif.)

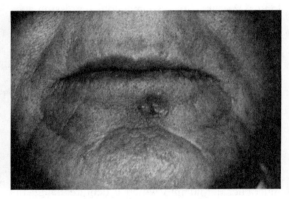

**Fig. 6-13** Basal cell carcinoma in a 72-year-old man.

## Malignant lesions

*Basal cell carcinoma* (basal cell epithelioma, rodent ulcer) is probably the most common type of carcinoma in men. It occurs most often in elderly, blond, fair-skinned, blue-eyed men who have spent much of their lives outdoors.

Eighty-five percent of the cases of basal cell carcinoma occur in the head and neck. In a study of some 9000 cases, Cotran[13] found the incidence of metastasis to be only 0.1%, indicating the benign character of this tumor.

Clinically, the basal cell carcinoma usually be-gins as a small papule that ulcerates, heals, and ulcerates again. During growth, there are cycles of ulceration and healing. Eventually, the crusting ulcer, which appears superficial, develops a smooth, rolled border (Fig. 6-13). As the lesion continues to enlarge, it infiltrates adjacent lateral and deeper tissues and may invade cartilage and bone

Basal cell cancer never arises in the oral mucosa.

*Epidermoid carcinoma* (squamous cell carcinoma) is the most common malignant neoplasm in the oral cavity. Although it may occur anywhere in the mouth, some sites are more frequently involved than others.

The incidence of oral cancer in the United States

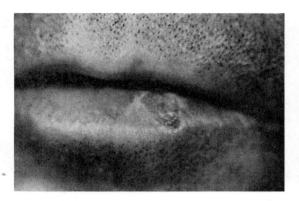

Fig. 6-14 Early lip cancer in a 55-year-old man who said he "pulled the skin off his lip" when a cigarette stuck to it. He smoked 3 packs a day for over 20 years.

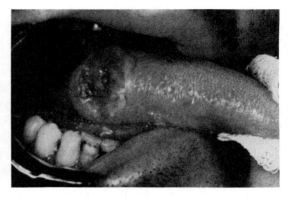

Fig. 6-16 Carcinoma of the lateral surface of the tongue. Patient is a 76-year-old man who claims the ulcer was painless and was present for over a year.

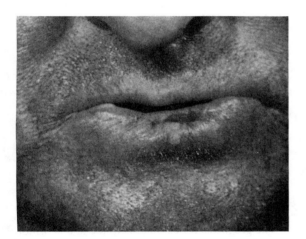

Fig. 6-15 Carcinoma of the lip in a 66-year-old farmer exposed to sun for many years. Notice the actinic elastoses on lower lip.

is about 20 per 100,000 population for men and 5 per 100,000 for women. There is also a great variation in sex incidence between various sites in the mouth and in geographic distribution. Krolls and Hoffman,[56] in a study of some 14,250 patients with oral carcinoma, found that 77% of the cases occurred on the lips, tongue, and floor of the mouth. When the cases of lip cancer were excluded, 68% of 8301 oral cancer cases occurred on the tongue and floor of the mouth. Thirty-two percent were in

the 70-year-old group, with 90% ranging in age from 40 to 99 years. It is of interest to note that oral cancer is the most common type of cancer of men in India, accounting for 40% of all cancers in one Bombay hospital[46] (Figs. 6-14 and 6-15).

*Carcinoma of the tongue* accounts for some 25% to 50% of all intraoral cancer. It is less common in women than in men, except in the Scandinavian countries, where it is frequently associated with Plummer-Vinson syndrome. Carcinoma of the tongue is essentially a disease of the elderly, with less than 5% of reported cases occurring before 30 years of age.

Clinically this carcinoma usually presents as a painless mass or ulcer on the lateral or ventral surface of the tongue (Fig. 6-16). Lesions on the lateral border are usually equally distributed between the base, the midportion, and the anterior third of the tongue. The specific site of origin of tongue cancer, however, is important. Lesions of the base and posterior portion of the tongue are usually of a higher grade of malignancy, metastasize earlier, and have a poorer prognosis than those occurring on the middle or anterior portion.[87]

In all cases of carcinoma of the tongue, metastases occur with great frequency, being present in some 70% of patients at the time of hospital admission.[25]

*Carcinoma of the floor of the mouth* represents about 15% of all intraoral cancers. It occurs primarily in elderly men.[3] As in all oral cancers, tobacco use, especially pipe and cigar smoking, along with heavy alcohol use, are said to be etiologic factors. The leukoplakia previously mentioned as occurring in this location seems to show more frequent epithelial dysplasia and malignant transformation than it does in other intraoral locations.[87]

Clinically, cancer of the floor of the mouth appears as an indurated ulcer of varying size on one side of the midline. It occurs much more frequently in the anterior portion of the floor of the mouth than in its posterior area.

This carcinoma frequently metastasizes to the submaxillary lymph nodes. Because the primary lesion may occur near the midline, bilateral or contralateral metastasis often occurs. Distant metastases are relatively rare.

*Carcinoma of the buccal mucosa* is relatively rare in the United States.[56] It occurs primarily in elderly men. Leukoplakia is a common predecessor of carcinoma of the buccal mucosa, which is associated with the use of chewing tobacco. There is some evidence that carcinoma of the buccal mucosa in smokeless-tobacco users develops in the area against which a quid of chewing tobacco was habitually carried.[87]

A special form of buccal mucosal cancer is the "verrucous carcinoma," which seems to occur exclusively in tobacco-chewing elderly men and women (Fig. 6-17).

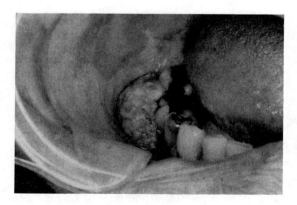

**Fig. 6-17** Verrucous carcinoma of buccal mucosa in a 65-year-old tobacco chewer of long duration. (Courtesy Drs. Sidney Epstein, San Francisco, and Paul Jacobs, Palo Alto, Calif.)

Clinically there is a painful, ulcerative lesion that develops along or inferior to a line opposite the plane of occlusion. The incidence of metastases is relatively high, occurring in about 50% of the cases at the time of initial evaluation.

*Carcinoma of the gingiva* accounts for about 10% of oral cancers. Because it may mimic dental infections, diagnosis may be delayed for a considerable time, leading to a poorer prognosis. Like all oral cancers, gingival carcinoma is primarily a disease of elderly men.

Clinically, carcinoma of the gingiva initially appears either as an area of ulceration or as an exophytic, granular, or verrucous lesion. It may look so benign that malignant disease may not be a part of the differential diagnosis.

The lesion may occur on either maxillary or mandibular gingiva, arising more commonly but not always in edentulous areas. The fixed gingiva is more frequently the site of the primary lesion than the free gingiva.[87] The periosteum and bone are frequently invaded by these tumors. Although cancer of the mandibular gingiva metastasizes more frequently than cancer of the maxillary gingiva, both frequently metastasize to the submaxillary or the cervical lymph nodes.

The prognoses for all intraoral carcinomas is not good. However, it does vary with such factors as location, duration before treatment, and presence or absence of metastases at initial evaluation. Carcinoma of the lip has a good prognosis, with a cure rate of over 80%, no matter what type of treatment is used.

The prognosis for carcinoma of the tongue is not favorable. The 5-year cure rate is somewhat less than 25% in most studies reported. The prognosis for carcinoma of the floor of the mouth seems to be somewhat better, though studies of this lesion report 5-year survival rates of between 21% and 43%. The prognosis for carcinoma of the buccal mucosa depends on the presence or absence of metastases. The 5-year survival rate for carcinoma of the buccal mucosa is about 50%. Carcinoma of the gingiva has a very poor prognosis if metastases are present at initial examination but may be as high as 25% if no metastases are present. The verrucous carcinoma has the best prognosis of all the intraoral cancers. It is very slow growing and only superficially invasive.

In summary, any lesion that occurs in older persons probably occurs in young ones, but the changes in the immune system, the endocrine system, and all other organ systems may change the direction and severity of the reaction. Understanding the biology of aging in general and the oral biology of aging and the aged in particular will provide a basis for the appropriate treatment of the elderly patient.

Medicine is currently dominated by the sheer number of sick, aging persons. Kohn points out "that problems caused by the aging population can only get worse as the number and proportion of older people increase. The great amount of information available on aging and age-related processes indicates more specifically what kind of problems can be expected in dealing with aging individuals."[5]

We in dentistry have not yet faced the problems of dealing with an aging population. We will and very soon. Will we be ready? That is the challenge to dentistry. That is the challenge to oral pathobiology in the coming decade.

## REFERENCES

1. Adler WH, Jones KH, and Brock MA: Aging and immune function. In Behnke JA, Finch CE, and Gairdner BM, editors: The biology of aging, New York, 1979, Plenum Press.
2. Arlot M, Edouard C, Meunier PJ, et al: Impaired osteoblast function in osteoporosis: comparison between calcium balance and dynamic histomorphometry, Br Med J 289:517, 1984.
3. Ballard BR, Suess GR, Picksern JW, et al: Squamous-cell carcinoma of the floor of the mouth, Oral Surg 45:568, 1978.
4. Barker BC: Relation of the alveolus to the cement-to-enamel junction following attritional wear in aboriginal skulls: an inquiry into normality of cementum, J Periodontol 46:357, 1975.
5. Bennet CG, Kelin EE, and Biddington WR: Age changes of the vascular pattern of the human dental pulp, Arch Oral Biol 10:995, 1965.
6. Bevelander G and Benzer S: Morphology and incidence of secondary dentin in human teeth, J Am Dent Assoc 30:1075, 1943.
7. Boyd E: The weight of the thymus gland in health and in disease, Am J Dis Child 43:1162, 1932.
8. Buckley CG, Beckley EG, and Dorsey FC: Longitudinal changes in serum immunoglobulin levels in older humans, Fed Proc 33:2036, 1974.
9. Biedtz-Jörgensen E: Denture stomatitis. III. Histopathology of trauma- and *Candida*-induced inflammatory lesions of the palatal mucosa, Acta Odontol Scand 28:551, 1970.
10. Burnet M (Sir): An immunological approach to aging, Lancet 1:358, 1970.
11. Claycomb CK, Summers GW, and Dvorak EM: Oral collagen biosynthesis in the guinea pig, J Periodont Res 2:115, 1967.
12. Coolidge ED: The thickness of the human periodontal membrane, JAMA 24:1260, 1937.
13. Cotran RS: Metastasizing basal cell carcinomas, Cancer 14:1036, 1961.
14. Diaz-Jouanen E, Williams RC Jr, and Strickland RG: Age-related changes in T and B cells, Lancet 1:688, 1975 (letter).
15. Dreizen S, Levy BM, Stern MH, and Bernick S: Human lingual atherosclerosis, Arch Oral Biol 19:813, 1974.
16. Emerit I and Cerutti PA: Tumor promoter phorbol 12-myristate 13-acetate induces a clastogenic factor in human lymphocytes, Proc Natl Acad Sci USA 79:7509, 1982.
17. Fejerskof O and Nyvad B: Pathology and treatment of dental caries in the aging individual. In Holm-Pedersen P and Löe H: Geriatric dentistry, Copenhagen, 1986, Munksgaard.
18. Fejerskof O and Thylstrup A: Pathology of dental caries. In Thylstrup A and Fejerskof O, editors: Textbook of cariology, Copenhagen, 1986, Munksgaard.
19. Finch CE and Schneider EL, editors: Handbook of the biology of aging, ed 2, New York, 1985, Van Nostrand Reinhold Co.
20. Freedman PO, Kerpel SM, Begel H, and Lumerman H: Solitary intraoral keratoacanthoma, Oral Surg 47:74, 1979.
21. Freeman BA and Crapo JD: Biology of disease: free radicals and tissue injury, Lab Invest 47:412, 1982.
22. Gargiulo AW and Grant D: Aging changes in the periodontium, Ill Dent J 42:780, 1973.
23. Gargiulo AW, Wentz FM, and Organ T: Mitotic activity of human oral epithelium, exposed to 30 percent hydrogen peroxide, Oral Surg 14:472, 1961.
24. Ghadially FN, Barton BW, and Kerridge DF: The etiology of keratoacanthoma, Cancer 16:603, 1963.
25. Gibbel MI, Cross JH, and Ariel IM: Cancer of the tongue: review of 330 cases, Cancer 2:411, 1949.
26. Gilchrest BA: Skin and aging processes, Boca Raton, Fla, 1984, CRC Press.
27. Götze W: Über Alternsveränderungen des Parodontiums (Volumenbestimmung der Gewebeanteile nach Hennig), Dtsche Zahnaerztl Z 20:465, 1965.
28. Gran JA: Notes on the teeth and gingiva of Central Australian Aborigines, Aust Dent J 2:277, 1957.
29. Hall DA, Blackett AD, Zajac AR, et al: Changes in skinfold thickness with increasing age, Age Ageing 10:19, 1981.
30. Hall N, McGillis J, and Goldstein AL: Activation of neuro-endocrine pathways by thymosin. In Cooper EL, editor: Stress, immunity and aging, New York, 1984, Marcel Dekker, Inc.
31. Hallgren HM, Buckley CE III, Gilbertsen VA, and Yunis EJ: Lymphocyte phytohemagglutinin responsiveness, immunologlobins and autoantibodies in aging humans, J Immunol 111:1101, 1973.
32. Halliwell B, editor: Oxygen radicals and tissue injury. Bethesda, Md, 1988, Federation of American Societies for Experimental Biology.

33. Halliwell B and Gutteridge JMC: Free radical in biology and medicine, Oxford, Engl, 1985, Clarendon Press.
34. Hardman FG: Keratoacanthoma of the lips, Br J Oral Surg 9:46, 1971.
35. Harmon D: Aging: a theory based on free radical and radiation chemistry, J Gerontol 11:298, 1956.
36. Harmon D: Free radical theory of aging: effect of free radical inhibitors on the mortality rate of $LAF_1$ mice, J Gerontol 23:476, 1968.
37. Harmon D: Free radical theory of aging: the "free radical" diseases, Age 7:111, 1984.
38. Harmon D: Role of free radicals in aging and disease. In Johnson HA, editor: Relations between normal aging and disease, Aging Series vol 28, New York, 1985, Raven Press.
39. Harmon D: Free radical theory of aging: role of free radicals in the organization and evolution of life, aging and disease processes. In Johnson JE, editor: Free radicals, aging and degenerative diseases, New York, 1986, Alan R. Liss.
40. Heckler E, Fusenig NE, Kunz W, et al, editors: Effects of tumor promoters, New York, 1982, Raven Press.
41. Hill TJ: Pathology of the dental pulp, J Am Dent Assoc 21:820, 1934.
42. Horton JE, Leikin S, and Oppenheim JJ: Human lymphoproliferative reaction to saliva and dental plaque deposits: an in vitro correlation with periodontal disease, J Periodontol 43:522, 1972.
43. Ivanyi L and Lehner T: Lymphocyte transformation by sonicates of dental plaque in human periodontal disease, Arch Oral Biol 16:1117, 1971.
44. Joris F and Girard JP: Immune response in aged and young subjects following administration of large doses of tuberculin, Int Arch Allergy Appl Immunol 48:584, 1975.
45. Jozat R: Ueber Veränderungen des Periodontiums durch Entlastung, Dtsche Zahnaerztl Wochenschr 36:155, 1933.
46. Ju DMC: On the etiology of cancer of the lower lip, Plast Reconstr Surg 52:151, 1973.
47. Kardochi BJ and Newcomb GM: A clinical study of gingival inflammation in renal transplant recipients taking immunosuppressive drugs, J Periodontol 43:307, 1978.
48. Karring T and Löe H. The effect of age on mitotic activity in rat oral epithelium, J Periodont Res 8:164, 1973.
49. Kay RF, Rasmussen DT, and Beard KC: Cementum anular counts provide a means for age determination in Macaca mulatta, Folia Primatol 42:85, 1984.
50. Kenney RA: Physiology of aging: a synopsis, Chicago, 1982, Year Book Medical Publishers, Inc.
51. Klein A: Systematische Untersuchungen über die Periodontalbreite, Zeitschrift für Stomatologie 26:417, 1928.
52. Kligman AM: Perspectives and problems in cutaneous gerontology, J Invest Dermatol 73:39, 1979.
53. Klingsberg J and Butcher EO: Comparative histology of age changes in oral tissues of the rat, hamster and monkey, J Dent Res 39:158, 1960.
54. Kohn RR: Principles of mammalian aging, New York, 1978, Prentice-Hall Inc.
55. Kohn RR: Aging and age-related diseases: normal processes. In Johnson HA, editor: Relations between normal aging and disease, Aging Series vol 28, New York, 1985, Raven Press.
56. Krolls SO and Hoffman S: Squamous cell carcinoma of the oral soft tissues: a statistical analysis of 14,153 cases by age, sex and race of patients, J Am Dent Assoc 92:571, 1976.
57. Lavelle CLB: The effect of age on the proliferative activity of certain epithelial tissues, J Periodont Res 3:212, 1968.
58. Levy BM, Dreizen S, and Bernick S: Effect of aging on the marmoset periodontium, J Oral Pathol 1:61, 1972.
59. Levy BM, Robertson RB, Dreizen S, et al: Adjuvant induced destructive periodontitis in nonhuman primates: a comparative study. J Periodont Res 11:54, 1976.
60. Löe H and Karring T: The three-dimensional morphology of the epithelial-connective tissue interface of the gingiva as related to age and sex, Scand J Dent Res 79:315, 1972.
61. MacKay IR: Aging and immunological function in man, Gerontologia 18:285, 1972.
62. Mackenzie IC, Holm-Pedersen P, and Karring T: Age changes in the oral mucous membrane and periodontium. In Holm-Pedersen P and Löe H, editors: Geriatric dentistry, Copenhagen, 1986, Munksgaard.
63. Mackler BF, Altman LC, Wohl S, et al: Blastogenesis and lymphokine synthesis by T and B lymphocytes from patients with periodontal disease, Infect Immun 10:844, 1974.
64. Maidhof R and Hornstein OP: Autoradiographic study of some proliferative properties of human buccal mucosa, Arch Dermatol Res 265:165, 1979.
65. Marks F and Furstenberger G: Tumor promotion in skin: Are active oxygen species involved? In Spies H, editor: Oxidative stress, New York, 1985, Academic Press, Inc.
66. Marx JL: The immune system "belongs in the body," Science 227:1190, 1985.
67. McCord MC and Fridovich I: Superoxide dismutase: an enzymatic function for erythrocuprein (hemocuprein), J Biol Chem 24:6045, 1969.
68. Meyer J, Marwah AS, and Weinmann JP: Mitotic rate of gingival epithelium in two age groups, J Invest Dermatol 27:237, 1956.
69. Mijor I: Age changes in the teeth. In Holm-Pedersen P and Löe H, editors: Geriatric dentistry, Copenhagen, 1987, Munksgaard.
70. Montagna W and Carlisle K: Structural changes in aging human skin, J Invest Dermatol 73:47, 1979.
71. Nyvad B and Fejerskof O: Root surface caries: clinical, histopathological and microbiological features and clinical implications, Int Dent J 32:312, 1982.
72. Oberly LW and Oberly TD: Free radicals, cancer and aging. In Johnson JE Jr, Harmon D, Walford R, and Miguel J, editors: Free radicals, aging and degenerative diseases, New York, 1986, Alan R. Liss, Inc.
73. Oota K, Makinodan T, Masome I, and Baker L, editors: Aging phenomena: relationship among different levels of organization, Adv Exp Med Biol, vol 129, New York, 1980, Plenum Press, Inc.
74. Osterwies M, Solomon F, and Green M: Bereavement reactions, consequences and care, Washington, DC, 1984, National Academy Press.

75. Papic M and Glickman I: Keratinization of the gum and gingiva in the menstrual cycle and the menopause, Oral Surg Oral Med Oral Pathol 3:504, 1950.

76. Pearl R: The rate of living, New York, 1928, Alfred A Knopf.

77. Pearl R: Studies in human biology, Baltimore, 1924, The Williams & Wilkins Co.

78. Pindborg JJ: Pathology and treatment of diseases in oral mucous membranes and salivary glands. In Holm-Pedersen P and Löe H: Geriatric dentistry, Copenhagen, 1986, Munksgaard.

79. Plewig G: Regional differences of cell sizes in the human stratum corneum, J Invest Dermatol 54:19, 1970.

80. Popp DM and Popp RA: Genetics. In Kay M and Makinodan T, editors: CRC handbook of immunology in aging, Boca Raton, Fla, 1980, CRC Press.

81. Pryor WA: The free-radical theory of aging revisited: a critique and a suggested disease-specific theory. In Warner HR, Butler RN, Sprott RL, and Schneider EL, editors: Modern biological theories of aging, New York, 1987, Raven Press.

82. Richman MJ and Abarbanel AR: Effects of estradiol and diethylstilbestrol upon the atrophic human buccal mucosa with a preliminary report on the use of estrogens in the management of senile gingivitis, J Clin Endocrinol 3:224, 1943.

83. Robertson PB, Mackler BF, Wright TE, and Levy BM: Periodontal status of patients with abnormalities of the immune system. II. Observations over a two year period, J Periodontol 51:70, 1980.

84. Ryan EJ, Toto PD, and Gargiulo AW: Aging in human attached gingival epithelium, J Dent Res 53:74, 1974.

85. Scott J, Valentine JA, St. Hill CA, and Balasooriya BA: A quantitative histologic analysis of the effects of age and sex on human lingual epithelium, J Biol Buccale 11:303, 1983.

86. Severson JA, Moffett BC, Kokick V, and Selipsky H: A histological study of age changes in the adult human periodontal joint (ligament), J Periodontol 49:189, 1978.

87. Shafer WG, Hine MK, and Levy BM: A textbook of oral pathology, Philadelphia, 1983, WB Saunders Co.

88. Sharav Y and Massler M: Age changes in oral epithelia, Exp Cell Res 47:132, 1967.

89. Ship II, Cohen DW, and Laster L: A study of gingival, periodontal and oral hygiene examination methods in a single population, J Periodontol 38:638, 1967.

90. Shklar G: The effects of aging upon oral mucosa, J Invest Dermatol 47:115, 1966.

91. Silberberg E: Cancer statistics, 1982, CA 32:15, 1982.

92. Siskind GW: Aging and the immune system. In Warner HR, Butler RN, Sprott RL, and Schneider EL, editors: Modern biological theories of aging, Aging Series vol 31, New York, 1987, Raven Press.

93. Sloga TJ, Klein-Szanto AJP, Triplett LL, et al: Skin tumor-promoting activity of benzoyl peroxide, a widely used free radical–generating compound, Science 213:1023, 1981.

94. Sohol RS: Metabolic rate, aging and lipofuscin accumulation. In Sohol RS editor: Age pigments, Amsterdam, 1981, Elsevier/North Holland Biomedical Press.

95. Sohol RS and Allen RG: Relationship between metabolic rate, free radicals, differentiation and aging: a unified theory. In Woodhead AD, Blackett AD, and Hollaender A, editors: Molecular biology of aging, New York, 1985, Plenum Press.

96. Stahl SS, Tonna EA, and Weiss R: The effects of aging on the proliferative activity of rat periodontal structures, J Gerontol 24:447, 1969.

97. Stahl SS and Tonna EA: H³-proline study of aging periodontal ligament matrix formation: comparison between matrices adjacent to either cemental or bone surfaces, J Periodont Res 12:318, 1977.

98. Stott GG, Sis RF, and Levy BM: Cementum annulation as an age criterion in the common marmoset *(Callithrix jacchus),* J Med Primatol 9:274, 1980.

99. Stott GG, Sis RF, and Levy BM: Cemental annulation as an age criterion in forensic dentistry, J Dent Res 61:814, 1982.

100. Ten Cate AR: Oral histology: development, structure, and function, St. Louis, 1980, The CV Mosby Co.

101. Thuringer JM and Katzberg AA: The effect of age on mitosis in the human epidermis, J Invest Dermatol 33:35, 1959.

102. Tindall JP: Geriatric dermatology. In Reichel W, editor: Clinical aspects of aging, ed 2, Baltimore, 1983, The Williams & Wilkins Co.

103. Tollefsen T, Koppong HS, and Messelt E: Immunosuppression and periodontal disease in man: histological and ultrastructural observations, J Periodont Res 17:329, 1982.

104. Tonna EA, Weiss R, and Stahl SS: The cell proliferative activity of parodontal tissues in aging mice, Arch Oral Biol 7:969, 1972.

105. Toto PD, Rubenstein AS, and Gargiulo AW: Labelling index and cell density of aging rat oral tissue, J Dent Res 54:553, 1975.

106. Tso POP, Caspary WJ, and Lorentzen RJ: The involvement of free radicals in chemical carcinogenesis. In Pryor WA, editor: Free radicals in biology, vol 3, New York, 1977, Academic Press, Inc.

107. Waldron CA and Shafer WG: Current concepts of leukoplakia, Int Dent J 10:350, 1960.

108. Waldron CA and Shafer WG: Leukoplakia revisited: a clinico-pathologic study of 3256 oral leukoplakias, Cancer 36:1386, 1975.

109. Walford RL: The immunological theory of aging, current status, Fed Proc 33:2020, 1974.

110. Walford RL, Weindruch RH, Gottesman SRS, and Tam CF: The immunopathology of aging. In Eisdorfer C, Starr B, and Cristofalo VJ, editors: Annu Rev Gerontol Geriatr vol 2, New York, 1981, Springer-Verlag (NY) Publ Co.

111. Warner HR, Butler RN, Sprott RL, and Schneider EL, editors: Modern biological theories of aging, Aging Series vol 31, New York, 1987, Raven Press.

112. Wentz FM, Maier AW, and Orban B: Age changes and sex differences in the clinically "normal" gingiva, Periodontology 23:13, 1952.

113. WHO Collaborating Centre for Oral Precancerous Lesions: Definition of leukoplakia and related lesions: an aid to studies on oral precancer, Oral Surg 46:518, 1978.

114. Williams CHM: Present status of knowledge concerning the etiology of periodontal disease, Oral Surg Oral Med Oral Pathol 2:729, 1949.

115. Zedeck MS and Lipkin MS, editors: Inhibition of tumor induction and development, New York, 1981, Plenum Press.

116. Zimmerman ER and Zimmerman AL: Effects of race, age, smoking habits, oral and systemic disease in oral exfoliative cytology, J Dent Res 44:627, 1965.

# PART TWO

# Clinical Care

# 7

# Assessment of the Older Adult

*Douglas B. Berkey*
*Ronald L. Ettinger*

The delivery of quality-based oral health care to the older adult population requires the effective utilization of assessment and evaluation skills by the dental professional.[1,2,7] Clinical decision making, patient management, and appropriate care interventions for the elderly require that the practitioner has an understanding of the patient that surpasses a specific chief complaint or diagnosis.[11,12] It is essential that the care provider retrieve and ultimately integrate a wide range of patient-related information. Many older adults have multiple medical and dental problems, creating a situation where physical, mental, pharmacologic, functional, and social domains are closely interrelated.[3] Dental health professionals must evaluate these multiple areas as well as the patient's perceived oral needs and attitudes in order to provide optimal dental care interventions.[6]

## GENERAL ISSUES AND CHALLENGES IN ASSESSMENT

The process of assessment has been described as the keystone to geriatric practice.[19] The dental assessment should generate a comprehensive data base, which includes all significant mitigating factors that may influence comprehensive dental care. Unfortunately, both students and practitioners often neglect this important phase of the diagnostic evaluation. Problems typically seen include:

1. Appointment scheduling with inadequate time allocation to perform a thorough assessment

2. Conducting the interview in an inappropriate setting: where there are many distractions and it is difficult to generate a warm and trusting atmosphere

3. Recording assessment data in an inconsistent manner without a systematic approach

4. Failure to direct the assessment beyond the traditional brief medical history, chief complaint, and a complete oral examination

5. Failure to understand the likelihood of inaccurate or incomplete patient-reported histories

6. Excessive reliance on open-ended questions to understand the patient's perceptions and desires

7. Inadequate updating of appropriate assessment data on a frequent and recurring basis

## COMMUNICATION CONCEPTS

It is extremely important to establish good patient-and-provider communication ties to build a trusting relationship. Effective communication requires patience, perception, and insight with many older adults.

The patient should be encouraged to talk freely, not only about his or her chief complaint, but also about other possible symptoms, feelings, and fears. Some older adults, in their anxiety to not forget items of importance, may take the opportunity to recite a long list of symptoms. (It is generally appropriate to permit the patient to continue for awhile and then retrace one's steps.) Clarification should be requested when the dentist is uncertain

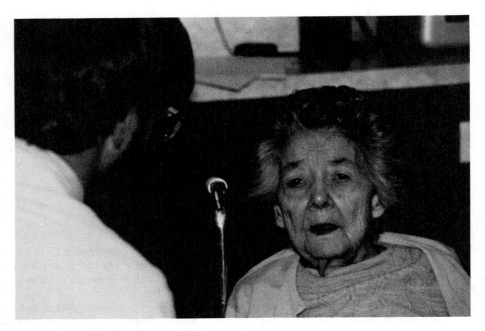

**Fig. 7-1** A doctor-patient interaction demonstrating appropriate provider positioning and eye contact.

of intended meanings and, whenever possible, should paraphrase what the patient has stated to confirm comprehension. Skillful and direct questioning, with utilization of patient-oriented nontechnical language, can greatly improve both the quality and quantity of the data obtained. Occasionally, the duration and history of the chief complaint and previous medical episodes are difficult for patients to recall accurately. It may be helpful to ask the patient to reference problems in terms of seasonal events or birthdays. An older adult may present with some mental confusion. If a patient is rambling or ambiguous, use of a mental-status questionnaire should be considered.

The environment in which the initial interview takes place can also play an important role in facilitating the communication process. If possible, the assessment should be performed in a consultation room or private office where the patient is seated comfortably and the furnishings are warm and less threatening than the dental operatory. Although auxiliary personnel may be asked to routinely record certain preliminary information, the history taking should be performed by the den-

tist. This emphasizes to the patient the importance of this evaluation procedure and provides important clues to the dentist interviewer. The dentist should position himself or herself in front of the patient at the same level and should speak slowly and clearly (Fig. 7-1). A caring and interested attitude should be exhibited with avoidance of a hurried, impatient, and unsympathetic approach. This is most important in gaining patient trust and confidence. The dentist should be an active listener, exhibiting empathetic responses when appropriate.

## NECESSARY ELEMENTS OF AN OLDER ADULT PATIENT ASSESSMENT

Assessment of the patient should begin the moment that the patient enters the office. A first impression of the patient's physical appearance, nutritional state, gait, posture, attitude, and behavior should be noted by the practitioner and staff. These impressions can provide important clues during the assessment and diagnosis process. The assessment of the elderly dental patient should be detailed and comprehensive with emphasis beyond resolving the patient's reported chief complaint (see box).

The patient history should include identification data, sources of information (such as patient, friend, relative, or physician), past medical history, review of systems, chief complaint or complaints and related history, social and family history, and past dental history.

### Patient identification data

The patient is requested to provide this information before the first appointment or recall examination. The receptionist or another auxiliary staff member should assist the patient to accurately and completely perform this task. The information includes name, date, age, birth date, address, telephone number, third-party information, social security number, and the name, address, and telephone number of a relative, not living with the patient, for emergency purposes. It is also important to note whether this patient was referred to the practice and by whom, so that appreciation and, when appropriate, consultation results can be forwarded. The name, address, and telephone number or numbers of the patient's other health care provider or providers should be routinely recorded to facilitate consultation and referral when necessary.

### Medical history and physical evaluation

Two approaches are generally employed to gather the required medical history information. One involves the use of a variety of closed-ended questionnaires (specific choice of answers) available from commercial sources, the American Dental Association, or a custom-designed form created by the practitioner. The breadth of these forms varies considerably, and some are less appropriate for use with the older patient. The second method involves an open-ended patient interview between the patient and the doctor. This dialog-oriented approach allows the practitioner to become better acquainted with the patient's mental status through observation of both verbal and nonverbal cues pertaining to evasiveness, anxiety, apathy, and confusion.

The most accurate and authoritative approach is a combination of both the questionnaire and an interview with the information recorded in ink on the forms. The University of Colorado Dental Geriatric Program has utilized this format. A large-print medical history was designed to be completed by the older dental patient (Figs. 7-2 and 7-3). A separate modified medical review interview format (Fig. 7-4) was created to facilitate an accurate summarization of the patient-completed questionnaire.

### PATIENT QUESTIONNAIRE

Essential patient medical data required from all patients before any dental procedure is performed, as stated by Little and Falace,[21] is listed below:

1. Under the present care of a physician
2. Previous hospitalizations
3. Current medicines (including nonprescription)
4. Allergy history
5. Heart disease, heart murmur, high blood pressure, or rheumatic fever history
6. Diabetes
7. Tuberculosis and other lung disease
8. Hepatitis or other liver disease
9. Kidney disease
10. Bleeding problems or blood disorders
11. Sexually transmitted diseases
12. Acquired immune deficiency disorder (AIDS)
13. Pregnancy

Additional questions pertaining to signs and symptoms (review of systems) were deemed im-

# MEDICAL / DENTAL HISTORY

NAME _____

DATE _____

1.  Are you now under the care of a physician?.................................... Yes ____  No ____
    Doctor's name _____
    Phone number _____
    Address _____

2.  Have you ever had excessive bleeding from wounds
    or tooth removal?............................................................ Yes ____  No ____

3.  When you walk up stairs or take a walk, do you usually
    have to stop because of:
    . . . pain in your chest?........................................................ Yes ____  No ____
    . . . or shortness of breath?................................................. Yes ____  No ____
    . . . or because you are very tired?..................................... Yes ____  No ____

4.  Are your ankles often swollen?.............................................. Yes ____  No ____

5.  Do you get dizzy or faint easily?........................................... Yes ____  No ____
    . . . use more than 2 pillows to sleep?................................. Yes ____  No ____
    . . . ever wake up from sleep short of breath?.................... Yes ____  No ____

6.  Has a physician ever told you that you had kidney or
    bladder trouble?............................................................... Yes ____  No ____

7.  Have you lost or gained much (7-8 pounds) weight
    in the past year?............................................................... Yes ____  No ____

8.  Have you had chemotherapy or X-ray treatment for
    any health problem?.......................................................... Yes ____  No ____

9.  Are you taking or have you taken cortisone?...................... Yes ____  No ____

10. Please list any other medicines (including non-prescription)
    you are taking at the present time.

    _____        _____
    _____        _____
    _____        _____
    _____        _____

**Fig. 7-2** Large-print medical history to be completed by the patient (page 1).

NAME _____

11. Are you sensitive or allergic to any medicines?.................................Yes ___    No ___

   _____
   (specify)

12. Have you had any of the following? (Check all that apply)

a) __ Rheumatic fever
b) __ Scarlet fever
c) __ Pneumonia
d) __ Emphysema/bronchitis
e) __ Tuberculosis (TB)
f) __ Asthma
g) __ Heart disease or attack
h) __ Stroke
i) __ High blood pressure
j) __ Heart murmur
k) __ Artificial heart valve

l) __ Prosthetic joint
   (artificial)
m) __ Angina pectoris
n) __ Pacemaker
o) __ Bruise easily
p) __ Anemia
q) __ A.I.D.S.
r) __ Venereal disease
   (syphilis, gonorrhea)
s) __ Diabetes
t) __ Frequent urination

u) __ Kidney trouble
v) __ Nervousness
w) __ Thyroid disease
x) __ Hepatitis (A or B)
y) __ Yellow jaundice/liver
   disease
z) __ Pain in jaw joints
aa) __ Epilepsy/seizures
bb) __ Cold sores
cc) __ Arthritis/rheumatism
dd) __ Cancer or tumor
ee) __ Dry mouth

13. Have you ever had an unusual reaction to
    Novocain or any other local anesthetic?   .......................... Yes ___    No ___

14. Have you ever been hospitalized?..................................... Yes ___    No ___
    Date  _____  Reason  _____
          _____          _____
          _____          _____

15. Have you ever had any major surgery?.............................. Yes ___    No ___
    Date  _____  Reason  _____
          _____          _____
          _____          _____

16. List any other medical/dental health problems, or other concerns not listed above.

    _____
    _____

To the best of my knowledge, all of the preceding answers are true and correct. If I ever have any change in my health, or if my medications change, I will inform this dentist/dental office at my next appointment without fail.

_____     _____
Date           Signature of Patient or Guardian

**Fig. 7-3** Large-print medical history to be completed by the patient (page 2).

NAME _____
DATE _____
COMPLETED BY _____
(resident/faculty)

**Medical Review**                          (check one)   Describe:

1. CNS                                        __ Yes __ No  _____
2. Cardiovascular                             __ Yes __ No  _____
3. Rheumatic Fever History                    __ Yes __ No  _____
4. Organic Heart Murmur                       __ Yes __ No  _____
5. Prosthetic Devices (heart valves, joints, etc.)  __ Yes __ No  _____
6. Pulmonary                                  __ Yes __ No  _____
7. G.I.                                       __ Yes __ No  _____
8. Hepatic                                    __ Yes __ No  _____
9. Renal                                      __ Yes __ No  _____
10. Bleeding Disorders/Problem                __ Yes __ No  _____
11. Malignant Disease                         __ Yes __ No  _____
12. Chemo/Rad Therapy - current or history    __ Yes __ No  _____
13. Antibiotic Prophylaxis Required (type)    __ Yes __ No  _____
14. Under Physician Care                      __ Yes __ No  _____
15. Other (please specify)                    __ Yes __ No  _____
                                                             _____
                                                             _____

**Mobility**

____ Ambulatory    ____ Wheelchair    ____ Assisted    ____ Other _____
                                                                        (specify)

**Mental Status**

____ Excellent/Good:    memory, judgment intact
____ Slightly impaired:    memory impaired, judgment intact, makes decisions
____ Severely impaired:    memory or judgment impaired, guardian makes decision
____ Other _____
            specify (e.g., depression, uncooperative, etc.)

**Medications & Dosages**

_____    _____    _____
_____    _____    _____
_____    _____    _____

**Drug Allergies**

_____    _____    _____

Adverse Drug Reaction Concerns _____
                                (e.g., possible allergy, hypotension,
                                 bleeding, xerostomia, etc.)

**Vital Signs:**

_____    _____    _____    _____
BP/date      BP/date      BP/date      BP/date

Other _____    _____    _____    _____

**Summary and Significant Findings:**

**Fig. 7-4** Assessment form utilized by the dentist to summarize, clarify, and provide additional information for the patient record.

portant for inclusion on the University of Colorado forms given the relatively high prevalence rates of many chronic diseases and their importance to safe patient management or successful treatment outcomes. This is important, since many older adults may be unaware of their complete health status. Indeed, recent national data[28] indicate that more than one third of all persons 65 years and older will present with either a history of heart disease or hypertension, or both. Additional questions helpful in diagnosis determination include:[23]

1. When you walk upstairs or take a walk, do you have to stop because of pain in your chest, or shortness of breath, or because you are very tired?
2. Are your ankles often swollen?
3. Do you become dizzy or faint easily?
4. Do you use more than two pillows to sleep?
5. Do you ever awaken from sleep short of breath?

Affirmative responses to these queries may assist in disclosing previously undiagnosed cardiovascular problems such as congestive heart failure and cardiac arrhythmias as well as more general issues of cardiac and pulmonary functional reserve capacity. These questions may also be helpful in establishing the presence and degree of renal or liver disease, pulmonary disease, and hypoglycemia.

Specific emphasis should be placed on expansion of the typical medical history. For example, more attention should be given to pronounced weight loss or gain. This may have an important relationship with nutritional status, malabsorption, neoplasia, ulcerations, diabetes mellitus, thyrotoxicosis, depression and dementia, other cancers, chronic infections associated with subacute bacterial endocarditis and tuberculosis, and drug-induced anorexia (such as digitalis). Other areas of detailed information should include inquiries on chemotherapy and radiotherapy, cortisone history, chronic obstructive pulmonary disease (emphysema, bronchitis), nervousness, thyroid disease, jaw joint pain, epilepsy and seizures, herpetic oral lesions, heart murmurs, prosthetic joints, osteoarthritis and rheumatoid arthritis, and pacemakers.

Upon completion of the questionnaire the patient or responsible party should sign a statement that attests to the accuracy of answers and his acknowledgment that when any changes occur in his health or medication status he will inform the dentist or dental office at the next appointment.

## PATIENT INTERVIEW AND SUMMARY

When the patient has finished the medical questionnaire, the dentist should review the document for completeness, affirmative responses, and discrepancies.

### Medical review

The information should be transferred and summarized. Specific symptoms noted in the history or other indications may further initiate a more detailed review of various organ systems (Table 7-1). This approach is important because patients may not associate particular symptoms to a disease

**Table 7-1** Important clinical signs associated with organ systems*
(A review of systems may allow detection of many problematic clinical signs.)

| Organ system | Clinical signs |
|---|---|
| Central nervous system | Fainting, convulsions, headache, dizziness, tremors, paralysis, paresthesias, anesthesia |
| Cardiovascular | Exertion-caused chest pain, heart palpitations, ankle swelling, dyspnea, and orthopnea |
| Pulmonary | Cough, sputum (amount, color, odor, blood), wheezing, infections |
| Gastrointestinal and hepatic | Appetite level, nausea, vomiting, dysphagia, heartburn (pyrosis), indigestion, pain, jaundice, food intolerance |
| Renal | Dysuria, nocturia, polyuria, hematuria, frequency, difficulty associated with starting the stream, infections |
| Hematopoietic | Bruising, bleeding, anemia, radiation or toxic agent exposure |

or abnormality and therefore neglect to describe them unless specifically questioned. The medical review also highlights antibiotic prophylaxis concerns with specific summary categories for rheumatic heart disease, organic heart murmurs, and prosthetic devices. The type of prophylaxis required for patients at risk should be prominently noted. Space is also available to summarize social history issues (occupations, residences, socioeconomic status, drugs such as coffee, alcohol, and cigarettes), the functional status of the individual, and family history (cancer, high blood pressure, heart disease, diabetes, tuberculosis, bleeding disorders, alcoholism, strokes, and so forth). Nondental signs and symptoms of nutritional deficiencies may also be highlighted (weight loss or gain, dermatitis, eyelid inflammation, angular conjunctivitis, and dimness of vision).

## Vital signs

It is important to routinely record a base-line blood pressure for all patients, especially for the older adult. Because of the high prevalence of hypertension in the elderly, provision of this important medical screening for the patient (for possible medical referral of this generally asymptomatic condition) is essential and the information obtained can be a basis for diagnostic comparisons during dental care. If the patient is hypertensive, blood pressure should be taken before each appointment to determine if it is adequately controlled. Careful attention to technique is important to minimize errors, especially in the elderly. Sound patterns may be difficult to hear in the frail elderly person. Avoid rapid deflation of the cuff, which may artificially elevate diastolic readings and lower systolic readings. If uncertain, repeat the procedure several times and change arms if necessary. If repeated measurements are taken, be careful to deflate the cuff to zero between each assessment to avoid the iatrogenic elevation of blood pressure, venous congestion, and pain.

There are no specific dividing lines between normal and elevated blood pressures, particularly for the older adult. Typically, systolic pressures will be slightly increased with chronologic age most likely because of the effect of arteriosclerosis. No age-related concomitant rise in diastolic pressure is expected and sustained elevation may lead to renal damage. Because of the stressful nature of

dentistry for many persons, normotensive older adults may have slightly elevated readings. It is prudent to record additional readings on other appointment days for confirmation of blood pressure status (accept the lowest as base-line value). Although it is unclear regarding specific hypertension definitions for older adults, diastolic pressures of 95 to 105 mm Hg may require medical treatment, 105 to 120 mm Hg will predictably require treatment, and 120 mm and higher are suggestive of severe, uncontrolled disease and no routine dental treatment should be provided without close collaboration with the patient's physician (Fig. 7-5).

Other vital sign measurements should include recording the *pulse rate* (a rate under 60 or one over 110 should be investigated) and *rhythm* (most favorably at the carotid artery—consultation is advised for a totally irregular pulse or premature ventricular contractions exceeding 5 per minute in a patient with cardiac disease), *respiration rate* (if it exceeds 20 per minute, it should be followed up), and *temperature readings* (96.8° to 98.6° F are within normal limits).

## Mental status

Affective and organic mental disorders occur frequently in older adults and therefore make this another important component of the assessment. Pfeiffer's Short Portable Mental Status Questionnaire (SPMSQ) can be helpful when the cognitive status of the patient is unclear (see box). When one is screening for dementia, warning signs are deficits in memory, judgment, intellect, and orientation, and possibly a flat affect. The classic signs and symptoms for depression include sadness, decreased appetite, weight loss, confusion, difficulty in decision making, dissatisfaction, and irritability. Many older adults, however, present with a less dramatic level of actual sadness and frequently have apparent cognitive impairment (especially memory deficits) and therefore differentiation from dementia is important[13] (Table 7-2). Depression may also accompany a wide variety of physical illnesses (cardiovascular disease, cancer, and so forth)[8,26] and may be the primary cause of somatic complaints, including oral discomfort.[16]

## Mobility

The assessment should involve describing the mobility status of the patient (ambulatory, wheelchair,

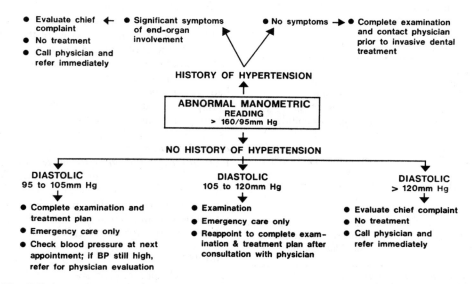

**Fig. 7-5** An assessment and treatment algorithm pertaining to an elevated blood pressure measurement.

## SCREENING QUESTIONNAIRE FOR AN ORGANIC BRAIN DEFICIT

**Short portable mental status questionnaire**

1. What is the date today (month/day/year)? Score all three.
2. What day of the week is it?
3. What is the name of this place?
4. What is your telephone number? If no telephone, what is your street address?
5. How old are you?
6. When were you born (month, day, year)? Score all three.
7. Who is the President of the United States now?
8. Who was the President just before him?
9. What was your mother's maiden name?
10. Subtract three from twenty and keep subtracting three from each new number all the way down. Whole series needed to score.

Error rate (out of 10): Add one if educated beyond high school; subtract one if black; subtract one if not educated beyond high school.

Scoring: 0-2 errors: intact intellectual function

3-4 errors: mild intellectual impairment

5-7 errors: moderate intellectual impairment

8-10 errors: severe intellectual impairment

From Pfeiffer E: A short portable mental status questionnaire for the assessment of organic brain deficit in elderly patients, J Am Geriatr Soc 23(10):433, 1975; reprinted with permission from the American Geriatrics Society.

**Table 7-2** Signs and symptoms associated with differentiation of depression and dementia

| Dementia | Depression |
|---|---|
| Insidious onset | Abrupt onset |
| Long duration | Short duration |
| Fluctuating mood | Constant mood |
| "Near-miss" answers | "Don't-know" answers |
| Conceal disability | Highlights disabilities |
| Stable cognitive loss | Fluctuating cognitive |
| Memory loss occurs first | loss |
| Associated with: | Depressed mood occurs |
|   Unsociability |   first |
|   Uncooperativeness | Associated with: |
|   Hostility |   Depressed or anxious |
|   Emotional instability |    mood |
|   Confusion |   Sleep disturbance |
|   Disorientation |   Appetite disturbance |
|   Reduced alertness |   Suicidal thoughts |

assisted, and other). This information warns the dentist that particular patient management will be required such as appointment-scheduling alterations and assistance in obtaining access to the dental office.

**Drug history**

A preexamination request for the patient to bring the containers of all current medications contributes significantly to correct drug and dosage charting. Particular attention should also be paid to identifying possible or current adverse drug reaction or reactions, other medication effects, and issues relating to patient management. These might include allergies, orthostatic hypotension, bleeding, xerostomia, sialorrhea, psychiatric disturbances, movement disorders, gastrointestinal upset, soft-tissue reactions, need to minimize vasoconstrictor use, decreased ability to tolerate stress, altered host resistance, and gingival hyperplasia.[20,24] An attempt should be made to determine the patient's compliance with the prescribed medication regimen. Problems may include misinterpretation of written instructions (such as "Take with meals" or "take two times a day"), access to the medication container,

and conscious deviations from recommendations (using "old" medications, drug trading, nonusage, and so forth). It has been estimated that nearly one fourth of all hospital admissions of the elderly are attributable to problems related to noncompliance with medications, and greater than one in five older consumers reported never filling prescriptions they had recently been prescribed.[22]

Important aids to assist the dentist in comprehending the important medical and dental issues associated with different medications are *Physicians' Desk Reference*,[25] *Facts and Comparisons*,[18] *USP DI Drug Information for the Health Care Provider*,[27] and the *AMA Drug Evaluations*.[4] Computer drug programs are also becoming available to provide information regarding indications, warnings, interactions with other drugs, side effects, and special precautions for dental care (Fig. 7-6).

**Updates**

Before each appointment, the dentist should inquire regarding any recent medical change. Given the possible tenuous physiologic and situational status of many frail and functionally dependent elderly, it is advisable to formally review the nondental patient evaluation every 6 months to 1 year.

## DENTAL HISTORY
**Chief complaints**

A determination of the major reasons for the dental visit should be thoroughly investigated. It may be recorded either in the patient's language or as a simple phrase describing the complaint, its duration and chronology, and any exacerbating factors. The emotional response associated with the chief complaint and patient expectations regarding appropriate interventions and their likelihood for success should also be noted. Interrupting the patient should be avoided if possible, as well as correcting inappropriate logic or inaccurate use of technical terms.

**Important dental questions**

The requisite dental history information for older adults differs only slightly from younger persons. Questions should be directed toward frequency of dental service utilization, date and location of last dental visit, date of last full-mouth radiographic series, current perceived dental needs, and an account of dental symptoms. To overcome the ten-

**TRADE NAME:** LOPRESSOR HCT
**GENERIC NAME:** METOPROLOL AND HYDROCHLOROTHIAZIDE
**MANUFACTURER:** Ciba-Geigy
**TYPE OF DRUG:** Beta-adrenergic blocking agent & thiazide diuretic
**ACTION:** Antihypertensive

INDICATIONS:
* Hypertension

CONTRAINDICATIONS:
* Should not be used if the following medical conditions exist:
  - Bronchial asthma
  - Sinus bradycardia
  - Cardiogenic shock
  - Heart block
  - Overt cardiac failure
  - Not indicated in patients

WARNING & PRECAUTIONS:
* Caution if following conditions exist:
  - Studies in animals have shown embryotoxicity and fetal resorption
  - Elderly patients may be less sensitive to the effects of beta-
    blockers
  - Patients with congestive heart failure controlled by digitalis and
    diuretics
  - Asthma patients requiring general anesthesia

INTERACTIONS WITH OTHER DRUGS:
* Digitalis glycosides - may result in excessive bradycardia and
  possible heart block
* Insulin or oral hypoglycemics - may reduce or increase blood glucose
  levels
* MAO inhibitors - increased risk of increased hypertension
* Phenothiazines - may result in increased plasma concentrations of the
  medication
* Barbiturates - may result in altered response to beta-blockers
* Oral contraceptives - may increased the beta-blocker response
* Apresoline (hydralazine) - response to medication may be altered
* Isuprel (isoproterenol) - these drugs are mutually antagonistic
* Aldomet (methyldopa) - increased risk of hypertensive episodes
* Nonsteroidal anti-inflammatory analgesics - antihypertensive effect of
  beta-blockers may be decreased

SIDE EFFECTS:
* Some effects that  may require medical attention:
  - Dizziness or light-headedness (hypotension)
  - Dry mouth
  - Unusually slow heartbeat
  - Increased thirst
  - Weak pulse
  - Breathing difficulty in patients with predisposition to
    bronchoconstriction
  - Mental confusion in the elderly
  - Reduced alertness
  - Mental depression
  - Cardiac arrhythmia

PRECAUTIONS FOR DENTAL CARE:
* Concurrent use with local anesthetics containing epinephrine may
  result in significant hypertension and excessive bradycardia and
  possible heart block
* Lidocaine - may slow liver metabolism and increase the risk of
  toxicity of lidocaine

**Fig. 7-6** A medication printout from the Automated Drug Information System (ADIS) developed
jointly by the University of Texas at San Antonio Health Sciences Center and SRC Systems, San
Antonio, Texas.

dency of many elderly to underreport health complaints and their effect upon daily functioning, one should utilize a closed-ended list of specific problems to accumulate important patient data.[5] Specific inquiry should be made regarding:

1. General discomfort of mouth
2. Specific discomfort of tongue, gums, or lips
3. Dry mouth
4. Bad or altered taste sensations
5. Bad breath
6. Temporomandibular joint pain, popping, or deviation
7. Bleeding of gums or other soft tissues

For patients with remaining natural teeth, inquiries should include:

8. Food entrapment around teeth
9. Tooth pain or sensitivity
10. Mobile teeth
11. Cavities, broken fillings, or broken teeth

For patients with removable prostheses, questions should include information on the occurrence of:

12. Denture slippage
13. Denture discomfort
14. Food entrapment under dentures

The patient should also be asked to describe his or her satisfaction with esthetics and chewing function. The regularity of performance of preventive dental behaviors such as brushing and flossing should be indicated. Specific inquiries should be made regarding possible patient fears or anxieties as well as specific concerns about potential cost of treatment.

## EXTRAORAL EXAMINATION

A visual inspection of the person should follow the patient history. The following areas should be examined for the following characteristics:

1. Skeletal form (symmetry, enlargement, Angle's classification)
2. Neck (evidence of thyroid enlargement, use of accessory muscles of respiration, jugular vein distension)
3. Skin (character, cyanosis, pallor, flushing, petechiae, eruptions, evidence of jaundice or pigmentation)
4. Hair (texture and amount)
5. Eyes, conjunctivas, and scleras (evidence of jaundice, pallor, petechiae, or exophthalmos)
6. Hands and fingers (tremors, finger clubbing, nail bed cyanosis)
7. Ankles (swelling, stasis, dermatitis)
8. Chest (prolonged or wheezing expirations, breathing rate)
9. Abdomen (ascites)
10. Ears (pain: referred mandibular molar pain, myofascial pain dysfunction syndrome)
11. Lymph nodes (enlargement, tenderness, mobility)
12. Salivary glands (enlargement, symptomatic)
13. Paranasal sinuses (pain: referred maxillary molar and premolar pain)
14. Temporomandibular joint and the muscles of mastication (tenderness, crepitus, clicking, deviation of the mouth on opening and closing, trismus)
15. Breath (halitosis: local causes being poor oral hygiene, periodontal disease, and large carious lesions; systemic disease concerns of diabetes, uremia, upper respiratory disease; and external factors like alcohol, drugs, and garlic)

## INTRAORAL AND PERIORAL SOFT-TISSUE EXAMINATION

A standardized oral examination approach should be pursued to ensure completeness. Good illumination and appropriate patient positioning should be utilized. Regions that are inaccessible to direct visualization or where texture differentiation is important (such as lymph nodes, lips, buccal mucosa, tongue, and floor of mouth) should be palpated. Palpation technique should include the use of one hand for feeling while the other hand provides tissue support (bimanual), rolling and pressing soft tissue between two fingers (bidigital), comparison of both sides (bilateral), and bound or supported tissue pressure (compression). *Remember: When looking for lesions, many older adults present asymptomatically and oral cancers are most frequently diagnosed during the sixth and seventh decades of life.*

### Oral soft tissues

Typically, the *lips and corners of the mouth* are initially examined. Ulcers, areas of enlargement

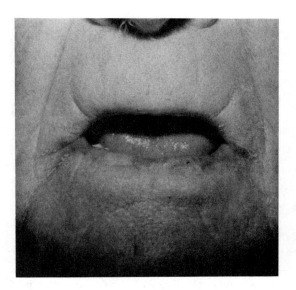

**Fig. 7-7** Clinical signs of angular cheilosis.

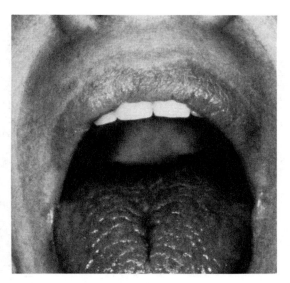

**Fig. 7-8** Fissuring of the tongue and partial loss of papillae associated with a dry mouth.

or swelling, and evidence of actinic cheilitis (degenerative changes especially in the vermilion of the lower lip) need to be noted. Corners of the mouth may appear inflamed with redness, a crusty appearance or fissures suggestive of angular cheilitis (a condition often associated with nutritional deficiencies), extension of oral infections, loss of vertical dimension, drooling, and local habits (Fig. 7-7). Atypical findings might also include squamous cell carcinomas, trauma, herpes simplex, chancres, and systemic pigmentation in conjunction with Addison's disease and Peutz-Jeghers syndrome.

The *buccal mucosa and mucobuccal folds* should be palpated to identify areas of tenderness and induration. Color, lesions, and salivary duct openings opposite the second maxillary premolar (Stensen's duct) need to be assessed. The presence of opportunistic *Candida albicans* tends to be associated with the long-term use of antibiotics, corticosteroids, and cytotoxic agents. Classically, these lesions have been described as soft, white, and slightly elevated nonfixed plaques; however, there are often areas of erythroplakia. When in doubt relative to the causative agent, one should take a culture. Eroded, painful, variable-sized areas surrounded by the characteristic radiating white striae

are diagnostic of erosive lichen planus, which may be infected with *Candida*.

The *dorsal and ventral surfaces of the tongue* should be closely inspected for atypical color, size, and papillae, as well as coatings, tremors or movement, and lesions. A gauze square should be used to handle the tongue to inspect and palpate the dorsal, lateral, and ventral surfaces. The floor of the mouth and contiguous structures should be examined and palpated. It is important to remember that the lateral border and base of the tongue are the most frequent sites of oral carcinoma in the U.S. population, and they represent over half of all the intraoral carcinomas. When examining the tongue and bordering structures, one should note evidence of mouth dryness.

A reduction of *salivary flow,* either acute or chronic, is a frequent finding in the elderly. The normal flow rate for resting saliva is $0.3 \pm 0.2$ ml/min, and values less than 0.1 ml/min are abnormal. Clinical features highlighting a possible dry mouth include generalized dryness and a pale or red or atrophic tissue appearance. The tongue may also be devoid of papillae, fissured, or inflamed (Fig. 7-8). The patient may complain of a dry or burning sensation, have some difficulty with speaking, eating, or tasting of foods, present with mucosal infections, have difficulty using dentures, and appear with multiple carious lesions, especially at the gingival margins. Palpation, or "milking," the major salivary glands may be helpful in clinical assessment of function. At the duct entrance (that is, Wharton's and Stensen's), look at both the quantity and quality (such as viscosity, pus, and casts). In the identification of dry mouth, subjective complaints may not be very predictive of patients with gland dysfunction. Helpful questions that may assist the dentist in distinguishing persons with salivary problems include the following:[9]

1. Is your mouth dry when eating a meal?
2. Do you have problems swallowing foods?
3. Do you drink liquids to aid in swallowing dry foods?
4. Is the amount of saliva in your mouth too little most of the time, or don't you notice it?

Mouth dryness is most likely associated with drug use. Other possible causes include radiotherapy, mechanical blockage, dehydration from chronic diarrhea or diuretic drugs, emotional stress, salivary gland infection or malignancy, surgery, avitaminosis, diabetes, anemia, collagen vascular diseases, inflammatory exocrinopathy (Sjögren's syndrome), and congenital factors (ectodermal dysplasia).

The *palate (both hard and soft)* should be palpated and viewed for symmetry and lesions. The tissue covered by a prosthodontic appliance should be inspected for redness. If either a smooth or granular appearance exists, it is suggestive of a denture stomatitis. The soft palate should also be evaluated for strength of motion.

The *oropharynx,* which begins at the distal end of the soft palate, can be better visualized by depression of the tongue with a tongue blade or mirror. Color, exudate, masses, and the gag reflex should be evaluated. The palatine tonsils should not be enlarged, and there should be no signs of inflammation.

### Alveolar ridge and periodontium

Extensive changes in the *alveolar bone* of partially to fully edentulous elderly are likely. The loss of mandibular alveolar crest height can often approach 1 cm (Fig. 7-9). Alveolar ridge characteristics (size, shape, alveolar mucosa integrity, degree of

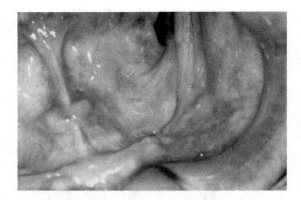

**Fig. 7-9** Extensive mandibular ridge resorption and atrophy.

bony resorption associated with tooth loss, tuberosities, interarch distance) should be determined and recorded. This information may be very helpful in determining needed surgical therapies as well as establishing the likelihood for future hard- and soft-tissue changes and the prognosis for proposed prosthesis.

The presence of *severe periodontal disease* in older adults is perhaps less common than might be expected.[15] Teeth with considerable loss of the supporting bone frequently can be maintained with conservative periodontal management for long periods of time. Several parameters should be considered when one is performing a thorough periodontal examination. The location, clinical signs, and degree of gingival inflammation and bleeding as well as the associated soft plaque and hard calculus buildup should be noted (such as slight, moderate, or heavy). The teeth should be examined and charted for the relative positioning of opposing and proximal teeth and inadequate proximal contact and marginal ridge relationships. Food-impaction areas will help to identify these areas. Periodontal probings (6 to 8 readings per tooth) and recession and attachment loss should be recorded for all remaining natural teeth. Additionally, mobility of all teeth should be assessed according to the following classification scheme:

**M1** Tooth can be moved 1 mm horizontally, an indication of moderate mobility

**M2** Tooth can be moved up to 2 mm horizontally, an indication of severe mobility

**M3**  Greater than 2 mm horizontal tooth movement or the tooth can be depressed vertically in the socket, an indication of very severe mobility

Anterior teeth may be tested by placement of the handles of a dental mirror on both the labial and lingual surfaces to transmit alternating directional force. Pressure on the incisal or occlusal surface will elicit vertical displacement. Posterior teeth may be assessed by utilization of a large sickle scaler to exert directional force.

With multirooted teeth, bone loss precipitating bifurcation or trifurcation involvement should also be noted (Fig. 7-10). These may be classified as:

**Incipient**  Slight bone loss
**Class 1**  Definite bone loss
**Class 2**  Moderate to severe bone loss extending deeply under the tooth
**Class 3**  Very severe bone loss extending from one furcation to another

The level of supporting bone is also ascertained by periapical and bite-wing radiography. Closely inspect the lamina dura (thin radiopaque line), which surrounds the roots of the teeth. A lack of continuity is suggestive of periodontal disease, and a widening at the apex and contralateral side is suggestive of traumatic occlusion. Mobile teeth will also present with wide periodontal spaces. A diagnosis of horizontal bone loss is made if bone levels are lower than 1.5 mm apical to the cementoenamel junction and may be attributed to calculus or faulty restoration margins. A specific periodontal diagnosis should be entered in the patient's chart (such as normal, gingivitis, or periodontitis/early or moderate or advanced). Information on mucogingival defects; purulent, serous, or bloody discharge upon palpation; and additional evidence of periodontal abscess formation (buccal or lingual swelling) should also be recorded for involved teeth and gingival regions.

#### Caries, restorations, and tooth structure loss

*Dental caries (both coronal and root)* are a prevalent problem in the older population. Incidence data from the Iowa Study[14] demonstrated that 77% of the dentate participants experienced either a new coronal or root lesion in 3 years. Several factors may contribute to this high caries rate. These include faulty restorations, malaligned and shifting

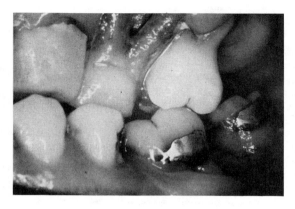

**Fig. 7-10** Severe periodontal disease with class 2 and class 3 furcation involvement of posterior teeth.

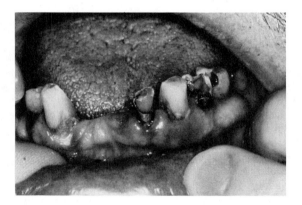

**Fig. 7-11** Extensive coronal and root caries.

teeth, mouth dryness, recession of gingival tissues, diet change, medications, poor oral hygiene, and partial denture clasps or design. Careful examination, utilizing radiography, is important for identification of many of these carious lesions. Identification of frank lesions (gross cavitation) presents few problems in diagnosis (Fig. 7-11). Incipient lesions, however, are more difficult to identify without radiographic confirmation. The presence of only stain or pigmentation does not confirm an active caries process. Pit-and-fissure lesions should be recorded not only when the explorer catches in the groove or grooves, but also when there is softness at the area base and adjacent enamel or opacity suggestive of undermining or demineralization. For smooth surface lesions, evidence of softness (explorer penetration or scraping away of enamel with an explorer) is necessary above and beyond visual evidence of demineralization (decalcification or white lesion). For proximal surfaces, seek to identify a discontinuity of enamel allowing an explorer confirmation of softness.

Transillumination can be helpful in identification of anterior proximal lesions. Coronal lesions are fairly equally divided between failing restorations and nonrestored surfaces, whereas root caries are more typically found on virgin cemental surfaces exposed by gingival recession but may also be associated with previous restorations.

Root lesions predictably develop coronally to the present gingival margin and predominantly occur on buccal and proximal surfaces. There are only a few lesions that are found solely in the gingival pocket. Marginal gingivitis might provide a clue to the location of these subgingival root caries proximal to the inflammation. Initially they appear as small and round lesions that frequently spread laterally and coalesce to form a collar around the tooth. These lesions typically do not directly affect the outer enamel but will undermine this enamel creating a ledge. The more advanced lesions facilitate enamel fracture creating the impression that the caries developed both in the coronal and the root portion of the tooth. Although they are frequently found under moderate-to-heavy accumulations of plaque, they are only infrequently found under calculus deposits. It is also important to understand that this decay is atypically associated with areas of abrasion or erosion because of typically good hygiene associated with these areas. The color of the lesions may also be helpful in diagnosis of active versus arrested lesions. Root caries that are yellow-orange, tan, or light brown in color are more likely to be active than the darker lesions. Modification of the standard coronal caries detection approach should be considered when you are evaluating possible root carious lesions. Cementum is less dense than enamel and will therefore provide a tactile sensation of yielding to the explorer tip upon firm pressure. In order to differentiate sound from carious cementum, feel for a greater comparative softness associated with the lesion along with easy explorer removal (no sticking or withdrawal resistance) after explorer penetration. Carefully examine all exposed root surfaces.

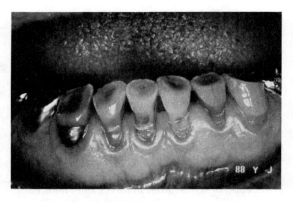

**Fig. 7-12** Generalized abrasion and attrition.

*Charting* should be performed for all *missing teeth, portions of residual teeth,* and *existing restorations. Nonerupted teeth* located on radiographs should be highlighted on the chart. Existent restorations are typically depicted by size and shape with a blue lead pencil. Amalgams may be colored with a solid representation, composites or glass ionomers utilizing a blue outline, and blue cross-hatch drawn for cast restorations. Defective restorations can be demonstrated by use of a red lead pencil in areas of recurrent caries, overhanging or failing margins, fractures, discoloration associated with silicates, poor proximal contact, or marginal ridge discrepancies.

The loss of tooth structure associated with occlusal wear and tear (*attrition*) as well as nonocclusal frictional factors (*abrasion*) is certainly prevalent in older adults (Fig. 7-12). In a recent study, as many as 75% of community-dwelling older adults examined had at least one tooth that had all the occlusal or incisal enamel lost to attrition, with 4% having at least one tooth worn down to the gingiva. Additionally, 30% had notable tooth structure loss associated with abrasion.[3] Significant areas of attrition and abrasion as well as chemical-induced tooth loss (*erosion*) and *tooth fractures* should be noted during the dental examination. In review:

1. Attrition may be related to bruxism or predominate use of selected tooth segments such as the use of anterior teeth when posterior teeth are absent.

2. Abrasion is often caused by hard tooth-

brushes, abrasive dentifrices, and excessive brushing pressures.

3. Erosion has been associated with acidic substances from drinks, especially when used before bedtime, sucking citrus fruits, candies, or medicines or chronic vomiting or regurgitation.

4. Tooth fracture may be caused by trauma and necrotic pulp.

Exact causes should be determined and the conditions brought under control in order to minimize occlusal problems, temporomandibular joint dysfunction, and the loss of structural integrity of the tooth.

**Occlusion**

The *occlusal examination* should include a clinical as well as a laboratory component. Maxillary and mandibular midlines should be checked for deviations and deflections during opening and closing of the mouth. With a Boley gauge (normal range of 40 to 60 mm) one can measure maximum opening, overbite (vertical overlap of maxillary and mandibular incisors), overjet (horizontal overlap of maxillary and mandibular incisors), and intraocclusal distance (difference between vertical dimension of rest position and vertical dimension of maximum intercuspation). Two to 3 mm are considered adequate for proper function, but the spacing can range from 0 to 11 mm in normal adults. Angle's molar relation classification (Class 1/normal, Class 2/disto-occlusion, and Class 3/mesio-occlusion), anterior and posterior crossbites, end-to-end relationships, open bites, and centric relation–centric occlusion discrepancies should also be noted. Dysfunctional occlusion can be identified through:

1. Tooth mobility and tooth migration
2. Pain in the temporomandibular joint, periodontium, or tooth
3. Lamina dura alterations
4. Periodontal membrane space widening
5. Atypical occlusal wear

It may be difficult, however, to accurately determine actual chewing impairment in the presence of these mitigating factors (Fig. 7-13). This may be best accomplished when one asks questions such as, "Are you able to chew foods such as hard bread or apples?"

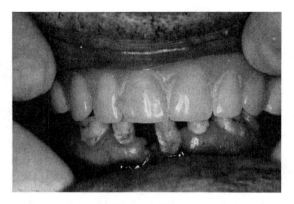

**Fig. 7-13** Partially edentate occlusion, which may present with varying levels of chewing dysfunction.

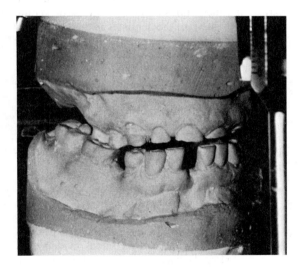

**Fig. 7-14** Diagnostic casts mounted on an adjustable articulator to demonstrate occlusal discrepancies and tooth relationships.

The use of mounted diagnostic casts should be utilized in the oral assessment of most older adults. They permit closer study of tooth position, size, and shape; the occurrence of occlusal facets; and supporting tissue architecture. Utilizing a face-bow transfer and an adjustable articulator, one can determine deflecting contacts, wear patterns, and tooth-to-arch relationships not obvious by clinical examination (Fig. 7-14).

## Diagnostic aids

One of the more important diagnostic tools in oral assessment is the *radiographic evaluation*. When coupled with the case history and clinical examination, radiographs play a critical role in identifying caries, periapical pathosis, periodontal disease, and intraosseous lesions. They are also useful in the evaluation of the sinus, identification of trauma, preprosthetic assessment, and detection of other abnormalities. In the older adult, recognizing recurrent (secondary) caries can be at times difficult because a radiopaque restoration may mask new lesion activity. Care should be exercised to utilize proper vertical angulation to gain diagnostic radiographs. Root caries may be identified as an ill-defined radiolucency that has a "cupped-out" or "notched-out" appearance. Occasionally, however, cervical burnout may be misinterpreted as cemental caries, and meticulous clinical examination should be utilized whenever the dentist is in doubt. Greater attention should also be paid to the radiographic presentation of the pulp, which may have calcifications, diminished chamber size, evidence of resorption, and periapical lesions. Radiographic evidence of chronic periodontal disease (resorption of alveolar bone on the mesial and distal surfaces) and occlusal trauma (thickened periodontal ligament space) may be also visualized. Recommendations regarding the radiographic assessment are the following:[17]

1. Radiographic examinations should be individualized and based on high-yield selection criteria (such as previous periodontal or endodontic therapy, history of pain or trauma, presence of implants, clinical evidence of periodontal disease, deep carious lesions, swelling, tooth mobility, and large or deep restorations).

2. Given the incomplete diagnostic yield, radiographs should never supplant a complete history and clinical examination.

3. Panoramic radiographs are usually less effective than intraoral radiographs when one is evaluating restorative and endodontic needs; they are about equally effective in periodontic applications but may play a more important role of screening for pathologic conditions before complete denture fabrication.

4. The initial dental examination for dentate patients typically requires posterior bitewings and selected periapicals, whereas the edentate patient should receive a full-mouth intraoral radiographic or panoramic examination.

5. Dentate recall patients who are at high risk for developing caries should have posterior bitewings at the 12- to 18-month interval, and the lower risk patients should have them at the 24- to 36-month interval.

6. Periodontal recall patients should have an individualized examination utilizing periapicals or bitewings for areas where clinical periodontal signs are present.

*Assessment of the pulp* is required when the patient complains of pain, where radiographs demonstrate periapical radiolucencies, soft-tissue swellings, or fistulas. It is also necessary where tooth discoloration has occurred and before crown preparation or abutment designation for fixed or removable prostheses. Percussion sensitivity usually is suggestive of an acute apical lesion but infrequently may implicate a chronic pathologic condition. Thermal testing (both hot and cold) may also contribute to a diagnosis of moderate and advanced pulpalgias, though it is of little value when diagnosing periapical problems. In the younger age groups, electric pulp testing is perhaps the best means for determining pulp vitality. The positive and negative predictive value (likelihood that the tooth is vital when it tests positively and likelihood that the tooth is nonvital when it tests negatively) of pulp testing is less consistent for older adults. Older adults may have vital teeth that give a nonvital response when tested because of sclerosed pulp chambers. Teeth with large restorations or full-coverage crowns may also make measurement difficult. To establish a proper diagnosis, it is important that the dentist utilize several different tests, observations, and radiographs.

*Laboratory testing* is an additional diagnostic tool that may be incorporated in the assessment of the older patient. Building on the chairside recognition of local and systemic pathologic processes, laboratory tests can provide valuable information when the dentist is uncertain about a differential diagnosis. The broad classification of these tests include:

1. Microbiologic testing—direct examination of oral specimens, antibiotic sensitivity tests, throat cultures, oral candidiasis cultures, caries activity tests, and root canal and root apex cultures
2. Blood tests—hematology, serology, blood chemistry, and immunohematology
3. Urinalysis—diabetes mellitus, hyperparathyroidism, and renal diseases
4. Contact allergy testing
5. Oral exfoliative cytology
6. Oral biopsy—excisional and incisional with aspiration.

The most accurate method of diagnosing soft-tissue pathosis is by *biopsy*. If the dental professional does not wish to perform this procedure, the patient should be referred to an appropriate dental or medical colleague. Although a large specimen is not necessary for the oral pathologist to determine a definitive diagnosis, excisional biopsy should be considered the best procedure for relatively small, well-defined lesions. For larger or diffuse lesions, multiple incisional biopsies may be indicated. Aspiration, oral exfoliative cytology, and toluidine blue staining may also be utilized for diagnostic purposes.

During the course of the broad-based health assessment of the elderly patient, the dentist should identify areas of information that need *clarification from a physician, dental specialist, other health care professionals,* or additional *care givers.* Many times, this may be handled by use of a multiple-copy consultation-request form. The referring practitioner can relate a specific patient history and identify important questions to be answered and the consultant can respond with information on physical findings and recommendations (Fig. 7-15). It is preferable that the practitioner arrange for the consultation on behalf of the patient and provide the necessary information including the health history, radiographs, diagnostic casts, and laboratory findings. It is important to remember that the referring dentist is not obligated to accept all of the consultant's recommendations and sometimes may seek a second opinion or choose a course contrary to the consultant's recommendations. Occasionally the need may arise to terminate the examination procedure for direct medical referral to the patient's physician (such as uncontrolled hypertension). The

dentist may also initiate a telephone consultation. This approach is more expedient and allows a more direct exchange of information and discussion regarding treatment approaches. When telephone contacts are made, the practitioner should summarize the conversation and recommendations of the consulting physician in the patient's chart. When necessary, assistants may be asked to monitor the telephone conversation and countersign the signed dental chart entry.

## PROSTHESES

*Evaluation of the existing prostheses* is also an important part of the examination. Before the intraoral inspection, particular attention should be directed to patient speech patterns and esthetics. Phonetic problems with *s* sounds as well as whistles and clicks may be indicative of poorly constructed dentures.[10] Poor esthetics associated with an artificial appearance (teeth too lightly colored or too straight) or inappropriate tooth positioning (smile lines, vertical dimension) should be noted. The dentures should be removed and cleaned. Denture defects (cracks, missing teeth, worn teeth, or worn denture base resin), use of denture adhesive, and the presence or absence of denture labeling should be noted. The clinical examination should include identification of soft tissue–related problems with the prostheses (angular cheilitis, stomatitis, traumatic ulcers, inflammatory papillary and peripheral hyperplasia, and level of alveolar ridge resorption). Upon reinsertion of the dentures, stability (resistance to pressure applied in a horizontal direction), retention (resistance to pressure applied in a vertical direction), vertical dimension of occlusion, the amount of interocclusal distance available, and occlusal contacts should be evaluated.

The patient should also be *queried regarding satisfaction* with *denture esthetics, chewing function, history of prosthesis use,* and associated *discomfort,* as well as an *interest in* receiving *prosthodontic treatment* to rectify noted deficiencies. These subjective responses are very important considerations for the dentist. It is conceivable that objective prosthodontic needs may be overruled in the treatment-planning process by important modifying factors (such as patient satisfaction in relation to perceived need as well as objective findings of severe residual ridge resorption, significant

**5A**

**SCHOOL OF DENTISTRY
UNIVERSITY OF COLORADO
HEALTH SCIENCES CENTER**

4200 EAST NINTH AVENUE
DENVER. COLORADO 80262
BOX C-284

**MEDICAL CONSULTATION REQUEST**

DATE: _____

_____ is planning to receive dental treatment at the University of Colorado Health
(Name of Patient)
Sciences Center School of Dentistry.

Patient relates a history of:                    Questions to be answered:

_____          _____

_____          _____

_____          _____

_____          _____

_____          _____

_____          _____

If prophylactic antibiotics are necessary. we will follow the most recent recommendations of the American Heart Association
and the American Dental Association.

_____          _____
Student Signature                              Faculty Signature

**PHYSICAL FINDINGS AND RECOMMENDATIONS**

_____

_____

_____

_____

_____

_____

_____          _____
Consult Date                                   Physician's Signature

Please keep Blue copy for patient's dental record. White and Green copy to physician. Physician to return White copy,
Green copy for physician's records.

**Fig. 7-15** Multiple-copy dentist-to-physician consultation form utilized at the University of Colorado.

physical or cognitive impairment, mouth dryness, or neuromuscular disorders).

## REFERENCES

1. Anderson F: An historical overview of geriatric medicine: definition and aims. In Pathy MSJ, editor: Principles and practice of geriatric medicine, Chichester, 1985, John Wiley & Sons.
2. Baum B: Alterations in oral function. In Andres R, Bierman E, and Hazzard W, editors: Principles of geriatric medicine, New York, 1985, McGraw-Hill Book Co.
3. Beck JD and Hunt RJ: Oral health status in the United States: problems of special patients, J Dent Educ 49(6):407, 1985.
4. Bennett DR, McVeigh S, and Rodgers B: AMA drug evaluations, ed 6, Philadelphia, 1986, WB Saunders Co.
5. Berkey DB: Clinical decision making for the geriatric dental patient, Gerodontics 4:321, 1988.
6. Berkey DB and Holtzman JM: Oral health. In Ham R, editor: Geriatric medicine annual 1987, Oradell, NJ, 1987, Medical Economics Books.
7. Ettinger RL: Clinical decision making in the dental treatment of the elderly, Gerodontology 3:157, 1984.
8. Finlayson RE and Martin LM: Recognition and management of depressions in the elderly, Mayo Clin Proc 57:115, 1982.
9. Fox PC, Bush KA, and Baum BJ: Subjective reports of xerostomia and objective measures of salivary gland performance, J Am Dent Assoc 115:581, 1987.
10. Gordon SR and Jahnigen DW: Oral assessment of the edentulous elderly patient, J Am Geriatr Soc 31(12):797, 1983.
11. Gordon SR and Sullivan TM: Dental treatment planning for compromised or elderly patients, Gerodontics 2:217, 1986.
12. Grembowski D, Milgrom P, and Fiset L: Factors influencing dental decision making, J Public Health Dent 48:159, 1988.
13. Ham R: Alzheimer's and the family. In Ham R, editor: Geriatric medicine annual 1987, Oradell, NJ, 1987, Medical Economics Books.
14. Hand JS, Hunt RJ, and Beck JD: Coronal and root caries in older Iowans: 36-month incidence, Gerodontics 4:136, 1988.
15. Hunt RJ: Periodontal treatment needs in an elderly population in Iowa, Gerodontics 2:24, 1986.
16. Jarvik LF and Neshkes RE: Alterations in mental functions with aging and disease. In Andres R, Bierman E, and Hazzard W, editors: Principles of geriatric medicine, New York, 1985, McGraw-Hill Book Co.
17. Kantor ML, Zeichner SJ, Valachovic RW, and Reiskin AB: Efficacy of dental radiographic practices: options for image receptors, examination selection, and patient selection, J Am Dent Assoc 119:259, Aug 1989.
18. Kastrup EK and Olin BR: Facts and comparisons, St. Louis, 1989, JB Lippincott Co.
19. Knight K: Evaluation of the geriatric patient. In Reichel W, editor: Clinical aspects of aging, Baltimore, 1983, The Williams & Wilkins Co.
20. Levy SM, Baker KA, Semki TP, and Kohout FJ: Use of medications with dental significance by a non-institutionalized elderly population, Gerodontics 4(3):119, 1988.
21. Little JW and Falace DA: Dental management of the medically compromised patient, ed 3, St. Louis, 1988, The CV Mosby Co.
22. Lundin DV: Medication-taking behavior of the elderly: a pilot study, Drug Intell Clin Pharm 12:518, 1978.
23. McCarthy F: A new, patient-administered medical history developed for dentistry, J Am Dent Assoc 111(4):595, 1985.
24. Nelson JF, Barnes GP, Tollefsbol RG, and Parker WA: Prevalence and significance of prescription medication usage among gerodontic patients, Gerodontology 6:17, 1987.
25. Physicians' desk reference, ed 43, Oradell, NJ, 1989, Medical Economics Books.
26. Rosenberg GM: Neuropsychiatric manifestations of cardiovascular disease in the elderly. In Levenson AJ and Hall RCW, editors: Neuropsychiatric manifestations of physical disease in the elderly, New York, 1981, Raven Press.
27. USP Drug Information for the health care provider, vol 1, ed 9, Rockville, Md, 1989, The United States Pharmacopeial Convention, Inc.
28. US Senate Special Committee on Aging: Aging America—trends and projections, PL 3377:584, 1983.

# 8

# Treatment Planning for the Older Adult

*Ronald L. Ettinger*
*Douglas B. Berkey*

Certain diseases with which dentists must be concerned have no cure, and so the damage they inflict is predominantly irreversible. Only when one is dealing with acute diseases of the oral mucosa that can repair themselves can the diseases be cured. At this time such treatments do not make up the major work load of the dental profession. Historically, the majority of dentists treat the acute exacerbation of dental diseases (such as caries and periodontal disease) in relatively healthy children or adults.

In the past the restorative needs of children and adults have formed the bulk of dental practice.[22] However, the nature of the U.S. population and the character of dental practice have changed and are continuing to change.[3,4,39,55,77] There has been a dramatic reduction in the caries rates of children and young adults.[14,34,47] At present more older persons are retaining some natural teeth,[9,26,42,79] and until recently the dental needs of this segment of our population were somewhat ignored. The elderly generally were treated as a dependent, edentulous group, not as individuals with complex and special needs.[23] Chauncey et al.[17,17a] have pointed out that if coronal caries prevalence and incidence are considered in proportion to the number of teeth present older adults exhibit a high attack rate. The 1985-1986 study by the National Institute for Dental Research of Seniors[76] showed that coronal caries was a significant problem for older adults (mean DFS = 20.4). The National Study indicated that root caries occurred in 57% of the senior population and was nearly three times higher than the 21%

figure noted for employed adults 18 to 64 years of age.

A survey of noninstitutionalized elderly in two Iowa counties found that a high level of treatment needs existed[38,41,43]; 40% of the persons examined required at least one restoration, 16% needed at least one extraction, 27% needed prosthodontic treatment, and over 60% of the dentate subjects needed some periodontal treatment. These data are further complicated by the fact that younger cohorts of elderly persons[26] are more likely to be dentate and to have higher expectations of dentistry differing significantly from their older edentulous predecessors. This younger cohort usually will not accept the simple solution of the past, that is, the extraction of remaining teeth with the subsequent construction of complete dentures. Thus disease prevention must become a cornerstone of future dental treatment planning, and dentists must be skilled in clinical techniques required to care for the changed dental needs of their older patients. The process of decision making called treatment planning used by dentists to choose the appropriate treatment is the focus of this chapter. In this chapter the problems associated with planning treatment for healthy as well as frail older persons are explored and discussed and several philosophies are presented.

## THE AGING POPULATION

The elderly have been defined as that cohort of people 65 years of age or older. However, utilization of only a chronologic criterion for the categorization of these individuals is inappropriate because great variation in physical, medical, and mental condition exists among elderly persons. Regardless of age, if a person remains relatively healthy, he or she presents few treatment problems for the general practitioner. Functionally independent healthy older adults make up the majority (70%) of the aging population. The knowledge base required to manage the oral problems of elderly patients does not depend on the development of new technical skills but rather on the following:

1. An understanding of normal aging
2. An understanding of pathologic aging
3. The recognition of oral implications of systemic disease
4. A knowledge of drug-induced dental disease
5. Interpersonal skills
6. Special communication techniques with older persons who have sensory deficits
7. Decision-making skills

A definition of geriatric dentistry was therefore needed so that it would define the individual in terms of a functional assessment rather than by chronologic age. It has evolved with the consideration for provision of dental care for adult persons based on one or more chronic, debilitating physical, mental, or psychosocial problems.[25] It seems apparent that although many of these conditions are frequently associated with increasing chronologic age they are not always a consequence of aging. Therefore a "geriatric" dental patient was defined as a physically or mentally compromised older adult who may or may not be 65 years old.

Two further groups have been identified within the geriatric population—the frail person who although he or she is at risk still can live in the community if provided with adequate support services, and the functionally dependent persons who are persons who have lost their support systems and as a result have been institutionalized or are housebound.[25]

The value of these definitions is twofold: they delineate the several levels of training required to prepare the dentist to treat each specific functional cohort, and they help define the content of courses required to understand the overall problems of the elderly.

Frail individuals make up about 20% of the elderly population. Clinical training courses geared toward providing care to this group must include:

1. All the skills needed for treating the functionally independent elderly
2. Additional experience in the recognition and application of medicine in oral health care
3. Additional experience in the recognition of drugs and polypharmacy that may complicate and influence the patient's oral health
4. Practical experience in clinical decision making

Dentists who wish to treat older patients might seek some postgraduate training, such as a 1-year general practice residency, associated with an acute care hospital that treats both inpatients and outpatients. Either option will give the dentist practical experience at making appropriate decisions. At the undergraduate level in dental school a special care unit designed to treat frail adults is a possible approach to teaching them clinical decision-making skills.

Functionally dependent individuals have been estimated to represent approximately 5% of the elderly population and another 5% are homebound. Clinical treatment for this group requires a considerable amount of experience in rational decision making, and postgraduate training is extremely useful.

The bulk of dental care is still reconstructive, that is, the restoration of teeth and the restoration of function of the stomatognathic system with fixed and removable partial dentures.[22] The clinical techniques are usually similar to those needed for treatment of younger persons; however, more problems are encountered. For example, in recurrent caries the margins of interproximal restorations will need to be placed subgingivally with all the associated problems of bleeding, marginal adaptation of restorative materials, and finishing.

The decisions as to what constitutes appropriate care may vary for an older cohort of individuals because those decisions must include consideration of a variety of age-related and age-associated psychologic, social, biologic, and pathologic changes. Therefore it is essential that modifying factors be identified before a comprehensive treatment plan is formulated. Milgrom et al.[58] evaluated treatment plans of 346 dentists for seven elderly patients who posed no economic constraints and wanted the best possible dental care. At the end of this exercise the findings indicated that, in general, the 346 dentists may have had insufficient training or guidelines to make informed diagnostic decisions. Specifically, the dentists had difficulty reducing the clinical data and integrating it into a meaningful diagnosis and treatment plan.

Braun and Marcus[15] have suggested that the three most common and important variables encountered when making treatment decisions are the patient's financial constraints, periodontal health, and the dentist's perception of the patient's needs and the degree of treatment desired. Grembowski et al.[37] indicated that clinical decision making in dentistry was a "social process that included the dentist, the patient, and sometimes other family members and insurers as well." They further stated that within this process dentists were primarily responsive to technical and patient factors in formulating and prescribing therapy. A sample of 156 dentists' decisions were sought between paired alternatives (such as root therapy versus extraction). The dentists keyed on technical factors (such as age and medical history) rather than on a patient's considerations (such as a patient's preference and a patient's oral hygiene status) with only one third of the dentists considering the input of patient factors as being important in choosing treatment alternatives. The authors called for more research on clinical decision making to provide a better understanding of the factors that influence dentists' therapeutic preferences.

## REVIEW OF THE LITERATURE

Current clinical decisions in dentistry tend to be based on qualitative, subjective estimates that the benefit of a specific treatment modality should outweigh the harm that it may do. The traditional approach has been for the clinician to collect individual pieces of evidence to weigh and synthesize into a subjective treatment plan, based on personal clinical experience rather than on quantitative scientific evidence.[29]

Decision analysis frequently has been used in medicine[29,30,63,72] and is characterized as decision making under the conditions of uncertainty. In its simplest form, decision making is the systematic separation of complex and confusing problems into a series of sequentially linked smaller units. Each decision is then based upon research results and

incorporates an evaluation of the risk and consequences. Tulloch and Antczak-Bouckoms[74] described the use of such decision analysis applied to the problem of whether to extract asymptomatic mandibular third molars. The outcome measure used was the number of days of standard discomfort. The difficulty in developing these assessments arises as result of consideration of the multidisciplinary nature wherein one must take into account the patient's health status, the uncertainty of the risks as well as the benefits, and an awareness of the patient's preferences for various possible outcomes. Each decision was based on an evaluation of the risks and consequences.

Marcus et al.[56] examined dental treatment plans for patients 60 years of age or older and compared the decisions made to those recommended for younger patients with similar problems. This study found that prejudices exist in the way general dentists plan treatment for older patients. In particular, dentists were more likely to extract teeth and less likely to use fixed prostheses for older patients. Dentists also were more likely to modify their preferred treatment plans if the patients either had no insurance or had a limited ability to pay for care. Furthermore, if the patients were uncooperative or not readily available for treatment or came mainly for cosmetic reasons, the dentists were more likely to modify their treatment plan by substituting less expensive dental care. These findings support those of Bailit et al.,[5] who reported that when treating minority older patients and lower socioeconomic groups dentists were more likely to extract teeth rather than restore them. Weinstein et al.[78] found that the quality of restorative treatment was also related to the patient's health care values. Unfortunately, little is known about how dentists make clinical decisions relative to treatment planning.

## STRATEGY OF DECISION MAKING

Dental treatment planning, a decision-making process that culminates in the selection of treatment modalities, is a critical process about which relatively little information is available. Studies of medical practices[21,22,30,75] indicate that two conditions that might contribute to the variation in treatment plans are inherent in any decision-making situation: these are uncertainty and complexity. Decision-making uncertainty occurs when there is insufficient knowledge relative to the impinging variables and possible outcomes. The dentist may be uncertain about the nature of the dental problem and when, or even if, it should be treated. One example is an elderly patient who had recently relocated and was brought to the clinic by her son for a checkup. Routine radiographic evaluation revealed a central incisor that had had root canal therapy. This tooth had a well-circumscribed periapical lesion. When she was questioned, the tooth was asymptomatic and the patient was poor in giving a history. She was mildly confused and could not remember when the tooth had been treated. It was not possible to contact her previous dentist, who is deceased. Her present dentist could not be sure if this was an active process or a healing lesion. If it were an active process, the treatment of choice might have been to redo the root canal therapy; however, if it were a healing lesion, the patient should be examined at regular intervals. Uncertainty about the possible therapeutic treatment alternatives and whether resources are available to carry them out may occur also. If the patient were in good health, no particular problem would exist. However, if this patient had a history of early Alzheimer's disease, would it be more therapeutically correct to observe the tooth over a period of time? Because it is known that the patient will physically and mentally deteriorate over time, should the root canal therapy be redone or should the tooth be extracted? Specifically, the dentist may be uncertain about the prognosis for this patient.

This is the kind of problem a dentist is faced with daily when caring for older frail adults. However, a decision needs to be made and the son needs to be given guidance so that he can make an informed decision as to what is in the best interest of his mother. The recommendation in this situation would be to do nothing except to emphasize the need for regular recalls. The reasons for coming to this conclusion are as follows:

1. There are no apparent signs or symptoms that an active disease process exists.
2. The site is easy to see and check and the son needs to be informed to look for signs of change such as swelling or looseness of the tooth.
3. The worst-case scenario for this condition is a periapical abscess, which one can deal with by redoing the root canal or by doing an

apicectomy or even extracting the tooth.
4. The mother has a limited life span and the tooth seems healthy at this time.

Decision-making problem complexities occur when multiple relevant variables exist. These include consideration of a variety of treatment alternatives, as well as several criteria on which a decision will be based. Because dental diseases are not always associated with a specific curative therapy and because of recent improvements in dental materials, there are many more treatment options available.

For instance, in a patient with root caries, the treatment of these lesions must include an evaluation of the patient's ability to maintain his or her oral hygiene as well as any xerostomic drugs that may be used, the extent of the lesion, the status of the lesion, that is, active or arrested, access to the lesion, ability to keep the tooth dry during restorative procedures, proximity of the lesion to the cementoenamel junction, and esthetics. These factors determine which restorative approach should be used: (1) remineralization with topical fluorides, (2) recontouring to make the tooth self-cleaning, (3) utilization of appropriate restorative materials such as amalgam, glass-ionomer cements, or composite resin, or (4) extraction of the tooth or teeth.

There should be consideration of patient-related factors, which can directly affect the prognosis of the dental treatment to be rendered, such as health, neuromuscular ability, vision, and motivation, which add to the complexity of treatment planning decisions. Since the dentist must choose the best therapeutic alternative early and anticipate the consequences of that decision on later events such as the deterioration in the health of the patient as described here, the treatment planning situation can become even more complex.

## THE DILEMMA: IDEAL OR RATIONAL TREATMENT PLANNING

The ideal treatment plan has been described by Barsh[8] as "that leading to the best dental prognosis without taking modifying factors into account." Traditionally, this has been based on the application of morphologic concepts; that is, the dentist views that dentition and proceeds technically to evaluate how many teeth can be saved or replaced without evaluating any other limiting factors. This morphologically based approach has been described by Levin[50] as "the 28-tooth syndrome" and usually was compatible with healthy patients in a fee-for-service system. After reviewing the literature, Pilot[64] concluded that there is no scientific evidence available to support the advisability of routine prosthetic replacement of dental arches that have been shortened by tooth loss. Much of the information related to reduced dentition comes from cross-sectional studies. However, Kayser[48] followed 118 subjects with different degrees of arch reduction and showed that there was sufficient adaptive capacity to maintain adequate oral function when at least four posterior occlusal units remained, preferably in a symmetric position. Ramfjord and Ash,[66] in discussing the replacement of lost teeth, stated that "clinical experience indicates that satisfactory function and occlusion, as well as neuromuscular stability, usually can be established if all biscuspids and anterior teeth are present, even if these teeth have lost a considerable amount of periodontal support."

When caring for an aging population in which significant limiting, modifying factors are often significant, a patient-oriented approach, requiring rational decisions is realistic. Berkey[13] has suggested that the dentist should begin by asking several basic questions such as:

1. What is the patient's dental problem?
2. Why did it occur?
3. What can I do about it?
4. What will the outcome be?

Barsh[8] suggests that when conditions prevent the achievement of an ideal treatment plan, the dentist should collect more data, focus on each problem, and then distinguish between the ideal, realistic alternatives and an interim plan.

Based on the assumption that since persons become increasingly compromised because of various medical, social, and psychologic problems, several authors[31,46,57] have prepared a modification of the American Society for Anesthesiologists evaluation system. Using the system as a reference, they have suggested therapy modification and patient management approaches. This modified system provides an excellent guideline for the dental treatment of medically compromised patients requiring anesthesia.[57] Kamen[46] has further modified the system

by dividing the care provided into the four broad categories listed below:

**Class I**     Comprehensive treatment
**Class II**    Intermediate care (maintenance of dentition and prevention of disease)
**Class III**   Emergency care (alleviation of pain and infection)
**Class IV**   No treatment

Although this system provides a useful concept, it has faults that Gordon and Kress[32] describe by stating that "when applied to specific situations the system is somewhat simplistic in that many patients fall between categories. Also many choices remain even within one category." Ingber and Rose[44] have described a problem-oriented system and utilized organized lists of dental problems with factors that may influence dental care. They suggest prioritizing the problems but give no guidelines on how to integrate the various treatment plans.

In 1983, Ettinger and Beck[25] presented a flow diagram of decision making called the "rational dental care model." Although the relative influence of the various modifying factors was unknown, they hypothesized that the decision-making flow diagram was the mechanism by which dentists experienced in geriatric care made treatment-planning decisions. They suggested that this model could be incorporated into any dental practice because it specified a thought process that would be helpful for the diagnosis and treatment planning for all patients. Gordon and Sullivan[33] pointed out that none of these approaches "addresses the important step where treatment alternatives are formulated and compared."

One of the difficulties encountered in treatment planning is that dental treatment options are continuously evolving and new information and techniques are becoming available to the clinicians.

For example, an elderly female seeks treatment; the dentist detects a large carious lesion on the central incisor. The diagnosis is obvious. However, there is the question as to what treatment should be rendered. What modifying factors should be assessed before a rational treatment plan is developed?

Below are some of the more global patient-related factors that must be assessed:

1. **Patient attitude.** *To what degree does the pa-*

*tient desire dental treatment, and will she give informed consent to institute treatment?*

It must be recognized that oral health is defined not only by objective signs, but also by the subject's or patient's perceived symptoms. It has been shown that good communication with the older patient, as well as his or her family or significant others, is essential.

If the dentist is not skilled at communicating with older patients who have sensory deficits, the true nature of the patient's chief complaint may be missed. For example, the patient's younger sister has recently died from oral cancer, but the patient cannot openly vocalize her fears and walk into the dentist's office and ask the dentist to check her mouth for oral cancer. Rather, she comes to the dentist saying she has "lost a filling" hoping that during the examination the dentist will tell her that she does not have oral cancer. Berkey[13] has had some success using a closed-ended dental questionnaire that uses a series of specific questions that still leaves space for patients to write in concerns.

A complete and up-to-date medical and drug history is part of good communications. An oral review of the medical questionnaire with the patient or significant other person, or both, is imperative to clarify areas of importance such as medication use, positive disease findings, and symptom history. When the questionnaire has been completed and reviewed, consultation with the patient's physician may be necessary to clarify or amplify confusing information provided by the patient. The physician can help the dentist understand the nature of the patient's illnesses, and the physician may have recommendations for the appropriate use of sedatives or a prophylactic antibiotic regimen that may be required before dental treatment.

It is important that the dentist establish the degree of treatment desired by the patient and what they are willing to accept. If the patient is accompanied by family members or significant others, those persons should be present during all discussions of potential treatment, especially those related to surgery, cosmetic interventions, prosthodontic treatment, and finances. Written instructions should be provided the patient and should be discussed with the patient and concerned others to minimize misinterpretation.

2. **Quality of life.** *How much is the patient af-fected either physically or emotionally by the dental problem and how will she respond to the different levels of treatment?*

The potential loss of a carious central incisor may be interpreted by this patient as a significant negative life change. Therefore the dentist must explore the patient fears and treatment expectations.

It has been shown that the patient's perceived need for dental care and her ability to successfully tolerate dental procedures may be associated with her dental status.[13] Deteriorating oral health may signal important changes in the patient's ability to maintain adequate home care. This may be related to a treatable condition such as depression or may be the first sign of a disorder such as Alzheimer's disease.

3. **Limitations of treatment.** *How much do existing medical, psychologic, or social problems limit the patient's ability to benefit from treatment?*

The overriding rule for the older patient, as with all patients, is that the treatment rendered must benefit the patient and do no harm. A thorough assessment of the patient is the key to understanding treatment limitations.[13]

This elderly lady reported a history of hypertension controlled by a diuretic, adult-onset diabetes controlled by diet, weight control, and an oral hypoglycemic and osteoarthritis controlled by nonsteroidal anti-inflammatory agents. She has had one hip replaced with a prosthesis about 2 years previously. This medical history is not unusual, for national data reports[9,62] show that one in three persons over 65 years of age will have a history of heart disease or hypertension, or both. Other common problems in this population will be arthritis (46%) disorders of hearing (28%) and vision (14%) as well as diabetes (8%). This older segment of society represents 12% of the U.S. population and has a large number of medical problems. It has been shown that they buy more than 20% of all prescription medications. Many of these medications have the potential to cause adverse oral side effects such as xerostomia, lichenoid type of lesions of the mucosa, enlargement of the gingiva, as well as dyskinetic movements of the oral musculature.[6] It is imperative that the dentist not only take a careful medical and drug history, but also understand the oral implications of the histories.[22]

Patients with angina, congestive heart failure, and hypertension should be treated during early morning appointments because they are strongest after a night's rest. Their appointments should be kept short. They should not be left in a supine position for prolonged periods because they are susceptible to orthostatic hypotension.[68] Patients with osteoarthritis; with chronic respiratory diseases, such as emphysema, bronchiectasis, or chronic bronchitis; or with a colostomy should be seen in the late morning. Arthritic patients become stiff when sleeping and need time to unlimber. Patients with respiratory problems require time to clear their lungs of residual fluid after being supine during the night. Patients with a colostomy may need time for toileting after breakfast.

A small number of older patients may demonstrate inappropriate behavior unless they are premedicated. These are primarily functionally dependent older adults suffering from a variety of dementias, psychiatric disturbances, any of the choreas producing degenerative illnesses, senile cortical atrophy, or severe cerebral arteriosclerosis. The benzodiazepines, especially when administered orally, have been shown to have the lowest risk for the older patient when used for the management of inappropriate behavior. Diazepam (Valium) has often been used because of its ability to reduce preoperative tension and anxiety. However, this drug is transformed by the liver into other active forms, and although clearance of the drug in young persons may take as long as 20 hours, in the elderly it may take up to 90 hours. Thus a shorter-acting form such as oxazepam (Serax) should be used with older adults. The usual dosage for premedication is 10 to 15 mg one half hour before treatment. The patient should be under the supervision of a family member or caretaker for the next 24 hours because of the possibility of prolonged drug activity or idiosyncratic reactions.[36,70]

4. **Iatrogenic potential.** *How much possibility is there of creating iatrogenic problems, either a medical emergency, a drug reaction, or a dental problem associated with the treatment plan?*

Many frail and functionally dependent older patients tolerate stress poorly.[7] Many of these persons cannot sit for extended periods of time; others require antibiotic coverage when soft tissues are invaded because of their medical status as described earlier. Frail persons who are underweight may need special padding to sit and cannot tolerate procedures that will last longer than 1 hour. Some older persons have weakness of the bladder sphincter and are on regular schedules to use the toilet, which the dentist must be aware of if urinary incontinence is to be avoided during dental treatment.[24]

Premedication with antibiotics is required for all procedures that may cause hemorrhage such as deep scaling and minor oral surgery in the following patients: brittle diabetics, immunosuppressed patients, persons who have had a joint replaced with an artificial substitute,[60,61] persons with valvular defects of the heart or a very recent myocardial infarction, and persons with mitral valve prolapse[28,71] (Table 8-1). Persons receiving antineoplastic chemotherapeutic agents, immunosuppressive agents, radiation therapy, or long-term steroid therapy usually have an increased susceptibility to infection and should also be given antibiotic coverage. It is important to consult the patient's physician before proceeding with treatment. Where multiple appointments are necessary, it is advisable that at least 2 weeks be allowed to elapse before the patient is premedicated again.[49] The reason for this time lapse is to prevent antibiotic-resistant organisms from developing by repeated frequent exposures to the particular antibiotic.

The prevention of medical emergencies in the dental office is essential for porper treatment. Persons taking hypoglycemics should have their appointments scheduled in midmorning, when insulin level is not at its peak, after a normal breakfast and after taking their medication.[35] Persons suffering from episodes of anginal pain should have their nitroglycerin with them at their dental appointments, and if the appointment may be stressful or they are susceptible to frequent anginal attacks, they should take a prophylactic dose of 0.4 mg sublingually 3 to 5 minutes before beginning treatment.[61] For patients with cardiovascular disease, it is advisable to have short morning appointments, adequate anesthesia, and, if required, sedation to reduce stress, which increases the oxygen demand of the myocardium.

It is standard practice to record blood pressure and pulse rates for all new dental patients at the

**Table 8-1** Prophylactic regimens for dental procedures recommended by the American Hospital Association

| | |
|---|---|
| **Standard regimen\*** | |
| For dental procedures that cause gingival bleeding, and oral or respiratory tract surgery | Amoxicillin 3 g 1 hour before procedure and 1.5 g 6 hours later |
| **Special regimens\*** | |
| Parenteral regimen for use when maximal protection desired, as for high-risk patients with<br>1. Prosthetic valves<br>2. Recent history of endocarditis (within the past 5 years)<br>3. Intracardiac surgery (within the last 6 months) | Ampicillin 2 g IM or IV 30 min before procedure, plus gentamicin 1.5 mg/kg IM before procedure (not to exceed 80 mg) |
| Oral regimen for penicillin-allergic patients | Erythromycin‡ 1 g 2 hours before procedure and 500 mg 6 hours later |
| Parenteral regimen for penicillin-allergic patients | Vancomycin 1 g IV slowly over 1 hour starting 1 hour before; no repeat dose necessary |
| **Regimen for arthroplasty patients†** | |
| Oral regimen for arthroplasty patients | Penicillin 2 g 1 hour before, and then 1 g 6 hours after first dose |
| Oral regimen for penicillin-allergic patients | Erythromycin‡ 1 g orally 1 hour before and 500 mg 6 hours after the first dose |

\*Modified from Dajani AS, Karchmer AW, Little JW, et al: Prevention of bacterial endocarditis, JAMA (submitted).
†Modified from Nelson JP et al: J Bone Joint Surg 72A:1, 1990.
‡This timing applies only to the erythromycin ethylsuccinate formulation of erythromycin; other forms generally display delayed absorption.

initial appointment.[54] If patients report a history of hypertension, even if it is controlled by medication, their blood pressure should be monitored and recorded before treatment and before patient dismissal for each dental appointment.[59] If the patient is on anticoagulants and if deep scaling or minor oral surgery is to be performed, the patient's physician should be consulted so that dosages may be adjusted. Normal prothrombin time is 10 to 12 seconds; the convention used for deep scaling can be twice normal, but for an extraction it should not be more than 1½ times normal values. If the anticoagulant dose requires adjustment, it must be adjusted with the patient's physician.

A person with a recent myocardial infarction or cerebrovascular accident should not receive elective dental treatment for at least 6 months.[52] It has been suggested that some cardiologists, who are evaluating their post–myocardial infarction patients with stress tests 6 to 8 weeks after the initial episode, may authorize elective dental treatment earlier than the usual 6-month time limit.[20] However, when one is treating a patient earlier than the recommended timetable, it is imperative that the dentist seek a consultation with the patient's cardiologist before beginning dental treatment. It is generally believed that patients who have had coronary bypass surgery do not need prophylactic antibiotic coverage before dental care once the patient has survived the immediate postoperative period of 2 to 3 weeks.[51,52]

Dental office equipment, such as pulp tests, electrodesensitizing or electrosurgery equipment, ultrasonic scaling devices or cleaners, and occasionally motorized dental chairs, have been reported to be potential sources of electromagnetic interference and may adversely affect the functioning of certain types of older cardiac pacemakers. Thus it is important to avoid the use of these instruments and devices when patients wearing pacemakers present for treatment.

With patients on long-term steroid therapy (greater than 20 mg of hydrocortisone per day, or its equivalent), it may be necessary to have their steroid dosage increased for the day of the dental appointment as well as the following day. This also should be done with their physician. Usually the steroid levels are increased to the equivalent of 30 mg of hydrocortisone per day.[11,16,45]

Local anesthetics must be carefully selected for older patients. Local anesthetics are either esters or amides, with or without a local vasoconstrictor. The esters are cleared by enzymatic hydrolysis in the plasma, whereas the amides are detoxified by the liver. Residual unhydrolyzed esters are excreted via the kidney. The amount and type of anesthetic must be carefully chosen for older patients having a history of liver or kidney dysfunction. The majority of local anesthetics used today are amides. Holroyd and Requa-Clark[40] suggest the following regimen based upon duration of anesthesia desired.

1. **Less than 30 minutes:**
   Mepivacaine plain (3% Carbocaine)
2. **30 to 60 minutes:**
   Lidocaine (2% Xylocaine with 1:100,000 epinephrine)
   Mepivacaine (2% Carbocaine with 1:20,000 nordefrin HCl [Levonordefrin])
3. **60 to 90 minutes:**
   Prilocaine (4% Citanest)
   Prilocaine (4% Citanest Forte with 1:200,000 epinephrine)
   Lidocaine (2% Xylocaine with 1:100,000 epinephrine)

Rose et al.[68] have suggested that vasoconstrictors still may be used in combination with local anesthetics. For patients with cardiovascular disease the suggested limit is 0.036 mg of epinehprine, which represent two carpules of local anesthetic with 1:100,000 epinephrine. It is imperative that deliberate aspiration is used before anesthesia deposition. The use of local hemostatic agents, such as an epinephrine-impregnated gingival retraction cord, is considered as being dangerous and is contraindicated for all older patients. Patients on propranolol should not be given epinephrine because unopposed vagal stimulation can procude bradycardia and hypotension.[52,68] The long-term inhibition of monoamine oxidase (MAO) has been shown to result in accumulation of norepinephrine, epinephrine, serotonin, dopamine, tyramine, and tryptamine in various tissues. The use of local anesthetic with epinephrine is contraindicated in persons taking monoamine oxidase inhibitors (MAOI) because epinephrine may precipitate a hypertensive crisis.[69]

5. **Prognosis.** *What are the consequences of not treating the dental problem and how long should the treatment continue (risk per benefit)?*

In severely compromised or terminally ill patients reparative and curative treatment often is not possible. Dentists must learn the art of providing only palliative care without feeling guilty. In these instances their primary responsibility is to eliminate pain and control infection. In the elderly patient, pain thesholds and tolerance can vary greatly, and a differential diagnosis, especially in dentate persons, can be difficult. The sensation of pain is an extremely subjective experience when the dentist is making an evaluation. The dental practitioner is dependent on the patient's description of the site, intensity, duration, and quality of the pain. It is known that the intensity and duration of pain varies greatly between each person as well as within a single person depending on a variety of social, emotional, and medical factors.[67] Further, one rarely finds acute dental infection in older patients and even periapical infections can occur without pain or fever.[7] Acetaminophen is the drug of choice for the relief of pain in aging persons. Acetaminophen has been shown to be as effective as aspirin in relieving pain but has limited anti-inflammatory effects.[18] In one study acetaminophen (975 mg) was reported to be more effective than aspirin (650 mg).[2] Also, it has been found to be less irritating to the gastric mucosa and has no reported effect on platelet function nor does it interfere with uric acid excretion and has no effect on carbohydrate metabolism.[19] Adverse reactions are rare if acetaminophen is taken in the recommended therapeutic dose of 2 to 4 g/day.[67] It is therefore the drug of choice for persons who have a history of gastrointestinal disorders, persons receiving oral anticoagulants, persons with gouty arthritis, or diabetics receiving sulfonylurea.[19]

The next responsibility of the dentist is to ensure oral comfort for the patient. In many instances, this follows naturally on the elimination of pain and infection. In patients wearing dentures, it often can be achieved through the use of tissue conditioners and in dentate patients through the use of desensitizing agents on exposed root surfaces as well as zinc oxide and eugenol cements in carious teeth. When the patient is pain free and comfortable, the dentist can evaluate the patient and the dentition with regard to possible improvement of function through reconstruction of the dentition or occlusion.

There are few available research data documenting the consequences of not treating a particular oral condition. If a proximal or distal enamel lesion is observed on a routine radiograph, what are the consequences of not treating that lesion? How long will it take to penetrate into the dentin? Berkey et al.[12] in a 10-year longitudinal study found that it took an average of 73 months in healthy males 28 to 76 years of age. Lesions on molar teeth in the maxillary arch progressed faster. Men with more teeth and fewer restored teeth and who were younger had a slower caries progression rate. In older men lesion progression into the dentin was more rapid. For all ages, poor oral health was associated with more lesions and more rapid progression. Studies such as these are important in estimating the consequences of not treating a particular dental problem. At the moment, however, there are very few guidelines.

6. **Dentists' limitations.** *Does the dentist have the equipment, the skill, or the experience to provide the appropriate therapy at the appropriate site?*

Oral health care delivery for the elderly patient requires a multidisciplinary approach.[22] Consultation with physicians is often required to determine the degree, severity, nature of physical impairments, and the effect of these impairments on the oral cavity. Communication with a pharmacist may be helpful in determining the effects of medications on oral disease treatment modalities. Interaction with a social worker may be necessary to assist persons in gaining access to social networks to help with transportation, finances, and so forth.

By evaluating the previously discussed six global factors one could establish that it was appropriate and important to treat the dental problems of this elderly lady before beginning treatment of the large carious lesion of the central incisor. The following list of dentally related issues common to patients of all ages should be addressed:

1. What is the degree of the disease state and therefore the condition of the tooth? That is, how much usable tooth structure will be left when the caries has been removed?
2. What is the oral hygiene status of the patient?
3. What is likely to be the patient's ability to maintain or improve her daily oral hygiene?
4. What is the importance of this tooth to the function of her occlusion as well as her dentition?
5. What is the periodontal support for this tooth?
6. What is the caries experience of the patient?
7. What is the restorative experience of the patient?
8. What ability does the patient have to pay for the appropriate care?

If the patient was severely compromised medically or mentally, does one simply conservatively remove the decay and use a zinc oxide–eugenol dressing as palliative care, or does one refer the patient for tooth extraction? When does one decide that there has been a loss of tooth structure to the extent that a crown is an appropriate treatment modality. If the lesion is large and the tooth reacts to pulp testing and a crown is the treatment option selected, should elective endodontics be performed? Is a cast post and core better than a prefabricated post or should one try to rebuild the tooth with light-cured resins and pins? The available information on which to base these important clinical decision is ambiguous, at best, even for the restoration of a single tooth.

One can, however, combine the systems discussed and provide a modified concept of staging treatment planning as suggested by Bennet and Creamer.[10]

The first task is information gathering. The dentist must identify the reasons why the patient has come for treatment.

It may be:

1. A symptomatic emergency such as an abscess
2. An asymptomatic problem such as a broken restoration
3. An unrelated problem such as cancerophobia
4. A patient seeking a new dentist
5. A patient seeking a second opinion
6. A significant other bringing in a reluctant patient

In each of these situations unless the dentist is made aware of the motivation behind the care seeking, the potential for a misunderstanding or conflict exists. The second is to determine the patient's desire for care and the value he places on his dentition and on dentistry. To achieve these goals, the dentist must interpret both verbal and nonverbal communication and be able to put the patient at ease. Once the dentist has established effective lines of communication he or she can gather a detailed:

1. Medical history
2. Drug history and current medication
3. Past dental history, especially a history of tooth loss, pain and pain control, and restorative experiences.
4. Perception of current oral health
5. Attitude toward tooth loss, denture use, prevention, and esthetic needs
6. An estimation by the patient of the economic value of his or her dentition and dentistry

A thorough radiographic and dental examination can then be done to evaluate the teeth, periodontium, neuromuscular function, oral soft tissues, and occlusion.

## STAGED TREATMENT PLAN

When all requisite information has been gathered, including medical consultations, a staged dental treatment plan can be evolved.

### Stage I—emergency care

1. Life-threatening emergency—immediate referral to a hospital for care
2. Referral to a hospital for stressful elective care
3. Oral emergency—alleviation of pain and infection
   a. Perform biopsy of the lesion.
   b. Extract high-risk teeth.
   c. Perform pulpectomy of symptomatic tooth.
   d. Debride periodontal tissues and follow up with chemotherapy.
   e. Control caries with temporary dressing or stainless steel crowns for symptomatic teeth.
   f. Repair damaged denture or reline with a tissue conditioner.
      At this point the dentist should evaluate the long-term needs of the patient and undertake the following:

(1) Consider the potential life span of the patient.
(2) Undertake special investigations, such as blood tests.
(3) Consult with specialists.
(4) Evaluate mounted study casts.
(5) Evaluate need for stress reduction.

### Stage II—maintenance and monitoring care

1. Management of chronic infections
2. Required preprosthetic surgery
3. Root canal therapy
4. Root planing and curettage
5. Patient education to improve oral health (such as changes in dietary habits, plaque control, and use of topical fluorides)
6. Restoration of carious lesions
7. Reline, rebase, or remake dentures or construct new dentures as required

A further period of evaluation is required before one proceeds further.

### Stage III—rehabilitative phase

1. Orthognathic surgery or implants
2. Surgical endodontics
3. Surgical periodontics
4. Esthetic dentistry
5. Reconstruction of the occlusal plane and restoration of vertical dimension with fixed and removable prostheses

If the practitioner carefully stages his provision of dental care, the patient can receive the requisite treatment in increments that are appropriate to the resolution of the immediate problem. Once a critical dental problem is stabilized the dentist can consider undertaking the next appropriate step, which is providing comprehensive rational care.

Medical researchers have used several methodologies to evaluate diagnostic performance. Proshek et al.[65] described these methodologies as either the use of simulations in presenting data such as the patient management problems system,[1,53] or employing the individual naturalistic observation of expert clinicians.[59] Ettinger et al.[27] used the latter technique to evaluate similarities and differences among five dentists, experienced in caring for geriatric patients, who were asked to interview, examine, and plan treatment for an elderly man while they were being videotaped. The results suggested that previous experience was an extremely important factor in the decision-making process. The implications of this observation was that the smaller the range of clinical experiences a dentist has, the more limited his ability for appropriate treatment strategies. Therefore training programs in geriatrics should either teach decision making and treatment planning from a more theoretical perspective or provide students and dentists with sufficient time and a diversity of experience to permit them to gather a store of information upon which to base meaningful comprehensive decisions.

## SUMMARY

Treatment planning is a formal procedure undertaken by dentists to make relevant decisions about the provision of care to their patients. If a patient is relatively healthy and ambulatory, the factors involved in providing appropriate care relate primarily to oral disease severity, the patient's perception of his or her need, various technical problems associated with the restoration of maximal function and esthetics, and the patient's ability to pay for the care provided. However, if the patient is medically compromised, physically disabled, or mentally impaired, the planning of appropriate treatment necessitates inclusion of medical and sociologic variables. This chapter has explored the problems associated with treatment planning for healthy as well as frail older adults. It discusses rational oral health care planning with thoughtful consideration of a vast variety of modifying factors.

## REFERENCES

1. Adams H, Wills R, Shannon F, et al: Assessing clinical judgment in dentistry: practitioner evaluation of patient management problems, J Am Coll Dent 46:187, 1979.
2. Amadido P: Peripherally acting analgesics, Am J Med 77:17, 1984.
3. American Dental Association: Council publishes facts in dental prepayment plans, Am Dent Assoc News, Jan 6, 1988.
4. Bailit HL and Bailit JL. Corporate control of health care: impact on medicine and dentistry, J Dent Educ 52:108, 1988.
5. Bailit HL, Braun R, Maryniuk GA, and Camp P: Is periodontal disease the primary cause of tooth extraction in adults? J Am Dent Assoc 14:40, 1987.
6. Baker KA and Ettinger RL: Intra-oral effects of drugs in elderly persons, Gerodontics 1:111, 1985.
7. Banting D and Oudshoorn W: The clinical management of the aging patient: treatment concepts and procedures, Ont Dent 56:19, 1979.
8. Barsh LI: Dental treatment planning for the adult patient, Philadelphia, 1981, WB Saunders Co.
9. Beck JD and Hunt RJ: Oral health status in the United States: problems of special patients, J Dent Educ 49:407, 1985.
10. Bennett JS and Creamer HR: Staging dental care for the oral health problems of elderly people, J Oregon Dent Assoc 53:21, 1983.
11. Bennett RW, Gehlhausen JA, and Poulos JT: Glucocorticoids: a review, US Pharmacist 7:40, 1982.
12. Berkey CS, Douglass CW, Valachovic RW, and Chauncey HH: Longitudinal radiographic analysis of carious lesion progression, Community Dent Oral Epidemiol 16:83, 1988.
13. Berkey DB: Clinical decision-making for the geriatric dental patient, Gerodontics 4:321, 1988.
14. Bohannan HM: The impact of decreasing caries prevalence: implications for dental education, J Dent Educ 61:1369, 1982.
15. Braun RJ and Marcus M: Comparing treatment decisions for elderly and young patients, Gerodontics 1:138, 1985.
16. Byyny RL: Withdrawal from glucocorticoid therapy, N Engl J Med 295:30, 1976.
17. Chauncey HH, Kapur KK, House JE, and Rissen L: The incidence of coronal caries in normal aging male adults, J Dent Res 57(spec. issue A):148 (abstract 296), 1978.
17a. Glass, RL, Alman, JE, and Chauncey HH: A 10-year longitudinal study of caries incidence rates in a sample of male adults in the U.S.A, Caries Res 21:360, 1987.
18. Cooper SA: Comparative analgesic efficacies of aspirin and acetaminophen, Arch Intern Med 141:282, 1981.
19. Deuben RR: Nonopioid analgesics for patients with dental pain, Dent Clin North Am 28:401, 1983.
20. Elizardi DJ, Redding SW and Tullman MJ: Cardiovascular disease. In Tullman MJ and Redding SW, editors: Systemic disease in dental treatment, New York, 1982, Appleton-Century-Crofts.
21. Elstein AS: Clinical judgment: psychological research and medical practice, Science 194:696, 1976.
22. Ettinger RL: Clinical decision making in the dental treatment of the elderly, Gerodontology 3:157, 1984.
23. Ettinger RL: Oral disease and its effects on the quality of life, Gerodontics 3:103, 1987.
24. Ettinger RL: Dental care and management of the aging dental patient, J Tenn Dent Assoc 69:10, 1989.
25. Ettinger RL and Beck JD: Geriatric dental curriculum and the needs of the elderly, Spec Care Dent 4:207, 1984.
26. Ettinger RL and Beck JD: The new elderly: What can the dental profession expect? Spec Care Dent 2:62, 1982.
27. Ettinger RL, Beck JD, and Martin WE: Treatment planning for an older adult: a pilot study, Iowa Dent J 75:31, 1989.
28. Everett ED and Hirschmann JV: Transient bacteremia and endocarditis prophylaxis: a review, Medicine 56:61, 1977.
29. Feinstein AR: Clinical judgment, Baltimore, 1967, The Williams & Wilkins Co.
30. Feinstein AR: The purpose of prognostic stratification, Clin Pharmacol Ther 13:285, 1972.
31. Fellman S: Treatment of complete denture patients in a geriatric facility, J Prosthet Dent 35:512, 1976.
32. Gordon SR and Kress CG: Treatment planning in dental schools, J Dent Educ 51:224, 1987.

33. Gordon SR and Sullivan TM: Dental treatment planning for compromised or elderly patients, Gerodontics 2:217, 1986.
34. Graves RC and Stamm JW: Oral health status in the United States: prevalence of dental caries, J Dent Educ 49:341, 1985.
35. Gotthelf TS and Rose LF: Diabetes mellitus, dental correlations. In Rose LF and Kaye D: Internal medicine for dentistry, St. Louis, 1983, The CV Mosby Co.
36. Greenblatt DJ and Shader RL: Benzodiazepines, N Engl J Med 291:1011, 1974.
37. Grembowski D, Milgrom P, and Fiset L: Factors influencing dental decision making, J Public Health Dent 48:159, 1988.
38. Hand JS and Hunt RJ: The need for restorations and extractions in a non-institutionalized elderly population, Gerodontics 2:72, 1986.
39. Health Insurance Association: Sourcebook of health insurance data 1982-1983, Washington, DC, 1983.
40. Holroyd SV and Requa-Clark B: Local anesthetics. In Holroyd SV and Wynn RL, editors: Clinical pharmacology in dental practice, St. Louis, 1983, The CV Mosby Co.
41. Hunt RJ: Periodontal treatment needs in an elderly population in Iowa, Gerodontics 2:24, 1986.
42. Hunt RJ, Hand JS, Kohout FJ, and Beck JD: Incidence of tooth loss among elderly Iowans, Am J Public Health 78:1330, 1988.
43. Hunt RJ, Srisilapanan P, and Beck JD: Denture-related problems and prosthodontic treatment needs in the elderly, Gerodontics 1:226, 1985.
44. Ingber JS and Rose LF: The problem oriented system: an approach to managing a comprehensive hospital dental system, Dent Clin North Am 19:703, 1975.
45. Kalkwarf KL, Hinrichs JE, and Shaw DH: Management of the dental patient receiving corticosteroid medications, Oral Surg 54:396, 1982.
46. Kamen S: The resolution of oral health care for the institutionalized geriatric patient, Spec Care Dent 3:249, 1983.
47. Katz RV, Hazen SP, Chilton NW, and Mumma D: Prevalence and intraoral distribution of root caries in an adult population, Caries Res 16:265, 1982.
48. Kayser AF: Shortened dental arches and oral function, J Oral Rehabil 8:457, 1980.
49. Kilmartin C and Monroe C: The dental management of the cardiac patient requiring antibiotic prophylaxis, J Can Dent Assoc 1:77, 1986.
50. Levin B: 'The 28-tooth syndrome'—or should all teeth be replaced? Dent Surv 50:47, 1974 (editorial).
51. Little JW: Dental management of patients with surgically corrected cardiac and vascular disease, Oral Surg 50:314, 1980.
52. Little JW and Falace DA: Dental management of the medically compromised patient, ed 2, St. Louis, 1984, The CV Mosby Co.
53. Mackenzie RA: An instructional information exchange for dentistry in the United States: measurement of judgmental and decision processes, vol 7, no (HRA)75-79, DHEW Publication, 1975.
54. Malamed SF: Blood pressure evaluation and the prevention of medical emergencies in dental practice, J Prevent Dent 6:183, 1980.
55. Manning WG, Benjamin B, Bailit HL, and Newhouse, JP: The demand for dental care: evidence from a randomized trial in health insurance, J Am Dent Assoc 110:895, 1985.
56. Marcus M, Schoen MH, Mason DT, Sue GY, and Hwu W: Dentists' preferences for treatment planning and their relationship to oral health status: final report, University of California, Los Angeles, 1983.
57. McCarthy FM and Malamed SF: Physical evaluation system to determine medical risk and indicated dental therapy modifications, J Am Dent Assoc 99:181, 1979.
58. Milgrom P, Kiyak HA, Conrad D, et al: A study of treatment planning: periodontal services for the elderly, J Dent Educ 45:522, 1981.
59. Moskowitz AJ, Kuipers J, and Kassirer, JP: Dealing with uncertainty, risks, tradeoffs in clinical decisions: a cognitive science approach, Ann Intern Med 108:435, 1988.
60. Mulligan R: Late infections in patients with prostheses for total replacement of joints: implications for the dental practitioner, J Am Dent Assoc 101:44, 1980.
61. Mulligan R: Preventive care for the geriatric dental patient, J Calif Dent Assoc 12:21, 1984.
62. National Center for Health Statistics: Current estimates from the National Health Survey, United States, 1979, series 10, no. 136, 1981, DHHS Publ no (PHS) 81-1564, Hyattsville, Md.
63. Pauker SG and Kassirer JP: Decision analysis, N Engl J Med 316:250, 1987.
64. Pilot T: A plea against extending the shortened dental arches, Ned Tijdschr Tandheelkd 85:477, 1978.
65. Proshek JM, Loupe MJ, and Serunian JH: The process of dental diagnosis: an initial analysis, Presented at annual meeting of the American Education Research Association, New York, April 1977.
66. Ramfjord SP and Ash MM: Periodontology and periodontics, Philadelphia, 1979, WB Saunders Co.
67. Rhodes RS, Jahnigen DW, Rhodes PJ, and Piepho RW: Management of dental pain in the elderly, Gerodontics 1:264, 1985.
68. Rose LF, Godfrey P, and Steinberg BJ: Cardiovascular diseases: dental correlations. In Rose LF and Kayed D, editors: Internal medicine for dentistry, St. Louis, 1983, The CV Mosby Co.
69. Roth-Schechter BF: Psychotherapeutic drugs. In Holroyd SV and Wynn RL, editors: Clinical pharmacology in dental practice, St. Louis, 1983, The CV Mosby Co.
70. Shader RI and Greenblatt DJ: Clinical implications of benzodiazepine pharmacokinetics, Am J Psychiatry 134:652, 1977.
71. Schulman ST et al: Prevention of bacterial endocarditis, Circulation 70:1123A, 1984.
72. Statson WB and Weinstein MC. Allocation of resources to manage hypertension, N Engl J Med 296:732, 1977.
73. Streeten DHP: Corticosteroid therapy, pharmacological properties and principles of corticosteroid use, JAMA 232:944, 1975.
74. Tulloch JFC and Antczak-Bouckoms AA: Decision analysis in the evaluation of clinical strategies for the management of mandibular third molars, J Dent Educ 51:652, 1987.
75. Tversky A and Kahneman D: Judgement under uncertainty, Heuristics and Bias Science 185:1124, 1974.

76. US Department of Health and Human Services: Oral health of United States adults: national findings, NIH Publication no 87-2868, Aug 1987.

77. US Senate Special Committee on Aging: Aging America: trends and projections, PL 3377:584, 1983.

78. Weinstein P, Milgrom P, and Morrison K: Patient dental values and their relationship to oral health status, dentist perceptions and quality of care, Community Dent Oral Epidemiol 7:121, 1979.

79. Weintraub JA and Burt BA: Oral health status in the United States: tooth loss and edentulism, J Dent Educ 49:368, 1985.

# 9

# Management of Dental Caries in the Older Patient

*David W. Banting*

Dental caries is an infectious process that results in the destruction of the mineralized tooth tissues. Although uncommon, evidence of dental caries has been found in human skeletal remains dating back to Paleolithic times. The occurrence of dental caries in man increased dramatically during the Neolithic period and has remained at a relatively high level since.[69]

Early civilizations in Japan, India, Egypt, Mesopotamia, and Greece believed that dental caries was caused by worms. In fact, *caries* is a Latin word meaning 'rottenness' or 'decay'. Other theories that have been advanced regarding the cause of dental caries included humors, internal resorption, acids, parasites, acids and parasites together, proteolysis, proteolysis combined with chelation, and a few others.[70] It is presently accepted that dental caries is a chronic disease. It proceeds from the surface of the tooth toward the pulp, and the destruction is caused primarily through decalcification of the mineralized tissues. The caries process depends on three essential factors: the tooth and its environment, microorganisms, and diet. Many secondary factors associated with the host (age, sex, saliva, immune response, oral hygiene), the agent (type, number, and virulence of the microorganism), or the substrate (cariogenic potential or presence of fluoride in foods and beverages) may affect the rate of progression of dental caries. But, without the simultaneous presence of the three primary factors for a sufficient length of time, disease is unlikely.

Dental caries is usually classified according to anatomic location. In ancient man, dental caries was frequently found on the root of the tooth (root caries), whereas in modern man the crown portion of the tooth is more commonly attacked (coronal caries). Both coronal and root caries can be active and untreated, arrested without being treated, or restored as an outcome of dental treatment. Similarly, they can exhibit low activity (incipient) or high activity (rampant) and progress through the stages of decalcification (early lesion), cavitation (clinical lesion), or gross destruction of the tooth. Unfortunately, these terms are not mutually exclusive. If the dental caries occurs adjacent to a filling material on either the crown or the root of a tooth, the lesion is referred to as "secondary or recurrent caries."

The occurrence of dental caries in children and young adults has declined dramatically in the past decade in response to extensive efforts over the previous 30 years to prevent the disease through the widespread use of systemic and topical fluorides, better nutrition, more sophisticated mechanical oral hygiene procedures, and improved dental health education. This accomplishment will almost certainly result in an increased number of natural teeth being retained by older adults. In addition to continued coronal dental caries activity, carious lesions occurring on the roots of teeth have been increasingly documented, particularly for older adults in contemporary populations. Because this text is directed toward the older adult and so much has been published already about coronal caries, emphasis is placed on root caries in this chapter.

**141**

## THE ROLE OF MICROORGANISMS

It has been conclusively demonstrated that microorganisms are a prerequisite for the initiation and progression of coronal dental caries, that a single type of microorganism is capable of inducing caries, and that the ability to produce acid as a byproduct of metabolism is essential to the process.[70] However, not all acidogenic oral microorganisms induce caries, and virulence varies among those that do. Furthermore, there is interaction among different bacterial species, and only the microorganisms present at a localized site are considered to be important in the carious process at that site.

Bacterial specificity in the cause of dental caries has not been convincingly demonstrated; however, *Streptococcus mutans* is considered to be a major pathogen in coronal caries. It comprises a much greater proportion of all microorganisms grown on nonselective media when harvested from decayed as opposed to caries-free surfaces of teeth.[62] The initiation of dental caries on sound teeth is most often preceded by colonization with elevated levels of *S. mutans*.[44] However, the ability of *S. mutans* to colonize a site and achieve dominance depends on the immediate environment. *Lactobacillus* organisms have also been shown to be strongly associated with coronal caries but are considered to be less cariogenic than *S. mutans*, except perhaps in the presence of fluoride.[18] The precise roles of each of these microorganisms in the development of a carious lesion are unknown, but it is believed that *S. mutans* is more closely associated with incipient caries, whereas *Lactobacillus* tends to be associated with caries progression.[30]

Animal studies[48-49,83] led to the hypothesis that a microflora different from that implicated in coronal caries may be involved in the root caries process. Jordan and Hammond[47] were the first to culture samples of microorganisms from human root caries lesions on extracted teeth. Gram-positive filamentous bacteria such as *Actinomyces viscosus, A. naeslundii, A. odontolyticus, Rothia dentocariosa,* other unidentified *Actinomyces*-like organisms, as well as *Streptococcus mutans* were isolated from the lesions. Sumney and Jordan[86] extended this hypothesis by culturing surface deposits of plaque and carious debris from teeth freshly extracted because of periodontal disease. The microorganisms isolated included *S. mutans, S. sanguis, S. mitis,* and enterococci but many filamentous organisms of the genus *Actinomyces* and an anaerobic, diphtheroidal organism similar to the genus *Arthrobacter. S. mutans* was the predominant organism isolated from the plaque covering the surface of the lesion, and the organism resembling the genus *Arthrobacter* was isolated from the advancing front of the root caries.

Syed et al.[90] obtained plaque samples from active, untreated root caries lesions in patients before restorative treatment. *Actinomyces viscosus* was found to be the dominant bacterial species recovered on anaerobic culture and therefore was considered to be the primary agent. *Actinomyces naeslundii, Streptococcus mutans, Streptococcus sanguis* and *Veillonella* strains were also isolated but as lesser proportions of the total viable counts. *S. mutans* was believed to be important, but not all subjects yielded this microorganism from their root plaque.

Ellen et al.[32] were the first to compare the microflora colonizing sound and carious root surfaces. *A. viscosus* was the most frequently isolated microorganism. The proportions of the total cultivable anaerobic flora of plaque from intact and carious root surfaces represented by *S. mutans, Lactobacillus, A. viscosus, A. naeslundii,* and *Veillonella* were similar. However, only 20% of the total colony count from the nonselective media could be accounted for on selective media. Brown et al.[22] also compared the surface microflora of carious and intact root surfaces. No significant differences were seen between carious and intact root surfaces for *S. mutans* and *Lactobacillus* when measured as proportions of the total anaerobic cultivable flora. But intact root surfaces had significantly higher proportions of *Actinomyces* than carious root surfaces did. *S. mutans* made up the largest proportion (34%) of the total anaerobic count followed by *A. viscosus* and *Lactobacillus*. Furthermore, *S. mutans* represented a significantly higher proportion of the total anaerobic count in initial compared with advanced lesions.

Fure et al.[34] compared the proportion of *S. mutans, Lactobacillus, A. viscosus* and *A. naeslundii* in subjects with four or more root surfaces affected with caries (group 1) with subjects who were caries free or had, at the most, one affected root surface (group 2). The latter subjects also had moderate-to-severe periodontal disease. The proportions of *S. mutans* in group 1 were significantly higher than those of group 2 as were the proportions of *Lactobacillus*. There was no difference in the proportion of *Actinomyces* between the groups.

Keltjens et al.[55] compared the plaque taken from one to three carious root lesions in periodontal patients on maintenance care with contralateral, intact root surfaces. The root lesions were further classified as soft (active) or hard (arrested). *S. mutans* counts on the carious surfaces were significantly higher than those on the sound surfaces. This difference was attributed exclusively to the increased counts on the soft carious surfaces. *S. sanguis* and *A. viscosus/A. naeslundii* counts were not significantly different on carious and sound roots.

Van Houte et al.[94] characterized the microbial flora of the plaque and saliva from adult subjects (1) without root caries or restorations, (2) with one or more root lesions (with or without root restorations), and (3) with root restorations only. The prevalence and concentration of *S. mutans* cocci in root surface plaque was higher for subjects with root caries compared with subjects without root caries or restorations. *A. naeslundii* was elevated in subjects without caries and subjects with restorations only relative to subjects with lesions. In the same subject, *mutans* streptococci were only modestly more prevalent in plaque overlying advanced lesions compared with plaque overlying a sound root surface but considerably more prevalent in plaque from an incipient lesion compared with that from a sound surface. No additional positive correlations were observed between other acidogenic microorganisms in plaque and root caries. Although higher median salivary concentrations of *mutans* streptococci were found for subjects with root caries compared with subjects without root caries, a direct relationship between salivary concentrations of these microorganisms and the number of root caries lesions was not evident.

Keltjens et al.[57] and Salonen et al.[78] however, were able to demonstrate a direct, positive relationship between root caries prevalence and salivary bacterial counts. Periodontal surgery patients with high *S. mutans* levels and those with high counts of *S. mutans* and *Lactobacillus* together showed significantly higher root caries rates. In Swedish adults, the mean number of carious surfaces increased with the greater number of colony-forming units (CFU) of *mutans* streptococci in the saliva. Interestingly, the correlations were stronger for younger adults where most of the caries occurred on enamel than for older age groups where most of the caries was found on the roots of the teeth.

Only two studies have followed a group of subjects and taken repeated samples of plaque or saliva for microbiologic analysis. Ellen et al.[31] reported that the relative risk of a patient developing a carious lesion on a susceptible tooth root was five times greater if both *S. mutans* and *Lactobacillus* were present in the root plaque than when both were absent. High salivary counts of *Lactobacillus* and *S. mutans* were also found in patients who had the greatest number of new root caries lesions over an 8-year period.[74]

Animal models of the role of microorganisms in the caries process are conclusive. *S. mutans* is capable of inducing coronal and root caries in the presence of a carbohydrate source. *A. viscosus* is also capable of causing extensive destruction of the bony support of teeth and root caries. Human experimentation, however, has supported only in a general way the findings in animals. The existence of a cause-and-effect relationship between root caries and an unique microorganism has yet to be demonstrated. Jordan[46] reviewed the available knowledge relating to the microbiology of root caries and concluded that a wide array of organisms should be considered as causative agents. *S. mutans* has not been found to be consistently present in root caries plaque but, when present, may comprise a high proportion of the anaerobic cultivable flora. The presence of *S. mutans* and *Lactobacillus* together increases the risk of root caries. *A. viscosus* has been identified as the most numerous organism among the cultivable bacteria isolated from plaque overlying tooth roots, but the proportion of the cultivable flora represented by this organism is higher for intact than for carious roots. The microflora of root lesions probably changes with the state of the lesion or the stage of development of the lesion.[19] For instance, *S. mutans* has been recovered predominantly from initial lesions and *Lactobacillus* organisms are associated with advanced lesions—a situation not unlike enamel caries.

## DIETARY FACTORS

Any consideration of a microbial cause in root caries must include dietary factors if it is accepted that decalcification of the calcified components of the tooth is central to the formation of a lesion.[43,71] Acidogenic organisms use carbohydrates from the diet for metabolism and, in the process, produce acids, which destroy the inorganic portion of the tooth.

Root caries in people appears to be enhanced by dietary sugars. The frequency of both coronal and root caries coincided with the increased daily intake of sugar, especially when taken between meals, in the Vipeholm Dental Caries Study.[36] This study also demonstrated that caries activity in the younger age groups was much higher than in the older age groups supplied with similar high-sugar diets. In the older age groups, however, the carious lesions occurred most frequently on the tooth roots. Hix and O'Leary[42] observed that patients with moderate-to-severe periodontal disease who were affected by root caries had a significantly higher number of fermentable carbohydrate exposures per week than those without root caries did. This relationship was independent of whether the patient received periodontal treatment.

Further evidence of the important role of diet in the root caries process is presented by Papas et al.[72] Three-day food diaries were compiled for 175 elderly subjects, and the results were then compared with a dental examination for coronal and root caries. Positive correlations were found between dietary sugars and both coronal and root decay. Associations were also confirmed between the frequency of snacks and the presence of root caries.

Bowen et al.[20] have recently demonstrated that a sucrose substitute (sucralose) added to the feed of normal and desalivated rats infected with *Streptococcus mutans* significantly reduced root caries formation in comparison to similar rats fed a diet containing sucrose. The substitution of sucrose with noncariogenic sweeteners therefore may be an effective means of minimizing the prevalence and incidence of root caries.

## PREVALENCE AND INCIDENCE OF DENTAL CARIES

Dental caries experience is usually measured and reported as the number of decayed and filled tooth surfaces. The mean number of coronal and root decayed and filled (DF) surfaces by age for employed adults in the United States[68] is shown in Fig. 9-1.

It is clear that the prevalence of enamel caries rises until middle age and then moderates slightly. For root caries, there is a slow but progressive increase in prevalence with advancing age. Ninety-four percent of the coronal surfaces were restored compared to 48% of root surfaces.

Although approximately 97% of persons 18 years of age and over have experienced dental caries, most do not currently have active, untreated dental decay. Beck et al.[15] found that 55% of the adults had no untreated coronal or root caries, whereas about equal proportions had either one type or both types of untreated lesions (Fig. 9-2). Eighty-six percent of caries on the crowns of the teeth were recurrent around existing restorations, whereas the decay on the roots of the teeth was either initial or recurrent in approximately equal proportions.

Among older adults, root caries has attracted the most attention during the past decade. A composite picture of the observed occurrence of root caries for different age groups in contemporary adult populations is presented in Fig. 9-3. These populations represent healthy, ambulatory, urban adults and the occurrence of root caries falls between 3% and 70%, depending on age. This rate increases dramatically for special population groups such as primitive tribesman, the institutionalized, chronically ill patients, patients with destructive periodontal disease, and the elderly.

Several studies express prevalence as the proportion of roots at risk that were decayed or filled; two of these are illustrated in Fig. 9-4. Only tooth roots with gingival recession, as a consequence of periodontal disease or periodontal treatment, were considered to be at risk of root caries. The *root caries index* (RCI) represents the proportion of susceptible teeth or root surfaces that become carious.[51-52] The mean prevalence rates expressed in this manner are lower than the crude rates, ranging from 1.1% to 26.6% of root surfaces at risk. Approximately 60% of tooth root surfaces exhibit gingival recession and are exposed to the oral environment.[15,55,98] The RCI, however, actually is an overestimation of the prevalence of root caries because approximately 10% to 20% of root lesions occur on surfaces with no visible recession (prob-

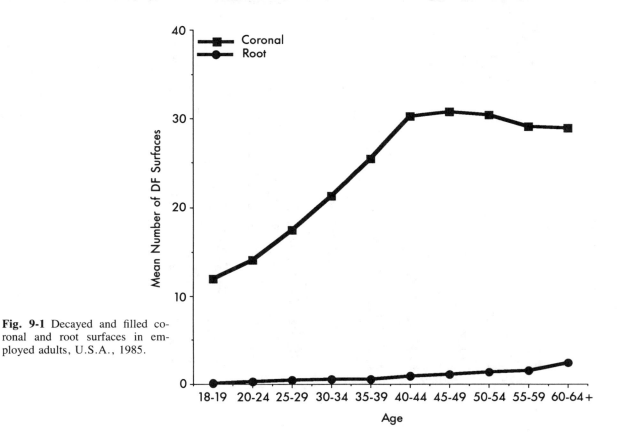

**Fig. 9-1** Decayed and filled coronal and root surfaces in employed adults, U.S.A., 1985.

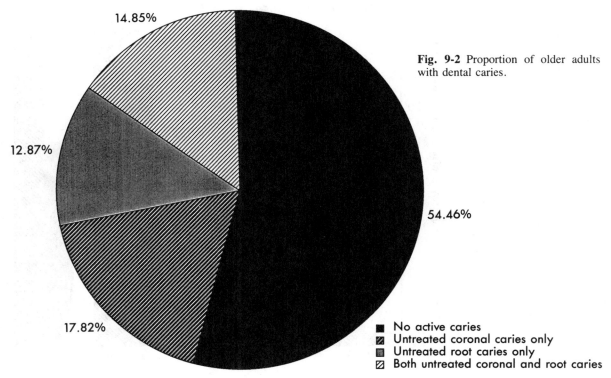

**Fig. 9-2** Proportion of older adults with dental caries.

No active caries
Untreated coronal caries only
Untreated root caries only
Both untreated coronal and root caries

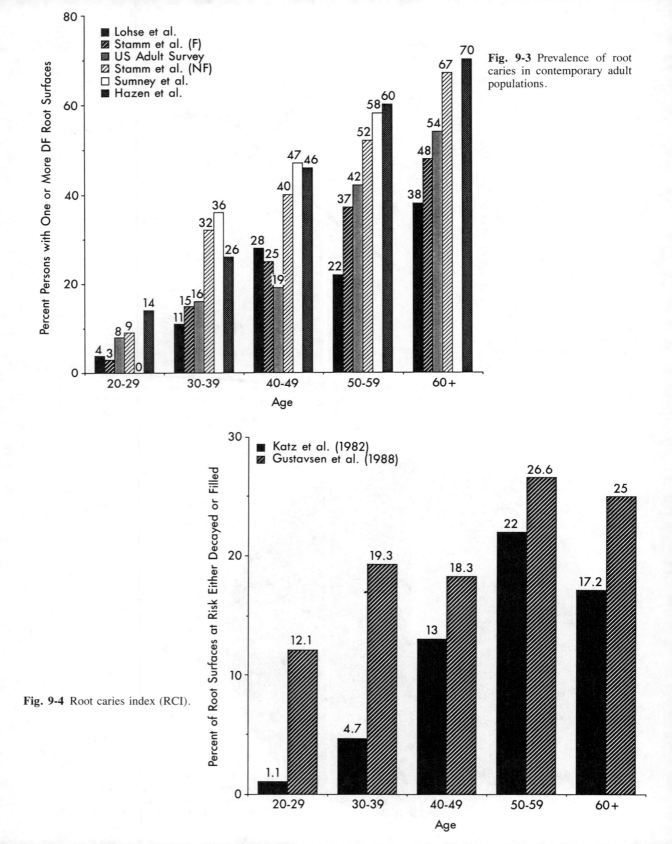

**Fig. 9-3** Prevalence of root caries in contemporary adult populations.

**Fig. 9-4** Root caries index (RCI).

ably because of gingival hypertrophy as a consequence of inflammation). Another 20% occur on surfaces that do not permit measurement of recession because of an obliterated cemetoenamel junction. Both of these types of surfaces are ignored in the RCI denominator.[23,61,84]

Subjects exhibiting root caries have an average of 3.7 affected surfaces. Primary root caries lesions were found to be almost six times more prevalent than secondary root lesions.[15] Mandibular molars have been shown to be the most frequently involved teeth with a decreasing susceptibility for premolars and incisors. In the maxillary arch, the anterior teeth have higher prevalence rates than the posterior teeth have.[55] Similar distributions have been observed for surfaces of teeth.[84] Although these investigators found uniformity in terms of the exposure of surfaces for each tooth type, the widely

variable root caries rates indicate that specific, local, intraoral factors may determine the pattern of root caries attack.

Considerable controversy has arisen regarding the tooth root surfaces most frequently affected by root caries. The evidence indicates that either facial or approximal surfaces may usually be affected followed by lingual surfaces.[8,87] A similar pattern is observed when tooth groupings are considered.[42] Katz et al.[55] compared the relative likelihood of different tooth root surfaces becoming carious by tooth type. The buccal surface of the mandibular molar, for example, is twice as likely to demonstrate root caries than the lingual or proximal surfaces of the same tooth would. The lingual surface of the maxillary molar is five times more susceptible than its buccal surface. Longitudinal studies of root caries incidence support the observations

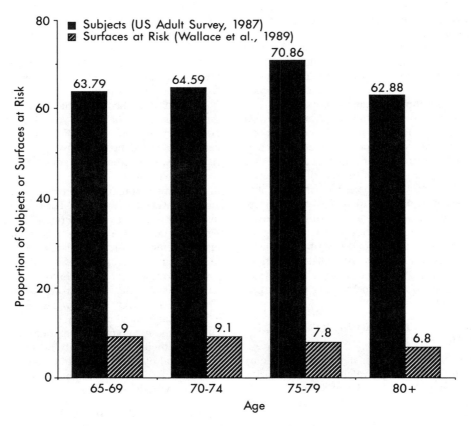

**Fig. 9-5** Prevalence of one or more decayed or filled root surfaces in seniors.

**Table 9-1** Incidence of root caries in contemporary adult populations

| Study | Average number of lesions per year | Rate per 100 surfaces at risk | Percentage of population with root caries over study period |
|---|---|---|---|
| Ravald et al., 1986[74] | Not available | 4.95 | 74 |
| Banting et al., 1985[9] | 0.25 | Not available | 36 |
| Emilson et al., 1988[33] | Not available | 4.5 | 69 |
| Hand et al., 1988[38] | 0.36 | 1.8 | 44 |
| Jensen and Kohout, 1988[45] | 0.14/0.43 | Not available | Not available |
| Ripa et al., 1987[76] | 0.12/0.14 | Not available | 36/43 |
| Leske and Ripa, 1989[60] | 0.15 | 0.87* | 19 |
| Wallace et al., 1988[98] | Not available | 1.1/1.4/1.6 | Not available |

*In subjects who developed root caries.

of the cross-sectional surveys with respect to surface distribution.[9]

The prevalence studies that have been limited to older adults reveal that the prevalence rate of root caries, whether measured by crude prevalence or by root surfaces at risk, remains relatively constant beyond 65 years of age[68,98] (Fig. 9-5).

The number of studies of the incidence rate of root caries is more limited compared to prevalence studies. Despite the fact that the populations observed were quite diverse, the observation periods varied, the criteria for determining root caries differed (particularly with respect to filled surfaces), and the methods of reporting incidence were not uniform; a useful estimate of the rate of occurrence of root lesions can nevertheless be made (Table 9-1). Anywhere from 19% to 74% of the subjects followed experienced root caries during the period of observation. Longer periods of observation generally resulted in a higher proportion of the subjects with new lesions. For every 100 surfaces at risk, between 1.1 and 4.95 became carious. The average number of root lesions per person per year ranged from 0.12 to 0.43.

## CHARACTERISTICS OF PERSON, PLACE, AND TIME

Virtually all the cross-sectional surveys have demonstrated an increased prevalence of root caries with advancing age. Prevalence rates for root caries, including root fillings, range from 3% to 14% for subjects 20 to 29 years of age, 9% to 36% for subjects 30 to 39 years of age, 15% to 47% for subjects 40 to 49 years of age, 22% to 64% for

subjects 50 to 59 years of age, and 38% to 70% for subjects over 60 years of age. The wide range of observed rates can be partially explained by factors such as fluoridation status, health, institutionalization, culture, and definition of root caries. A direct, positive association of root caries prevalence and age is also observed when one calculates the prevalence rate using in the denominator only teeth with gingival recession.[54-55,84,97-98]

Males have higher prevalence rates of root caries than females do for all 10-year age groups from 30 to 60 years and over.[87,96] However, when one calculates prevalence rates using only surfaces at risk, the sex difference disappears.[29,55]

Only two sets of data are available to permit a direct comparison of the prevalence rate of root caries between countries.[39,96] The occurrence of this disease is much lower in Finland than in North America; however, this may be attributable to cultural differences, or, more likely, the criteria used to determine the presence of root caries.

There are no data available to relate occupation and socioeconomic status to root caries experience. There are, however, special population groups that exhibit exaggerated prevalence rates of root caries. One common characteristic among these high-risk groups is their reduced ability or interest in maintaining oral hygiene at a level commonly accepted as being associated with the prevention of progressive periodontal disease.

## CLINICAL CONSIDERATIONS

The adjectives "cementum," "radicular," "senile," "cervical," and "radiation" have all been used to describe carious lesions on the roots of teeth. Interestingly, the terms "cervical caries" and "radiation caries" apply equally to the coronal and root surfaces of teeth. However, to describe decay involving the hard tissues of the tooth root, namely, cementum and dentin, the term "root caries" is preferred. Root caries must be differentiated from other conditions that result in destruction of the tooth root such as abrasion, erosion, and idiopathic root resorption.[40]

As early as 1879 a different type of caries involving the gingival margins was identified.[1] Soon after that Darby[25] wrote about caries at the gingival margins in cement and dentin that did not arrest itself and was only limited by the gingival margin.

Hecht and Friedman[41] observed a high prevalence of "cervical" dental caries in drug addicts. He described the lesions as being "leathery brown" in consistency and spreading "in a vertical direction, tending to undermine the enamel incisally, apically, and horizontally, to produce circular caries." In describing root caries among New Guinea natives, Davies[26] observed that they were commonly seen in adults with advanced periodontal disease. The lesions were characterized by a "primary attack of cementum which spread laterally along the cemento-enamel junction and advanced rapidly toward the pulp but left the enamel virtually intact." Lowenthal[63] also noticed a "peculiar type of carious lesion" during the course of examining thousands of residents at a correctional institution, many of whom were narcotic addicts. He noted that this atypical lesion "covers a larger area of the tooth than does the usual crescent-shaped, gumline cavity and is much darker in color than typical carious lesions, frequently being black. . . . Also, the lesion feels harder than conventional caries and clinically is less pain-producing upon probing." These early descriptions of the clinical picture of root caries characterize the more chronic and advanced forms of root caries found in special population groups and are most insightful from a clinical perspective.

Numerous epidemiologic surveys on root caries conducted in the 1970s and 1980s have collectively provided a clinical description of early and moderately advanced root caries. Table 9-2 presents a summary of the characteristics attributed to root caries from some selected clinical investigations. It is readily apparent that there is no consensus;

indeed, there is a difference of opinion with respect to whether lesions that involve the cementoenamel junction and the adjacent enamel should be classified as root or coronal caries. In the absence of definitive criteria, most epidemiologic surveys take a conservative approach with a preference to slightly underestimate the disease and therefore to be reticent in classifying lesions with any involvement of the enamel as root caries. Although root caries is commonly referred to as a "lesion," it is not at all clear whether cavitation or loss of surface continuity is involved in all cases. Furthermore, even though these investigators are in unanimous agreement about root caries being "soft," softness is a tactile phenomenon that is subject to wide interpretation, especially when the hard tissues involved in root caries are soft compared to enamel. In other words, how soft must an area of root surface be to be carious?

Billings[16] expanded the criteria to include surface cavitation so that root lesions can more objectively be assigned to treatment regimes. His root surface caries severity index takes into account surface texture, surface defect, and pigmentation as follows:

### ROOT SURFACE CARIES SEVERITY INDEX
*Grade I (incipient)*
1. Surface texture: soft, can be penetrated with a dental explorer
2. No surface defect
3. Pigmentation: variable, light tan to brown

*Grade II (shallow)*
1. Surface texture: soft, irregular, rough, can be penetrated with a dental explorer
2. Surface defect (less than 0.50 mm in depth)
3. Pigmentation: variable, tan to dark brown

*Grade III (cavitation)*
1. Surface texture: soft, can be penetrated with a dental explorer
2. Penetrating lesion, cavitation present (greater than 0.50 mm in depth), no pulpal involvement
3. Pigmentation: variable, light brown to dark brown

*Grade IV (pulpal)*
1. Deeply penetrating lesion with pulpal or root canal involvement
2. Pigmentation: variable, brown to dark brown

Regardless of the criteria used, to accurately measure the occurrence of root caries in individual patients and population groups, one needs to make two important clinical decisions. The first involves what root surfaces are at risk. Caries occurs on root

**Table 9-2** Criteria used to describe root caries

| Investigator | Location | Visual | Tactile |
|---|---|---|---|
| Hazen et al., 1973[40] | Anywhere on the root surface | Progressive lesion | Soft |
| Sumney et al., 1973[87] | On the root surface below the CEJ but not involving the enamel | Shallow, ill-defined cavitation, usually discolored | Softened |
| Hix and O'Leary, 1976[42] | On the root surface and may or may not involve the adjacent enamel | Well-established, discolored cavitation | Explorer point easily inserted with moderate finger pressure |
| Banting et al., 1980[8] | At the CEJ or wholly on the root surface | Discrete, well-defined, discolored soft area | Explorer enters easily and displays some resistance to withdrawal |
| Katz et al., 1982[55] | Totally confined to the root surface or involving the undermining of enamel | Progressive, destructive lesion | Soft |
| Vehkalahti et al., 1983[96] | More than half the lesion is located on the cementum | Lesion | Soft |
| Beck et al., 1985[15] | Half the lesion extends apically to the CEJ | Lesion | Soft and could be penetrated easily with an explorer |

*CEJ*, Cementoenamel junction.

surfaces only when there has been loss of periodontal attachment (that is, apical migration of the periodontal attachment from the cementoenamel junction. The *root caries index* proposed by Katz[51] defines a root surface at risk as one where the cementoenamel junction can be visualized. However, several investigators[23,61,84] have shown that 10% to 20% of root caries lesions occur subgingivally. Therefore, use of gingival recession as the criterion of risk results in an overestimate of the occurrence of root caries.

The second decision is whether to include roots with restorations present as being at risk. The root surface caries index does not specify whether root surfaces with restorations are at risk. It is obvious that the cementoenamel junction is not visible on these surfaces, yet they are exposed to the oral environment and are therefore at risk of primary or recurrent caries, most likely the latter. Although surveys of root caries can be found to both include and exclude restorations on the root surface in the computation of root caries rates, restorations on the root surface are at risk of recurrent caries and should be counted. Between 50% and 75% of decayed and filled root surface scores are accounted for by the filled component,[27,60] and many facial root restorations were likely placed because of abrasion rather than root caries. Failing to include restored root surfaces in counts of prevalence or incidence would seriously underestimate the disease.[84] However, inclusion of restored facial root surfaces must be carefully considered before one interprets them as root caries experience.[28] The effects of lack of consensus regarding the diagnosis of root caries is well illustrated in a recent review by Aherne et al.[2]

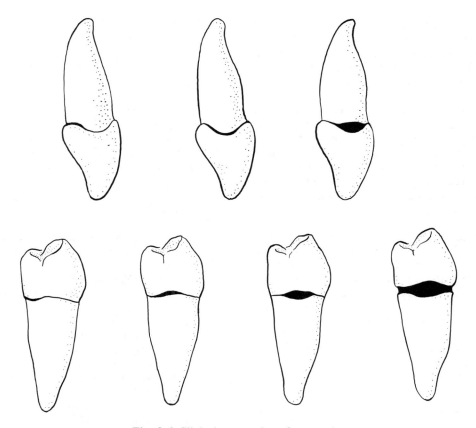

**Fig. 9-6** Clinical progression of root caries.

## CLINICAL DIAGNOSIS OF ROOT CARIES

Caries may occur on any tooth root surface where there has been loss of periodontal attachment (apical recession from the cementoenamel junction). Generally, caries on root surfaces occurs coronally to the gingival margin but approximately 10% to 20% of root caries are found in the gingival pocket. Although all exposed root surfaces are susceptible, it has been reported that caries predominantly occur on the proximal and buccal surfaces.

Root caries usually starts at or just below the cementoenamel junction (CEJ). Most commonly, early root caries lesions are small, round, shallow, pigmented defects on the root surface. However, they often spread laterally along the CEJ, sometimes coalescing with neighboring lesions to produce a gutter or even a collar of caries around the root (Fig. 9-6). Caries that begins on a root surface does not normally affect the adjacent enamel surface directly. Rather, it may undermine the cervical enamel but remain in coronal dentin, leaving a cervical enamel spur or ledge. If the caries process continues, pieces of this ledge may fracture, making it appear as if caries had originated in the enamel as well as the cementum. The opposite sequence can occur as well, with cervical coronal caries spreading apically to involve the CEJ and then the root surface.

## MEASURING ROOT CARIES

The Planning Committee, which is developing a national dental epidemiology project for Canada, has recommended an adaptation of Billings' root caries severity index for use in large population surveys. Using some suggestions from Katz,[53] the committee has developed guidelines for diagnosing and recording root caries. These guidelines take into consideration the practical issues and concessions required for clinical epidemiologic research.

When root caries is being assessed, each tooth is considered to have four root surfaces, irrespective of the number of roots. These surfaces are lingual, labial, mesial, and distal. All portions of a tooth's root surface should be carefully examined, including subgingival and restored areas. The most difficult areas to examine are approximal surfaces in posterior teeth, particularly those that contain restorations.

Third molars should not be included. As with coronal caries, the examination should start with the upper left central incisor and proceed distally through the second molar. The same procedure is followed in sequence for the upper right, lower left, and lower right quadrants. The examiner should examine the root surfaces in the following order: lingual, labial, mesial, and distal. Mobile teeth are to be scored in the usual manner.

The suggested clinical criteria for root caries are as follows:

### Active root caries

#### Incipient

1. Surface texture: soft, can be penetrated with a dental explorer
2. Cavitation: surface defect less than 0.50 mm in depth
3. Pigmentation: amber to brown

#### Gross lesion

1. Surface texture: soft, can be penetrated with a dental explorer
2. Cavitation: surface defect greater than 0.50 mm in depth
3. Pigmentation: amber to brown

### Arrested root caries

1. Surface texture: hard, smooth, polished appearance, not easily penetrated with a dental explorer, no resistance to removal
2. Cavitation: surface defect present
3. Pigmentation: brown to black

## SPECIAL CONDITIONS

The following conventions should be used when one is diagnosing and recording root caries:

1. When the coronal and root surfaces are both affected by a single lesion, it will be necessary to determine whether the lesion originated on the root or the crown. If more than half the lesion is below the CEJ, the site of origin is assumed to be on the root surface. If the site of origin is determined to be on the crown, no call is made for root caries. When the lesion appears to affect the root and coronal surfaces equally, both surfaces should be scored as being carious.

2. When there is a retained root, all four root surfaces should be recorded as being carious.

3. When a root surface contains both a carious lesion and a separate restoration, both are scored as being present. However, if the caries is contiguous with the restoration, "recurrent caries" is what it is called. It is possible but rare to have all three conditions on the same surface. For example, a root surface with a sound restoration, a new lesion, and a second restoration with recurrent decay would be coded for all three conditions. It is important to examine each filled surface for recurrent decay before one makes the final surface call.

4. When a filling or a lesion on a posterior tooth or a lesion on an anterior tooth extends beyond the line angle onto an adjacent surface, the adjacent surface is also included. However, a proximal filling on an anterior tooth is not considered to involve the adjacent lingual or labial surface unless it extends at least a third of the distance to the opposite proximal surface.

5. A deficiency in a root restoration (such as marginal defect) should not be scored as carious in the absence of definitive visual and tactile criteria for caries even though some restorative retreatment may be indicated.

6. If the diagnosis of caries—or filled—is uncertain, score the surface as sound.

7. When a coronal restoration extends onto the root surface more than 3 mm beyond the CEJ, the root surface is deemed to be filled. (Exception: cast crowns extending onto a root

surface are never recorded as filled for that root surface.)

8. Decay on the root surface associated with a coronal filling (such as a coronal restoration extending less than 3 mm onto the root surface) should be recorded as recurrent coronal decay.

9. Any root surface which appears sound but has more than 20% of its area inaccessible to clinical examination because of calculus or heavy plaque deposits shall be scored as unreadable.

## PREDICTORS OF ROOT CARIES

The absolute risk, or probability, of a disease is the number of new cases of the disease that appears in a population in a specified period of time.[35] The risk of root caries is therefore approximately 0.1 to 0.4 surfaces per person per year. However, clinicians and patients are usually more interested in explaining or predicting risk based on exposure to or possession of characteristics or factors, only some of which may be the source or cause of the disease. Many characteristics, both clinical and demographic, have been found to be associated with root caries, but Beck[13] makes the point that associations found between these variables and root caries as determined from prevalence surveys does not qualify them to be considered risk factors because they do not fulfill the requirements of causality. He prefers to label these variables as *potential* risk factors or risk indicators (that is, related but not causal). Table 9-3 presents the variables associated with the occurrence of root caries derived from several prevalence studies as determined by Beck.

Factors associated with root caries can be grouped according to their perceived mode of action. Banting[4] used a classification proposed by Susser[88] to group the variables associated with root caries into antecedent, intervening, moderating, and causal (Table 9-4). Grouping factors into these classifications helps in understanding where in the causal chain a given factor may exert its effect and the nature of the effect.

Multivariate statistical techniques have been employed in an attempt to determine the association or effect of a single factor or combinations of factors and to explain the variability associated with

**Table 9-3** Risk indicators for root caries from prevalence studies

| Risk indicators | Number of times measured | % factor found to be important |
|---|---|---|
| Age | 11 | 82 |
| Gender | 10 | 60 |
| Fluoride | 4 | 100 |
| Race | 2 | 50 |
| Microorganisms | 2 | 100 |
| Education | 3 | 67 |
| Income | 3 | 0 |
| Use of services | 3 | 100 |
| Brushing | 1 | 100 |
| Sugar consumption | 2 | 100 |
| Coronal caries | 4 | 75 |
| Plaque | 2 | 100 |
| Calculus | 2 | 100 |
| Loss of attachment | 2 | 100 |
| Number of teeth | 5 | 80 |

**Table 9-4** Factors associated with root caries by type

| Type | Factors |
|---|---|
| Antecedent | Oral hygiene and plaque |
| | Gingivitis |
| | Periodontal disease |
| | Coronal caries experience |
| | Root caries experience |
| | Number of teeth |
| | Systemic fluoride |
| Intervening | Diet |
| | Saliva secretion rate |
| | Saliva pH |
| | Saliva buffering capacity |
| Moderating | Age |
| | Sex |
| Causal | *Streptococcus mutans* |
| | *Lactobacillus* |

root caries prevalence rates. Banting et al.[8] used stepwise multiple regression to determine the influence of age, sex, number of retained teeth, number of retained roots, and decayed and filled coronal surfaces on the prevalence of decayed and filled root surfaces. The only significant partial regression coefficient was related to age, and only 9% of the variability of decayed and filled root surfaces could be explained by those particular variables. A discriminant function analysis was also performed on the same data. The number of retained teeth, decayed and filled coronal surfaces, and age each had had statistically significant ($p$ <0.05) discriminant function coefficients and could together correctly classify people with root caries experience and those without it 83% of the time.

Stepwise multiple regression procedures were used by Kitamura et al.[58] to test the relative effects of several potential risk factors. The variables with significant partial regression coefficients associated with root caries experience in the populations observed, using the root caries index as the outcome measure, were the number of teeth and the presence of calculus. These two variables accounted for 32% of the variance observed in root caries. The other four variables measured were domicile, oral hygiene, medications causing dry mouth, and number of medications taken daily. These four variables explained an additional 4% of the variation.

The dental component of the Mini–Finland Health Survey examined 5028 adults aged 30 years and over. A log linear model was used to define the importance of certain demographic and clinical factors relative to the prevalence of root caries.[94] Age, sex, region of domicile, number of teeth, and depth of periodontal pockets were defined as the predictor variables. Positive associations were found between root caries occurrence and age, region, and periodontal condition. However, interactions occurred among the variables such that root caries occurrence could not be determined reliably by use of each of the factors alone.

Burt et al.[23] developed a logistic regression model to examine potentially confounding effects among variables they measured and the presence or absence of root caries in subjects residing in communities with different levels of fluoride in the water supply. The potential risk factors measured were fluoride level, age, sex, ethnicity, education, number of teeth with recession, presence of plaque, presence of subgingival calculus and loss of periodontal attachment. The fluoride level, age, years of education, mean number of teeth with recession, and mean loss of periodontal attachment were determined to be statistically significant predictors of root caries ($p$ <0.05). Similar results were obtained with a linear regression model with use of the root caries index as the dependent variable.

Beck et al.[14] employed multivariate regression analysis to identify potential risk factors for root caries in a cohort of noninstitutionalized, older adults. A large number of independent variables gathered through personal interviews and clinical examinations were organized into physicomedical, social, behavioral, psychologic, and subsets of other dental conditions.

Multiple linear regression models were constructed separately for males and females with age and number of teeth with gingival recession forced into the equation. Factors that were not significantly related to root caries prevalence were removed from the model. The regression equation for males explained 33% of the variance in root caries with other dental conditions (number of teeth present and number of teeth with coronal caries) producing the largest partial regression coefficients. The regression model for females accounted for 51% of the variance in root caries. The variables with the largest effects were negative life events and the number of teeth with coronal caries. Regression models were also constructed by use of a dichotomized dependent variable (presence or absence of root decay). These models explained about the same amount of the variance for males but less of the variance for females. The variables that made the greatest contribution remained unchanged in both equations.

To be of practical use, predictive models of risk factors should explain at least 80% of the variability of root caries. According to this criterion only one of the models[14] was even close to being useful in terms of explaining the occurrence of root caries. It had a positive predictive value of 0.74 and a negative predictive value of 0.77.[13]

Incidence studies can estimate risk directly and, depending on the design, allow for the estimation of relative risk (that is, the risk in exposed persons compared to the risk in unexposed persons) or the degree of association of the causal and other factors with the occurrence of the disease. Existing data from animal models and in vitro experiments indicate that it is reasonable to hypothesize that root caries, like coronal caries, is a plaque-associated disease. Microbial plaque must colonize the root surface before the development of root caries.

Ellen et al.[32] sampled the dental plaque overlying noncarious roots of teeth and compared the isolation frequency and recovery of two suspected pathologic microorganisms—*Streptococcus mutans* and *Lactobacillus*— with the initiation of root caries over a 34-month period. The presence of both *S. mutans* and *Lactobacillus* organisms on the same tooth surface at the same time was the best discriminator between subjects who experienced new root caries and subjects who remained root caries free. More than 80% of root surfaces with both *S. mutans* and *Lactobacillus* present at the first plaque-sampling session belonged to subjects who subsequently developed root caries. The relative risk of root caries was found to be 0.88 when only *Lactobacillus* was present, 3.38 when only *S. mutans* was present, and 4.96 when both were present.

Differences between groups of subjects who developed root caries over an 8-year period and those who did not were measured for salivary *Lactobacillus* counts, salivary *Streptococcus mutans* counts, plaque scores, salivary secretion rate, salivary buffer rate, oral sugar clearance time, dietary habits, and age.[74] Salivary counts of *S. mutans* and *Lactobacillus,* plaque score, and dietary habits differed significantly between groups of subjects who had developed no root caries and those who developed root caries on more than 5% of the root surfaces at risk. A positive correlation was found between dental caries scores at the time of treat-

ment and the incidence of new root caries. At the 4-year examination, only the *Lactobacillus* counts differed significantly between the two groups.[73]

No primary risk factor was identified, and a causal relationship was not being tested in a study by Kohout et al.,[59] who analyzed incidence data derived from 447 older adult subjects followed for 18 months. Because sex was found to interact with many other variables, separate sex-specific regression equations were developed. The subject's age, number of root surfaces at risk, prior caries experience, fluoridation history, and examiner effects were controlled and three classes of other variables were entered into the equation. For males, the number of pockets, gingival bleeding, physical stress, angina, fingernail and toe problems, social contacts, anxiety, and use of smokeless tobacco were all significant ($p < 0.05$) effects and explained 60% of the variance of root caries. For females, number of periodontal pockets, amount of saliva, physical stress, phlegm production, and social participation were significant predictor variables accounting for 40% of the root caries variation.

The only study that provides information regarding true risk factors is by Ellen et al.[32] Banting[5] has further analyzed the data from this study limiting the analysis to a 24-month observation period. The incidence rate of root caries attributed to the presence of *S. mutans* in 45 subjects was 0.53. The association between the presence of the microorganism and the occurrence of the disease was statistically significant, and the odds of a subject experiencing root caries with the microorganism pres-

**Table 9-5** Incidence of root caries associated with the presence of selected microorganisms, 24 months

| Microorgansim | Present or absent | N | % with root caries | Fisher exact *p*-value | Odds ratio |
|---|---|---|---|---|---|
| *Streptococcus* | Present | 8 | 75 | 0.008 | 10.71 |
| *mutans* | Absent | 32 | 22 | | |
| *Streptococcus* | Present | 31 | 29 | 0.44 | 0.51 |
| *sanguis* | Absent | 9 | 44 | | |
| *Actinomyces* | Present | 37 | 32 | 1.00 | 1.44 |
| *viscosus* | Absent | 3 | 33 | | |
| *Actinomyces* | Present | 15 | 13 | 0.15 | 0.24 |
| *naeslundii* | Absent | 23 | 39 | | |
| *Lactobacillus* | Present | 12 | 42 | 0.48 | 1.79 |
| | Absent | 28 | 29 | | |

ent compared to someone who does not have the microorganism present was 10.7:1 (Table 9-5). When both *S. mutans* and *Lactobacillus* were recovered from the root surface, the odds ratio was 24.0. None of the other factors measured (age, sex, number of teeth, number of decayed and filled coronal surfaces, number of decayed and filled root surfaces, gingival pocket depth, gingival recession, gingivitis, between-meal snacks, and medications affecting salivary flow) were associated with the incidence of root caries in any clinically or statistically significant way.

Unfortunately, the above findings may not necessarily apply to the healthy, ambulatory adult patient in a private dental office. However, assuming that salivary microbiologic counts are correlated with root plaque microbiologic counts and that the oral microorganisms resident in the mouths of chronically ill patients do not differ significantly in virulence or pathogenicity from those of dental office patients, one can apply this information in a clinical situation to predict root caries.

There is now available a simple, chairside test for the presence of *S. mutans*.[50] The presence of this microorganism (particularly in high numbers) in a patient's saliva as determined by the test would indicate a high likelihood that the patient is at risk of root caries (Fig. 9-7).

The positive predictive value (that is, the proportion of subjects with a positive test who develop root caries) of root plaque yielding *Streptococcus mutans* is 0.75.[5] When two consecutive positive cultures are found, the positive predictive value of the test increases to 0.83. Jordan et al.[50] have already established a high correlation between a positive chairside test and a positive test using a standard selective medium for *S. mutans*. A positive saliva test (50,000 microorganisms or more) should invoke in the dentist a high index of suspicion regarding the patient's susceptibility to root caries. Other factors, such as oral hygiene, diet, and use of caries-preventive materials, would obviously reduce or intensify the risk.

## RESTORATIVE MATERIALS

There are several dental materials that are used to restore root caries. The critical factors that influence the choice of material include the patient's physical condition and compliance, esthetics, moisture control, the location and extent of the cavity preparation, and the patient's or caregiver's ability to perform adequate oral hygiene. Cost considerations are infrequently encountered because gold restorations on the roots of teeth are rarely prescribed for the older patient.

The materials currently suggested for use in restoring root caries are reinforced zinc oxide and eugenol cement, amalgam, composite resin, and glass-ionomer cement. The latter two materials can be used in combination.[3,89] The major advantages and disadvantages of these materials for restoring root caries are listed in Table 9-6.

The glass-ionomer cements are highly recommended for the restoration of root surfaces because of their ability to adhere to dentin through chelation

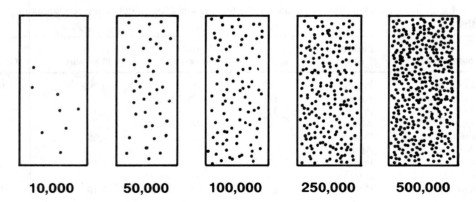

| 10,000 | 50,000 | 100,000 | 250,000 | 500,000 |

**Fig. 9-7** Cariescreen colony-density comparison chart.

**Table 9-6** Advantages and disadvantages of selected restorative materials for restoring root caries

| Material | Advantages | Disadvantages |
|---|---|---|
| Reinforced zinc oxide–eugenol cement | Easily placed<br>Stimulates pulpal repair<br>Anticariogenic | Limited durability<br>Unesthetic<br>Plaque retentive |
| Amalgam | Easy to manipulate<br>Stable | Unesthetic<br>Corrosive<br>Microleakage/secondary caries |
| Composite resin | Esthetic<br>Can bond to enamel<br>Smooth surface | Microleakage/secondary caries |
| Glass-ionomer cement | Chemical bond to dentin<br>Fluoride released | Technique sensitive<br>Extended maturation time<br>Low translucency<br>Brittleness<br>Poor abrasion resistance |

---

### GUIDELINES FOR THE TREATMENT OR RESTORATION OF ROOT SURFACE DENTAL CARIES

**Polishing only**

*Indications*: Grade I (incipient) lesions (no surface defect)

*Materials*: Flexible polishing disks and prophylaxis paste

*Advantages*: Noninvasive

*Limitations*: Access can be problematic, especially on interproximal surfaces

*Adjunctive treatment*: Topical fluoride

**Recontouring and smoothing**

*Indications*: Grade II (shallow) lesions (surface defect less than 0.50 mm)

*Materials*: Mounted abrasive points, fine diamonds, flexible polishing disks, prophylaxis paste

*Advantages*: Minimally invasive, no restoration required

*Limitations*: Access can be problematic, especially on interproximal surfaces

*Adjunctive treatment*: Topical fluoride

**Restoration**

*Indications*: Grade III (cavitated) lesions (surface defect greater than 0.50 mm)

*Materials*: Glass-ionomer cement, conventional finishing and polishing instruments and supplies

*Advantages*: Minimal preparation limited to removal of carious tissue, releases fluoride to surrounding tooth structure

*Limitations*: Access can be problematic, especially on interproximal surfaces and at margins of amalgam and cast restorations

*Adjunctive treatment*: Topical fluoride

---

and because they contain fluoride, which minimizes the risk of recurrent caries. These very desirable properties apply equally to all types of glass-ionomer cements. The categories of glass-ionomer cements include type I (luting and lining), type IIa (esthetic, low stress-bearing), type IIb (cores and high stress-bearing), type III (pit and fissure sealant) and type IV (light-cured).[92] Type IIb glass-

**Table 9-7** Restorative materials for root caries by cavity design

| Cavity design | Single material | Combinations |
| --- | --- | --- |
| Class III | Type II glass-ionomer cement | Type II glass-ionomer cement and microfilled resin |
| Class IV | Composite resin | Type II glass-ionomer cement and microfilled resin |
| Class V | Type II glass-ionomer cement | Type II glass-ionomer cement and microfilled resin |
| Proximal | Amalgam-ionomer mixture, or amalgam | Amalgam-ionomer mixture and amalgam |
| Recurrent | Type II glass-ionomer cement, or amalgam-ionomer mixture | None |

ionomer cements are combinations of metal fibers or powders, amalgam alloy powder, high-density sintered metal-glass powders, or mineral crystallites to glass-ionomer cement powder resulting in greater compressive and tensile strength and creep resistance where esthetics is not a primary consideration.[66,81] The recent introduction of light-cured glass-ionomer cements promises to further enhance the properties and manipulation of this restorative material. Some excellent reviews of glass-ionomer cements have just recently been published.[64-65,82,85,92-93]

In 1986, Billings[16] proposed restorative treatment guidelines for root caries based on the previously mentioned root surface caries severity index. He also advocated glass-ionomer cement for the restoration of root lesions (see box).

The recontouring and polishing of early lesions was first proposed by Banting and Ellen,[7] but subsequently Billings et al.[17] demonstrated that one can successfully manage minor root surface defects using topical fluoride alone. They also demonstrated that grade II (shallow) lesions that were treated by recontouring and polishing remained clinically sound for more than 4 years. The investigators make the point that it is neither necessary nor desirable to remove all stained dentin. The purpose of the recontouring and smoothing is to eliminate the soft, diseased dentin and leave a smooth, nonretentive surface.

Table 9-7 presents some recommendations for restorative material selection, either alone or in combination with other materials, for different cavity designs.

## CAVITY DESIGNS

Information on cavity design for root restorations is sparse. Al-Joburi and Jordan,[3] Suzuki and Jordan,[89] and Mount,[67] however, provide some description of a conventional cavity design for Class V restorations.

Most clinicians recommend conventional rotary instruments (slow and high-speed handpieces) with carbide or diamond burs to restore root-surface defects. Burs with long shanks facilitate the cavity preparation and caries removal in interproximal areas. However, a chemicomechanical method of caries removal has been successfully attempted on root surfaces.[91] With both methods, pain does not commonly accompany the caries-removal procedure even when the lesion extends well into the dentine.

Minimal removal of root tissue before placement of the lining and restoration is advocated for the restoration of root caries. Sheth et al.[80] recommend a shallow, nonretentive cavity form prepared with use of a spoon excavator to remove the soft decay followed by conservative caries removal with a round carbide bur in a high-speed handpiece using an air-water spray (Fig. 9-8).

They further suggest the use of beveled angles at both the enamel and dentin cavosurface angles. A light-cured dentin bonding agent is then applied in two coats to the dentin surface, and a light-cured, microfilled resin is used to restore the defect. These investigators followed 97 class V root restorations restored in this manner for 12 months and observed that only three (3.1%) had been lost and none showed any sign of recurrent decay. However,

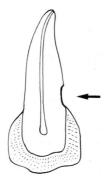

**Fig. 9-8** Nonretentive root preparation.

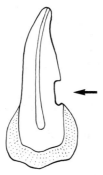

**Fig. 9-9** Retentive root preparation.

when significant dislodging forces are expected, they suggest undercutting the dentin and etching the adjacent enamel before placement of the restorative material (Fig. 9-9).

All the materials used in the restoration of root caries perform better if they are placed in a dry field. Use of a rubber dam is the preferred method of moisture control, but application of a rubber dam is often not possible, particularly when a root lesion is subgingival. For class V lesions Al-Joburi and Jordan[3] and Suzuki and Jordan[89] recommend the use of a No. 212 clamp stabilized with compound. They also illustrate a composite resin restoration placed over a glass-ionomer cement lining after a 1-minute etching of both the glass-ionomer lining and the adjacent enamel with phosphoric acid. A bevel was suggested for the enamel cavosurface, whereas a butt joint was suggested for the dentin or cemental margin.

Battock et al.[12] and Rosen[77] provide some direction regarding the management of proximal root caries in posterior teeth. If a posterior tooth has no restoration involving the proximal surface or there is recurrent caries around in existing restoration extending onto the root below the cementoenamel junction, it may be more convenient and conservative to reach the lesion from the buccal or lingual aspect. After placing of a rubber dam secured by a No. 207 or 2A clamp, use a 170L bur to establish the initial outline form by guiding the bur perpendicular to the long axis of the tooth. The preparation is made into the form of a slot (Fig. 9-10).

Caries is removed with a spoon excavator or round bur, and undercuts are placed in the occlusal and gingival aspects of the slot for retention with use of either a 160L or smaller round bur. A flat wall should be maintained on the side opposite the access opening. Depending on the location and extent of the caries, the final outline of the preparation may vary (Figs. 9-11 to 9-13). Silver amalgam or a glass-ionomer cement containing amalgam, or both types, are recommended in these situations (see Table 9-7).

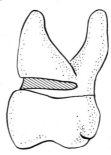

**Fig. 9-10** Mesial slot preparation for root caries.

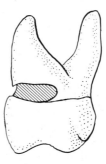

**Fig. 9-11** Mesial slot preparation involving more extensive root lesion.

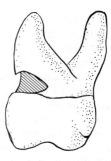

**Fig. 9-12** Root preparation involving adjacent surfaces, mesial view.

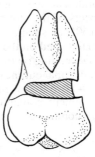

**Fig. 9-13** Root preparation involving adjacent surfaces, buccal view.

## PULP PROTECTION AND CONDITIONING OF HARD TISSUES

In all but the most minimal preparation, the pulp should be protected with a lining cement before placement of the permanent restorative material. Either calcium hydroxide or type III glass-ionomer lining cement, or both, can be used as root cavity liners. The advantage of the latter lining is that it can be etched to provide a better bond with a resin. If a type II glass-ionomer cement is used, no etching of the liner is necessary, but tooth sensitivity may be a problem.[24,85] Conditioning the dentin surface with 25% solution of polyacrylic acid for 10 seconds, or 10% polyacrylic acid for 20 seconds, removes the debris (smear layer) from the cut surface of the dentin leaving a clean, smooth surface, which maximizes the adhesive bond. A slurry of pumice applied with a rubber cup or a jet of water and cleaning powder followed by a thorough rinsing with water and moderate drying with an air

syringe also results in a smooth dentin surface and should precede the application of the conditioner.

If there is adjacent enamel and a resin is the material of choice, the enamel should be etched with 30% phosphoric acid for 30 seconds followed by a thorough rinsing with water.

## MATRICES

The finish of both composite resins and type II glass-ionomer cement is enhanced when a smooth matrix is employed. For light-cured materials, a Mylar strip or clear plastic crown form is necessary, but an opaque or soft metal matrix can be used with autopolymerizing materials. With type II glass-ionomer cement, the matrix should be held in place under light pressure for 3 to 5 minutes.

For interproximal restorations, the matrix should be stabilized with wooden or plastic wedges secured by compound or a pellet of cotton soaked in light-cured resin that is hardened after it is gently packed interproximally.

When the cavity preparation involves two or more root surfaces of posterior teeth, a hole cut into the middle of the matrix band will facilitate placement of the restoration (Fig. 9-14). Although this technique works well with amalgam and composites, which can be condensed or packed into the cavity preparation under pressure, it will obviously not work for light-cured materials or for type II glass-ionomer cements unless a syringe is used and the tip of the syringe is placed as deeply as possible into the preparation and slowly withdrawn as the material is expressed. The glass-ionomer cement begins to chelate immediately and will not flow readily. The glass-ionomer cements

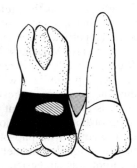

**Fig. 9-14** Matrix (with access window) placement for mesiobuccal root restoration in Figs. 9-12 and 9-13.

reinforced with amalgam are recommended for these types of restorations.

## FINISHING AND POLISHING

The finishing and polishing of type II glass-ionomer cements is critical to their esthetic appearance and durability. Because the maturation or setting of the material is prolonged, it is recommended that only gross flashing be removed at the insertion appointment. The final trimming and polishing should be delayed for at least 24 hours.

After the removal of the matrix, the glass-ionomer restoration should immediately be covered with a low-viscosity, light-activated composite resin and exposed to a curing light for 10 seconds to prevent moisture contamination and dehydration. After a 5-minute wait to allow for an initial setting of the material, any gross flashing can be removed with a gold-foil knife. The resin should be reapplied and the restoration left to mature for 24 hours. Final trimming of the restoration can be done with white stones lubricated with petroleum jelly[93] or an ultrafine diamond point under water spray. Flexible disks coated with aluminum oxide and lubricated with petroleum jelly can be used to produce a smooth surface where the restoration has been trimmed. The restoration should then be covered with a final coating of resin. The recommended procedures for glass-ionomer cement restorations for root caries are summarized in the box.

---

### SUMMARY PROCEDURES FOR GLASS-IONOMER CEMENT RESTORATIONS FOR ROOT CARIES

**Cavity preparation**

Use a stabilized rubber dam whenever possible.

Remove all caries with a large, round bur in the slow handpiece.

Undercut the gingival and occlusal borders (and mesial and distal borders if possible) for retention.

Bevel the enamel cavosurface margin and leave the dentin or cementum margin as a butt joint.

Clean the cavity preparation with a slurry of pumice followed by 10% polyacrylic acid applied for 20 seconds with a cotton pellet.

Rinse with water and dry (but do not dehydrate) the preparation.

**Lining**

Protect pulp with calcium hydroxide.

Clean dentin surface with pumice followed by polyacrylic acid.

Apply a type III glass-ionomer cement liner to all exposed dentin.

**Filling material**

Prepare a type IIa or IIb glass-ionomer restorative cement according to the manufacturer's instructions.

Insert the material into the preparation using the applicator syringe or spatula and secure with a Mylar or soft metal matrix applying light pressure.

Remove the matrix after 3 to 5 minutes and immediately cover the restoration with a low-viscosity, light-activated composite resin.

Expose to a curing light for 10 seconds.

Allow glass-ionomer material to cure for 5 minutes.

**Finishing**

Remove any gross flashing of material with a gold-foil knife and, if required, adjust occlusion with a round bur.

Immediately reapply resin.

Leave the restoration for at least 24 hours.

Trim the margins of the restoration with finishing burs (12 fluted and 30 fluted), white stones, or ultrafine diamond points under water spray or with lubrication.

Polish margins with flexible polishing disks lubricated with petroleum jelly.

Apply resin to the finished restoration and expose it to the curing light for 10 seconds.

NOTE: If a rubber dam is applied over an existing glass-ionomer restoration, it should be protected from dehydration with petroleum jelly (Vaseline).

## PREVENTION

Since the occurrence of root caries is largely dependent on the strength of the caries challenge (diet and bacteria) and the duration of that challenge, the approach to the prevention of dental caries in older adults involves three basic procedures: elimination of the parasite, increasing the resistance of the host, and reducing the availability of substrate for the parasite. Ideally, all three procedures should be initiated at the same time for maximum benefit, though the circumstances of the person will determine the sequence and which combination is actually employed.

Elimination of the parasite (the microflora attached to the tooth root surface) can most readily be achieved by use of either mechanical or chemical methods, or both. Toothbrushing and interdental flossing are the most commonly advocated measures of mechanical plaque control but are limited in the sense that the plaque is only temporarily removed or disrupted. The efficacy of these devices may be reduced when the older adult has a physical or mental disability such as arthritis, Parkinson's disease, or Alzheimer's disease. For many older adult patients who have not routinely used dental floss, the use of an interdental brush may be equally as efficacious and much easier to manipulate, particularly when there are large interdental spaces created as a consequence of gingival recession. Unfortunately, there are no studies reported to compare the efficacy of mechanical plaque control measures among younger and older persons. The clinical judgment of the dentist must determine whether mechanical plaque control is adequate or some form of supplementation is required.

Chemical plaque control is advocated as a supplement to mechanical plaque control in situations where the person cannot provide his or her own mouth care and must rely on a family member, friend, or health care worker for this component of personal care. The choice of agent and the period of application should be carefully determined based on the patient's physical limitations, ability to follow instructions, and accessibility to follow-up observation. Table 9-8 presents guidelines that can be helpful in making clinical decisions with regard to the need for and the type and length of application of chemical plaque control agents in older adults. The use of antibiotic drugs to control dental plaque

for other than exceptional cases is not advocated.

Clinical studies of the efficacy of chemical agents for dental plaque removal in adults, particularly older adults, are few in number. Banting et al.[6] reported a 35% reduction in supragingival plaque for adults using a twice-daily rinse containing 0.12% chlorhexidine over 2 years compared to controls. An even greater reduction in plaque scores was achieved in a 6-month study of a once-daily rinsing with 0.2% chlorhexidine in an institutionalized elderly population.[100]

Most older adults are quite capable of performing their own mouth care to an acceptable standard using conventional mechanical devices such as toothbrushes and dental floss. In specific cases, the introduction of special devices such as interdental brushes and floss holders will often facilitate mouthcare. However, there are occasions, particularly with institutionalized older adults, when mouthcare cannot be adequately performed by the patient. In these cases, the caregiver or a member of the patient's family must assume responsibility for this aspect of the patient's care. In these situations, the availability of chemical agents to assist with mouthcare is most helpful.

Occasionally an older adult patient will not be able to follow instructions concerning rinsing and spitting out. If a chemical agent is indicated as a supplement for mouthcare, it can be applied by the caregiver using a toothbrush cotton-tipped applicator or a foam-tipped applicator. However, care must be taken to ensure that the patient does not swallow large amounts of the material.

Increasing the resistance of the host usually refers to the fortification of the outer layers of the mineralized tooth tissues, namely, the cementum or dentin of the tooth root. Although there may be a role for a cementum or root-surface sealant, there is no commercially available product. Tooth resistance is most commonly enhanced through the application of fluoride either topically or ingested through the diet. Fluoride concentrates in the surface layers of the mineralized tooth tissues, particularly cementum, and decreases their solubility in weak acids.[10-11]

Although it has been demonstrated that cementum and dentin take up fluoride at an enhanced rate (when compared with enamel) resulting in a high surface layer concentration,[21] no statistically sig-

**Table 9-8** Guidelines for the use of chemical agents for dental plaque removal in older adult patients

| Situations | Amount and type | Duration |
|---|---|---|
| Subject is capable of performing his or her own mouth care adequately | No chemical agent is indicated | Not applicable |
| Subject is capable of performing his or her own mouth care, but results are poor and there is a chronic oral hygiene problem | 10-15 ml of 0.05% cetylpyridinium chloride or 0.06% thymol solution used as a mouth-rinse after assisted toothbrushing and interdental brushing | 20-30 seconds once daily for an indefinite period as a supplement to mechanical plaque removal |
| Subject is unable to perform his or her own mouth care because of a physical disability or mental incom-petence | 10-15 ml of 0.1% to 0.2% chlorhexidine digluconate used as a mouthrinse or brushed onto teeth using a toothbrush or interdental brush | 20-30 seconds once daily for an initial 3-month period, which may have to be continued indefinitely with close supervision |

nificant direct relationship has yet been shown between root surface fluoride concentration and the occurrence of root caries in persons.[75] However, the administration of fluoride, both topically onto the tooth root surface or systemically through the drinking water and diet, has been linked to lower rates of root caries in several populations. Ripa et al.[76] demonstrated an 18% reduction in the incidence of decayed and filled root surfaces over 3 years among employed adults 45 to 65 years of age using a daily 0.05% sodium fluoride mouthrinse. When only subjects deemed to be at high risk (that is, those with a previous history of root caries) were considered, significantly less (25%) new caries occurred in the mouthrinse group compared to the placebo group. A more dramatic reduction in root caries was shown by Jensen and Kohout[45] among volunteers 54 years of age and older who used a fluoridated dentifrice containing 1100 ppm fluoride on a daily basis. After 1 year, the test group had 67% less root caries compared to the group using the control dentifrice.

The beneficial effect of lifelong residence in a fluoridated community on the reduction of root caries prevalence has been clearly demonstrated. Burt et al.[23] compared the prevalence rates of root caries in adults who were born and had lived with only limited absences in optimally fluoridated (0.7mg/L) and high-fluoride (3.5 mg/L) communities. The root caries index (RCI) score was over 5 times greater in the optimally fluoridated community. Stamm et al.[84] observed substantially lower root caries rates among lifelong residents of a naturally fluoridated community (1.6 ppm F) compared with those living in a comparable nonfluoridated community (0.7 ppm F). A difference in root caries prevalence was found in virtually all age- and sex-specific groups. The proportion of subjects with root caries experience was 43% lower in the naturally fluoridated community.

Table 9-9 provides some guidelines for the use of topical fluoride preparations in caries-susceptible older adults. Initial and even advanced lesions can be arrested with topical fluoride therapy. The degree and location of remineralization, however, depends on the severity of the lesion.[79]

For patients with new or recurrent caries it is recommended that a saliva test be done at the baseline time and periodically thereafter to monitor the effectiveness of the therapy. If the *Streptococcus*

**Table 9-9** Topical fluoride regimes recommended for caries-susceptible older adults

| Clinical situation | Procedure | Vehicle and dose |
|---|---|---|
| No evidence of new or recurrent caries | No topical fluoride therapy indicated | Not applicable |
| Evidence of recurrent coronal caries | Semiannual topical fluoride with or without | 1.23% APF or 2.0% NaF gel |
| | Daily topical fluoride rinse | 0.2% NaF solution |
| Evidence of new or recurrent root caries | Semiannual topical fluoride with or without | 5.0% NaF varnish |
| | Daily topical fluoride | 0.2% NaF solution |
| Rampant coronal or root caries | Quarterly topical fluoride and | 5.0% NaF varnish |
| | Daily topical fluoride | 0.2% NaF solution |

*APF*, Acidulated phosphate fluoride; *NaF*, sodium fluoride.

*mutans* count is above 500,000, the use of a daily rinse containing 0.1 to 0.2% chlorhexidine digluconate is recommended for at least a 3-month period. If the bacterial count is dramatically reduced after 3 months, the chemical agent may be withdrawn. As the caries activity decreases, the more aggressive fluoride therapies can also be slowly but deliberately decreased. The judicious use of topical fluoride preparations combined with the appropriate chemical plaque-control agent will dramatically reduce the occurrence of root caries. When there is evidence of active caries, the use of a saliva test for *Streptococcus mutans* is highly recommended to monitor the efficacy of the preventive methods selected. Drastically reduced counts of colony-forming units (CFU) on the selective medium is normally associated with a reduced risk of caries. However, for any of the recommended procedures and agents to be optimally effective, all active caries (both coronal and root) must first be removed and replaced with permanent or temporary restorations, and all overhangs, defective margins of restorations, and other sites of plaque retention must be repaired.

The significant role that diet and reduced salivary flow can play in the caries process and the impact of these contributing factors should not be overlooked and should be carefully considered when one is implementing a program of preventive dentistry for older, adult patients. These topics are presented in considerable depth elsewhere in this publication.

## REFERENCES

1. Abbott F: Caries of human teeth, Dent Cosmos 21:177, 1879.
2. Aherne CA, O'Mullane D, and Barrett BE: Indices of root surface caries, J Dent Res 69:1222, 1990.
3. Al-Jabouri W and Jordan RE: Management of root surface caries. In Clark JW, editor: Clinical dentistry, Philadelphia, 1985, Harper & Row, Publishers.
4. Banting DW: Epidemiology of root caries, Gerodontology 5:5, 1986.
5. Banting DW: Factors associated with root caries initiation, doctoral dissertation, London, Ontario, 1988, University of Western Ontario.
6. Banting DW, Bosma M, and Bollmer B: Clinical effectiveness of a 0.12% chlorhexidine mouthrinse over two years, J Dent Res 86(spec. issue):1716, 1989.
7. Banting DW and Ellen RP: Carious lesions on the roots of teeth: a review for the general practitioner, J Can Dent Assoc 42:496, 1976.
8. Banting DW, Ellen RP, and Fillery ED: Prevalence of root surface caries among institutionalized older persons, Community Dent Oral Epidemiol 8:84, 1980.
9. Banting DW, Ellen RP, and Fillery ED: A longitudinal study of root caries: baseline and incidence data, J Dent Res 64:1141, 1985.
10. Banting DW and Stamm JW: Effect of age and length of residence in a fluoridated area on root surface fluoride concentration, J Clin Prevent Dent 1:7, 1979.
11. Banting DW and Stamm JW: Effects of age and length of exposure to fluoridated water on root surface fluoride concentration, Clin Prevent Dent 4:3, 1982.
12. Battock RD, Rhoades J, and Lund MR: Management of proximal caries on roots of posterior teeth, Oper Dent 4:108, 1979.
13. Beck JD: The epidemiology of root surface caries, J Dent Res 69:1216, 1990.
14. Beck JD, Kohout F, and Hunt RJ: Identification of high caries risk adults: attitudes, social factors and diseases, Int Dent J 38:231, 1988.

15. Beck JD, Hunt RJ, Hand JS, and Field HM: Prevalence of root and coronal caries in a noninstitutionalized older population, J Am Dent Assoc 111:964, 1985.

16. Billings RJ: Restoration of carious lesions of the root, Gerontology 5:43, 1986.

17. Billings RJ, Brown LR, and Kaster AG: Contemporary treatment strategies for root surface dental caries, Gerodontics 1:20, 1985.

18. Bowden GH, Milnes AR, and Boyer R: *Streptococcus mutans* and caries: state of the art. In Cariology today, Basel, 1984, S Karger, AG.

19. Bowden GHW: Microbiology of root caries in humans, J Dent Res 69:1205, 1990.

20. Bowen WH, Young DA, and Pearson SK: The effects of sucralose on coronal and root-surface caries, J Dent Res 69:1485, 1990.

21. Brewer KP, Retief DH, Wallace MC, and Bradley EL: Cementum fluoride uptake from topical fluoride agents, Gerodontics 3:212, 1987.

22. Brown LR, Billings RJ, and Kaster AG: Quantitative comparisons of potentially cariogenic microorganisms cultured from noncarious and carious root and coronal tooth surfaces, Infect Immun 51:765, 1986.

23. Burt BA, Ismail AI, and Eklund SA: Root caries in an optimally fluoridated and high-fluoride community, J Dent Res 65:1154, 1986.

24. Christiansen GJ: Glass ionomer as a luting material, J Am Dent Assoc 120:59, 1990.

25. Darby ET: The etiology of caries at the gum margins and the labial and buccal surfaces of the teeth, Dent Cosmos 86:218, 1884.

26. Davies GN: A comparative epidemiological study of the diet and dental caries in three isolated communities, Alabama Dent Rev 6:19, 1958.

27. DePaola PF, Soparkar PM, and Kent RL: The clinical profiles of individuals with and without root surface caries, Gerodontology 8:9, 1989.

28. DePaola PF, Soparkar PM, and Kent RLK: Methodological issues relative to the quantification of root caries, Gerodontology 8:3, 1989.

29. Donner A and Donald A: The statistical analysis of multiple binary measurements, J Clin Epidemiol 41:899, 1988.

30. Edwardsson S: Bacteriological studies on deep areas of carious dentine, Odontol Rev 25(suppl. 32):1, 1986.

31. Ellen RP, Banting DW, and Fillery ED: *Streptococcus mutans* and *Lactobacillus* detection in the assessment of dental root surface caries risk, J Dent Res 64:1245, 1985a.

32. Ellen RP, Banting DW, and Fillery ED: Longitudinal microbiological investigation of a hospitalized population of older adults with a high root surface caries risk, J Dent Res 64:1377, 1985b.

33. Emilson C-G, Klock B, and Sanford CB: Microbial flora associated with the presence of root surface caries in periodontally treated patients, Scand J Dent Res 96:40, 1988.

34. Fure S, Romaniec M, Emilson CG, and Krasse B: Proportions of *Streptococcus mutans*, lactobacilli and *Actinomyces* spp in root surface plaque, Scand J Dent Res 95:119, 1987.

35. Gordis L: Estimating risk and inferring causality in epidemiology. In Gordis L, editor: Epidemiology and health risk assessment, New York, 1988, Oxford University Press.

36. Gustafsson BE, Quensel C-E, Lanke LS, et al: The Vipeholm Dental Caries Study: the effect of different levels of carbohydrate intake on caries activity in 436 individuals observed for five years, Acta Odontol Scand 11:232, 1953.

37. Gustavsen F, Clive JM, and Tveit AB: Root caries prevalence in a Norwegian adult dental patient population, Gerodontics 4:219, 1988.

38. Hand JS, Hunt RJ, and Beck JD: Coronal and root caries in older Iowans: 36 month incidence, Gerodontics 4:136, 1988.

39. Hazen SP, Chilton NW, and Mumma RD Jr: The problem of root caries: 3. A clinical study, J Dent Res 51(special issue):no. 689, 1972.

40. Hazen SP, Chilton NW, and Mumma RD: The problem of root caries: 1. Literature review and clinical description, J Am Dent Assoc 86:137, 1973.

41. Hecht SS and Friedman JF: The high incidence of cervical caries among drug addicts, Oral Surg 2:1428, 1949.

42. Hix JO and O'Leary TJ: The relationship between cemental caries, oral hygiene status and fermentable carbohydrate intake, J Periodontol 47:398, 1976.

43. Hoppenbrowers PPM, Driessens FCM, and Borggreven JMPM: The demineralization of human dental roots in the presence of fluoride, J Dent Res 66:1370, 1986.

44. Ikeda T, Sandham HJ, and Bradley EL: Changes in *Streptococcus mutans* and lactobacilli in plaque in relation to the initiation of dental caries in Negro children, Arch Oral Biol 18:555, 1973.

45. Jensen ME and Kohout F: The effect of a fluoridated dentifrice on root and coronal caries in an older adult population, J Am Dent Assoc 117:829, 1988.

46. Jordan HV: Microbial etiology of root surface caries, Gerodontology 5:13, 1986.

47. Jordan HV and Hammond BF: Filamentous bacteria isolated from human root surface caries plaque, Arch Oral Biol 17:1333, 1972.

48. Jordan HV and Keyes PH: Aerobic, gram-positive filamentous bacteria as etiologic agents of experimental periodontal disease in hamsters, Arch Oral Biol 9:401, 1964.

49. Jordan HV, Keyes PH, and Bellack S: Periodontal lesions in hamsters and gnotobiotic rats infected with *Actinomyces* of human origin, Periodont Res 7:21, 1972.

50. Jordan HV, Laraway R, Snirch R, and Marmel M: A simplified diagnostic system for cultural detection and enumeration of *Streptococcus mutans*, J Dent Res 66:57, 1987.

51. Katz RV: Assessing root caries in populations: the evolution of the root caries index, Public Health Dent 40:7, 1980.

52. Katz RV: Development of an index for the prevalence of root caries, J Dent Res 63:814, 1984.

53. Katz RV: Clinical signs of root caries: measurement issues from an epidemiologic perspective, J Dent Res 69:1211, 1990.

54. Katz RV Newitter DA, and Clive JM: Root caries prevalence in adult dental patients, J Dent Res 64:293, 1985 (Abstr. no 1069).

55. Katz RV, Hazen SP, Chilton NW, and Mumma RD: Prev-

alence and intraoral distribution of root caries in an adult population, Caries Res 16:265, 1982.

56. Keltjens HMAM, Schaeken MJM, van der Hoeven JS, and Hendriks JCM: Microflora of plaque from sound and carious root surfaces, Caries Res 21:193, 1987.

57. Keltjens HMAM, Schaeken MJM, van der Hoeven JS, and Hendriks JCM: Epidemiology of root surface caries in patients treated for periodontal diseases, Community Dent Oral Epidemiol 16:171, 1988.

58. Kitamura M, Kiyak HA, and Mulligan K: Predictors of root caries in the elderly, Community Dent Oral Epidemiol 14:34, 1986.

59. Kohout FJ, Levy SM, Beck JD, and Hand JS: Predictors of root caries incidence in an elderly population, J Dent Res 66:325, 1987 (Abstr. no 1750).

60. Leske GS and Ripa LW: Three-year root caries increments: an analysis of teeth and surfaces at risk, Gerodontology 8:17, 1989.

61. Locker D, Slade GD, and Leake JL: Prevalence of the factors associated with root decay, J Dent Res 68:768, 1989.

62. Loesch WJ, Rowan J, Straffon LH, and Loos PJ: Association of *Streptococcus mutans* with human dental decay, Infect Immun 11:1252, 1975.

63. Lowenthal AH: Atypical caries of the narcotics addict, Dent Surv 43:44, 1967.

64. Lynch E and Tay WM: Glass-ionomer cements. Part III. Clinical properties II, J Irish Dent Assoc 35:66, 1989a.

65. Lynch E and Tay WM: Glass-ionomer cements. Part IV. Clinical properties II, J Irish Dent Assoc 35:75, 1989b.

66. McLean JW: Cermet cements, J Am Dent Assoc 120:43, 1990.

67. Mount GJ: Restorations of eroded areas, J Am Dent Assoc 120:31, 1990.

68. National Institute for Dental Research, US Department of Health and Human Services: Oral health of United States adults: national findings, NIH publ no 87-2868, 1987.

69. Newbrun E: Cariology, Baltimore, 1978, Williams & Wilkins Co.

70. Nikiforuk G: Understanding dental caries, Basel, 1985, S Karger, AG, pp. 60-82.

71. Nyvad B and Fejerskov O: Root surface caries: clinical, histopathological and microbiological features and clinical implications, Int Dent J 32:311, 1982.

72. Papas A, Palmer C, McGandy R, et al: Dietary and nutritional factors in relation to dental caries in elderly subjects, Gerodontics 3:30, 1984.

73. Ravald N and Hamp S-E: Prediction of root surface caries in patients treated for advanced periodontal disease, Clin Periodontol 8:400, 1981.

74. Ravald N, Hamp S-E, and Birkhed D: Long-term evaluation of root surface caries in periodontally treated patients, Clin Periodontol 13:758, 1986.

75. Retief DH, Wallace MC, Brewer KP, and Bradley EL: Relationship between cementum fluoride concentration and root caries experience, Gerodontics 4:28, 1988.

76. Ripa LW, Leske GS, Forte F, and Varma A: Effects of a 0.05% neutral NaF mouthrinse on coronal and root caries of adults, Gerodontology 6:131, 1987.

77. Rosen H: Repair of interproximal root surface caries in aging periodontal-prosthodontic patients, Int J Periodontics Restorative Dent 8:40, 1988.

78. Salonen L et al: Mutans streptococci, oral hygiene, and caries in an adult Swedish population, J Dent Res 69:1469, 1990.

79. Schupbach P, Guggenheim B, and Lutz F: Histopathology of root surface caries, J Dent Res 69:1195, 1990.

80. Sheth JJ, Jensen ME, Wefel JS, and Levy SM: Restoration of root caries with dentinal bonding agent and microfilled composite resin: 1-year clinical evaluation, Gerodontics 4:71, 1988.

81. Simmons JJ: Silver-alloy powder and glass ionomer cement, J Am Dent Assoc 124:49, 1990.

82. Smith DC: Composition and characteristics of glass ionomer cements, J Am Dent Assoc 120:20, 1990.

83. Socransky SS, Hubersack C, and Propas D: Induction of periodontal disease in gnotobiotic rats by a human oral strain of *Actinomyces naeslundii*, Arch Oral Biol 15:993, 1972.

84. Stamm JW, Banting DW, and Imrey PB: Adult root caries survey of two similar communities with contrasting natural water fluoride levels, J Am Dent Assoc 120:143, 1990.

85. Stanley HR: Pulpal responses to ionomer cements: biological considerations, J Am Dent Assoc 120:25, 1990.

86. Sumney DL and Jordan HV: Characterization of bacteria isolated from human root surface carious lesions, J Dent Res 53:343, 1974.

87. Sumney DL, Jordan HV, and Englander HR: The prevalence of root surface caries in selected populations, J Periodontal 44:500, 1973.

88. Susser M: Causal thinking in the health sciences, New York, 1973, Oxford University Press, pp. 111-135.

89. Suzuki M and Jordan RE: Glass ionomer–composite sandwich technique, J Am Dent Assoc 120:55, 1990.

90. Syed SA, Loesche WJ, Pape HL Jr, and Grenier E: Predominant cultivable flora isolated from human root surface caries plaque, Infect Immun 11:727, 1975.

91. Tavares M, Soparkar PM, and DePaola PF: Evaluation of a chemicomechanical method of caries removal in root surface lesions, Quintessence Int 19:29, 1990.

92. Tay WM and Lynch E: Glass-ionomer cements. Part I. Development, setting reaction, structure and types, J Irish Dent Assoc 35:53, 1989a.

93. Tay WM and Lynch E: Glass-ionomer cements. Part II Clinical properties I, J Irish Dent Assoc 35:59, 1989b.

94. Van Houte J, Jordan HV, Laraway R, et al: Association of the microbial flora of dental plaque and saliva with human root caries, J Dent Res 69:1463, 1990.

95. Vehkalahti MM: Relationship between root caries and coronal decay, J Dent Res 66:1608, 1987.

96. Vehkalahti MM, Rajala M, Tuominen R, and Paunio I: Prevalence of root caries in the adult Finnish population, Community Dent Oral Epidemiol 11:188, 1983.

97. Wagg BJ: Root surface caries: a review, Community Dent Health 1:11, 1984.

98. Wallace MC, Retief DH, and Bradley EL: Prevalence of root caries in a population of older adults, Gerodontics 4:84, 1988.

99. Wallace MC, Retief DH, and Bradley EL: Incidence of root caries in older adults, J Dent Res 67(special issue):147, 1989.

100. Yanover L, Banting DW, Grainger R, and Sandhu H: Effect of a daily chlorhexidine rinse on the oral health of an institutionalized elderly population, J Can Dent Assoc 54:595, 1988.

# 10

# Endodontic Considerations for the Older Adult

*Joseph I. Tenca*

It is universally accepted that in the future of dentistry, the number of geriatric, handicapped, and medically compromised patients seeking dental care will increase. Presently there are over 30 million people in the United States 65 years of age or older. The number is expected to increase to over 50 million in the next 30 years.[5] There have always been 70- and 80-year-old and even older persons, but there is now longer life expectancy to increasing numbers of people.[48] In addition, these older adults will in the future have more natural teeth than today's patient. This improvement will increase the demand and need for dental treatment. Dentists will be significantly affected by the modifications in treatment necessary for geriatric patients. These differences will become apparent upon initial contact with the patient whether by telephone or in person at the dentist's office. Time and length of appointments and accessibility to the office cannot be overlooked in the provision of service to these older patients.

Endodontic therapy, whether it is practiced by the specialist or the general practitioner, will be greatly affected by the projected increase in older patients. At present, approximately 85% of root canal therapy in this country is accomplished by the general practitioner. In the future, this percentage may be reduced because of more complex procedures, which will be treated by specialists. In this chapter, endodontic considerations for the older adult are discussed in order that the practitioner will be able to diagnose and treat endodontic problems in these patients successfully, thus providing them with quality care. Before endodontic treatment procedures in the older adult are discussed, it is necessary to understand the changes that take place in the dentin and pulp in aged teeth that will directly affect the endodontic treatment.

## DENTINAL AND PULPAL CHANGES IN THE OLDER ADULT

Chronologic aging of the dentin and pulp, as seen in the older adult, is similar to induced pulp aging that occurs mainly as a result of dental procedures and dental caries. Conditions such as abrasion, attrition, and erosion and periodontal disease may also contribute to induced pulp aging. Seltzer and Bender[37] have outlined the following age changes reported to occur in the dentin and pulp, all of which affect endodontic treatment:

*Decrease in cellular components.* The most prevalent cell in the intact uninflamed pulp is the fibroblast. As the pulp ages and circulation is reduced, these cells decrease in number. Odontoblasts exhibit degenerative changes as evidenced by more vacuoles in older cells. These cells eventually atrophy and disappear.

*Dentinal sclerosis.* Occlusion of primary dentinal tubules by aging is known as "sclerosis." With aging, it occurs consistently in the apical third of the root. Dentinal sclerosis also occurs because of caries and as a response to external irritations and drugs such as corticosteroids and calcium hydroxide.

*Decrease in number and quality of blood vessels and nerves.* The blood vessels of aged pulps

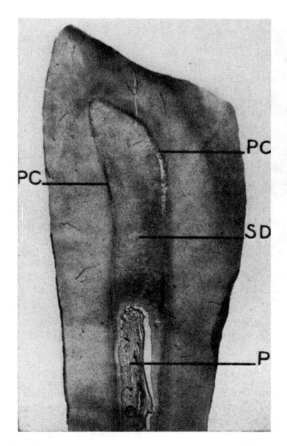

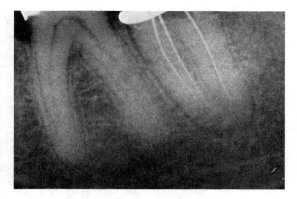

**Fig. 10-2** Mandibular first molar with secondary dentin formation resulting in a reduced pulp chamber. Second molar with apparent cementum deposition at the root apices.

**Fig. 10-1** Secondary dentin formation in mandibular incisor of older patient resulting in loss of pulp chamber and portion of root canal. *PC,* Original outline of pulp chamber; *SD,* secondary dentin; *P,* pulp. (From Boyle P: Kronfeld's histopathology of the teeth, ed 4, Philadelphia, 1955, Lea & Febiger.)

***Reduction in size and volume of the pulp.***
Secondary dentin formation, which is characterized by regular but fewer dentinal tubules, occurs throughout life and may eventually result in almost complete pulp obliteration (Fig. 10-1). This process may be accelerated by masticatory forces, which cause a mild irritation and could also result in dentin exposure. In maxillary anterior teeth the dentin is formed on the lingual wall of the pulp chamber,[30] whereas in molar teeth the greatest deposition occurs on the floor of the chamber.[40] The size of the pulp chamber is reduced in an occlusoradicular direction, which accounts for the loss of pulp horns in aged teeth (Fig. 10-2). As we shall see later, this directly affects endodontic access in the older adult.

Reparative dentin forms as a result of pulp injury, which may be attributable to caries, operative procedures, abrasion, and attrition. It is found in the root canals of all teeth that exhibit chronic pulpitis as well as teeth that are periodontally involved.[37] The tubules are irregular, decreased in number, or absent. These root canals become narrowed, but complete obliteration rarely occurs.

Pulp atrophy is characteristically seen in older adults because it occurs normally in aged pulps. Usually there is a relative increase in the number of collagen fibers, particularly in the radicular pulp, because of a decrease in the number and size of the cells.[7] Atrophy may also occur as a result of

often become arteriosclerotic resulting in a diminished blood supply, especially to the coronal pulp. These vessels can exhibit dystrophic changes such as deposition of free mineral deposits, which can result in complete obliteration.[3,4] There is also a decrease in the number of blood vessels in the teeth of older adults. Bernick[4] has shown that there is a pronounced reduction in the number of nerve branches in the aged pulp, especially in the coronal portion.

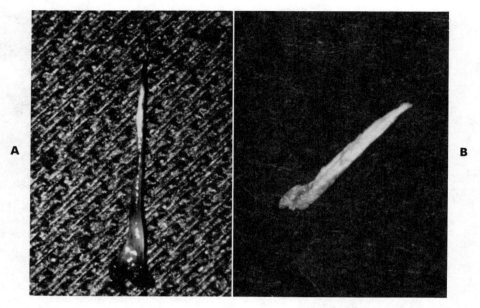

**Fig. 10-3 A,** Young pulp extirpated from maxillary anterior tooth. **B,** Mineralized, or "wooden," pulp removed from maxillary anterior tooth. (Courtesy National Naval Dental Center, Bethesda, Md.)

caries, operative procedures, and periodontal disease.

*Increase in the number and thickness of collagen fibers (fibrosis).* Fibrosis is increased in older pulps because of a reduction in pulp volume by the continuous deposition of secondary dentin.[47] It is also increased in the coronal pulp as a response to operative procedures, caries, and external irritants. In chronically inflamed pulps, fibrosis is increased and blood vessels are prominent and dilated.[37]

*Increase of pulp stones and dystrophic mineralizations.* Cellular degeneration and an increase in dystrophic mineralizations occurs in aged pulps because of alterations of the ground substance.[4] This probably occurs because of reduced circulation. The incidence of dystrophic mineralizations is also increased in pulps affected by caries, restorations, and periodontal disease.[3] A clinically completely mineralized pulp is hard and whitish and appears to be wooden in contrast to a young intact pulp (Fig. 10-3). In aged teeth, the condition is sometimes present in the apical portion of the pulp. During root canal therapy, it may completely block the canal and may be confused with blockage from debris or from dentin chips.

Now that we have seen the effect of aging upon the dentin and pulp, let us see how this affects endodontic treatment in the older adult.

## DIAGNOSIS AND TREATMENT PLANNING

History, clinical examination, clinical tests, and radiographs are essential elements in an accurate diagnosis. Accurate medical and dental histories are important, since elderly patients are prone to be medically compromised and usually have had more extensive dental treatment than younger patients do. A significant past medical history can alter the management or prognosis of an endodontic case. It is essential that the practitioner be aware of all medical complications including patient medications and that the necessary treatment precautions be undertaken. Drug interactions and exacerbation of chronic diseases must be avoided. Consultation with the patient's physician is more frequently necessary before beginning endodontic treatment.

A complete clinical examination is essential in older adults. The presence of sinus tracts must be noted, traced, and radiographed. The mobility of the involved tooth should be recorded. Pocket depth must be measured and documented because the probability of an endodontal-periodontal lesion is greater in the older adult. If present, the patient must be informed that the prognosis for a true combined lesion is not so good as that of an endodontic lesion with secondary periodontal involvement.

Pulp testing is an essential part of endodontic diagnosis. However, because of the pulpal changes in older adults as previously discussed, there may be no response to thermal stimuli or the electric pulp tester. Remember that the electric pulp tester tests the sensory nerve supply whereas vitality is dependent on blood supply. In the absence of other signs and symptoms, failure of the tooth to elicit a response does not necessarily indicate that the pulp is nonvital. Other factors that must be considered are radiographic changes, percussion sensitivity, and the presence of pain. A diagnosis of irreversible pulpitis, which is difficult in most patients, is more complicated in the geriatric patient. A chronologic record of dental procedures, history, duration and severity of pain, and method of onset are important in determining the need for endodontic treatment. It may be necessary to use so called last-resort tests such as the test cavity and the anesthetic test in determining the need for endodontic treatment.

Radiographs are an indispensable aid to an accurate diagnosis as well as to successful endodontic therapy. Although most pulp canals are wider buccolingually than mesiodistally in younger patients, this may not be true in older adults (Figs. 10-4 and 10-5). Often root canals in older adults tend to disappear apically on radiographs because of thinning of the canal and increased cementum deposition, which occurs throughout life. This should not be confused with the disappearance of a root canal radiographically when it splits into two canals

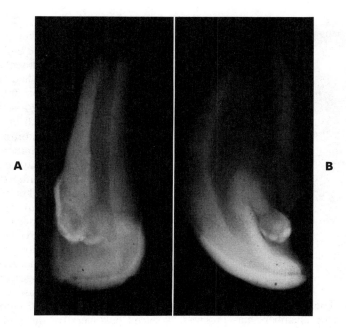

**Fig. 10-4** Extracted maxillary lateral incisor showing the narrow mesiodistal width of the pulp canal, **A,** compared with the broad buccolingual width, **B.** (Courtesy National Naval Dental Center, Bethesda, Md.)

A    B    C    D

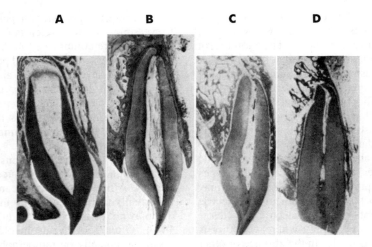

**Fig. 10-5** Narrowing of pulp canal system with advancing age. **A,** Age 8 years, open apex, wide pulp canal system. **B,** Age 14 years, root fully formed. **C,** Age 35 years, secondary dentin in incisal portion of chamber and narrowing of root canal system. **D,** Age 55 years. Advanced abrasion, secondary dentin deposition has narrowed the root canal system and reduced its length. (From Boyle P: Kronfeld's histopathology of the teeth, ed 4, Philadelphia, 1955, Lea & Febiger.)

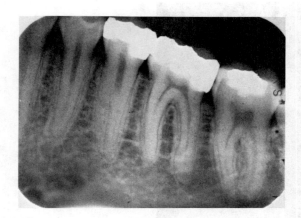

**Fig. 10-6** Disappearance of bicuspid root canal radiographically as tooth splits into two roots.

or roots (Fig. 10-6). The recession of pulp horns and the shrinking of pulp chambers may progress to the point where in older adults there is no radiographic evidence of any root canals, making diagnosis of pulpal conditions more difficult (Fig. 10-7, *A*). However, as previously mentioned, rarely is calcification complete and frequently the orifice can be found and instrumentation and filling of the canal can be accomplished (Fig. 10-7, *B* and *C*). Pulpal inflammation or pulpal necrosis, as evidenced by condensing osteitis, may be visible around the roots of teeth in elderly patients.[18]

Because of slight distortion of periapical radiographs, which makes interpretation difficult, the bite-wing radiograph may be a valuable diagnostic aid in the older adult with extensive prosthodontic coverage (Fig. 10-8). The use of a good magnifying glass is essential in viewing radiographs, especially when canals appear to be calcified.

Premedication for the older adult may be the rule rather than the exception. Elderly patients, who exert a great deal of energy coming to the dental office, will require longer appointments for endodontic therapy. The use of longer acting local anesthetics for profound pulpal anesthesia and reduced postoperative discomfort should be a consideration. One-visit root canal therapy may be preferable to multiple-visit endodontics in the older adult. After a careful review of various studies con-

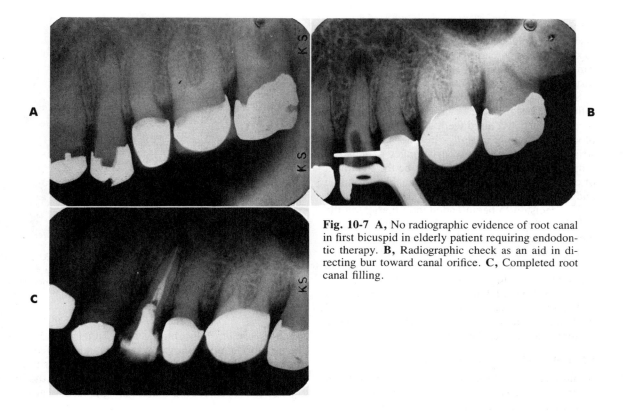

**Fig. 10-7 A,** No radiographic evidence of root canal in first bicuspid in elderly patient requiring endodontic therapy. **B,** Radiographic check as an aid in directing bur toward canal orifice. **C,** Completed root canal filling.

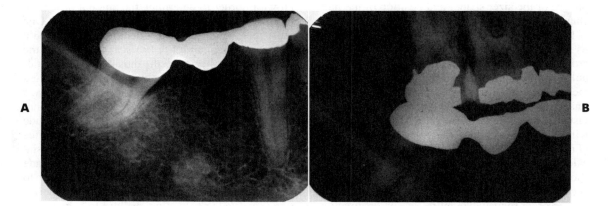

**Fig. 10-8 A,** Distorted periapical film of a symptomatic mandibular molar with pulp chamber partially occluded. **B,** Bite-wing radiograph of same tooth revealing large radiolucent area below the crown margin characteristic of carious lesion.

cerning one-visit versus multiple-visit endodontics, Osetek[29] concluded that there is sufficient evidence to support the contention that one-visit endodontics can be successful and that it does not necessarily result in a greater incidence of posttreatment pain.

Surgical endodontics in the older adult will be influenced by an increase in calcified canals, resorptions, and fractured teeth. Because of reduced blood supply, pulp cappings in older teeth are not so successful as are those in younger patients. A pulpotomy in the older adult may be the treatment of choice in a tooth that is not amenable to routine endodontic therapy.[18]

The decision to begin endodontic therapy in the elderly will more likely be influenced by other disciplines including prosthodontics, periodontics, and restorative dentistry. Certainly, consideration will be given to the restorability of the tooth to function and to the periodontal support necessary for successful endodontic therapy. The retention of endodontically treated teeth beneath dentures will be of major importance to the older adult in need of complete or partial dentures.

## ENDODONTIC ACCESS

A knowledge of pulp canal morphology is essential so that one design adequate endodontic access preparations. The preoperative radiograph must be examined very carefully, and a second radiograph taken from a different angulation may be necessary. Finally a bite-wing radiograph may give a truer picture of the size, shape, and position of the pulp chamber than a routine periapical film does.

In young teeth, the pulp chamber is large, and its shape is reflected in the external anatomy of the crown. In aged teeth, pulp horns are receded and pulp chambers are smaller in both buccolingual and mesiodistal direction because of the pulpal and dentinal changes of aging. The pulp chamber must be visualized in three dimensions. The outline form will be more ovoid than triangular in anterior teeth (Fig. 10-9). In all teeth with calcified or partially calcified pulp chambers, the direction of the root should be palpated. It may be advisable to begin access preparation before application of the rubber dam in order to visualize more clearly the direction of the canal in the root. Of equal importance in multirooted teeth is the usual procedure of directing the bur toward the largest canal first in hopes of gaining entrance to its orifice. The use of an irrigant

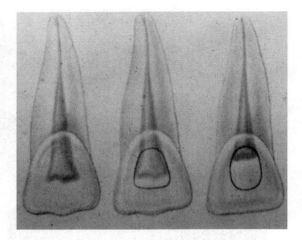

**Fig. 10-9** Outline form for endodontic access in older anterior tooth is more ovoid than triangular because of recession of pulp horns. (Courtesy National Naval Dental Center, Bethesda, Md.)

such as sodium hypochlorite is essential for adequate lubrication, removal of debris, and disinfection. Probing with a sharp endodontic explorer in the proper direction may be necessary to find the orifice to the canal. Additional radiographs may aid the operator in directing entry to the canal opening (Fig. 10-7, *B* and *C*).

For teeth with full-coverage crowns it may be helpful to remove the entire occlusal surface of the crown in order to determine the amount of natural tooth structure remaining beneath the crown. One must remove all secondary dentin within the pulp chamber being careful not to scar the floor of the chamber in posterior teeth, thus disturbing canal-orifice location. The objective of endodontic access preparation is to provide an unobstructed approach to all surfaces of the canal. Therefore access cannot be a static procedure.[49] Modifications may include enlarging the preparation and relocating the orifice in older curved posterior roots, such as the mesial roots of mandibular molars. The cuts are made away from the furca area allowing the operator to prepare curved canals with less danger of perforation and ledge formation. Failure to achieve the objective of unobstructed approach may result in incomplete débridement, improper shaping and disinfection, incomplete obturation of the canal space, and failure in therapy.

## ROOT CANAL PREPARATION AND FILLING

The objectives of eliminating all irritants from the root canal space and preparing the canal for filling in the older adult can be a challenging procedure. Because of the limited degree of opening in some older adults, it is wise to use a filling instrument of the shortest length possible in order to obtain the necessary path of insertion for proper canal negotiation. Tactile sense will also be improved by use of a shorter instrument. Because of limited openings it may be necessary to place the filing instrument in the canal orifice with the aid of a hemostat. Constant irrigation and suction and the use of a chelating agent, when necessary, will aid the operator in the instrumentation of fine canals. Rotary instruments such as Gates-Glidden drills should be used early in the preparation to widen the orifice and the coronal portion of the canal, thus facilitating the instrumentation and flaring of the canal. Binding of the upper half of an instrument in a thin canal will interfere with the reaming and filing action of the instrument in the critical apical third of the canal.

A step-back technique is essential for preparing curved canals, especially in the older adult. After the apical portion of the canal is prepared with curved instruments to at least a size 25, the next-sized instrument is placed in the canal 1 mm short of the working distance and worked in the usual manner with the aid of an irrigating solution. This procedure is repeated with the next-sized file working progressively away from the apex until preparation is complete. A return to the last file to the apex after each higher sized file and repeated irrigation will ensure patency. The canal will then be flared preparatory to filling.

The apical extent of root canal preparation and filling can be quite variable in older adults. The dentinocemental junction is formed by an invagination of cementum into the apical foramen, usually 0.5 to 1 mm from the anatomic apex. The ideal termination of a root canal filling is at this dentinocemental junction. In the intact uninflamed pulp, this is the narrowest diameter of the canal and is known as the "apical constriction." Several studies[9,17,23] have shown that the percentage of major foramina deviating from the anatomic apices is more than 50%, and this deviation of the apical foramen may be as much as 2 mm from the anatomic apex (Fig. 10-10).[17] Another study[25] has shown that in more than one third of the deviations the apical foramen opened on the buccal or lingual surface (Fig. 10-11). This location can be determined only with tactile sense. Grady and Clausen[16] have shown that the anatomic apex and the radiographic apex may not be the same (Fig. 10-12). Preparing and filling to the radiographic apex will

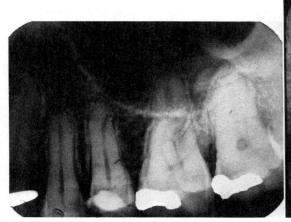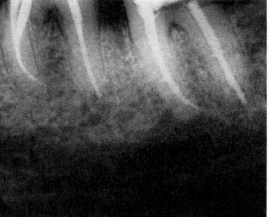

**Fig. 10-10 A,** Radiograph of maxillary second bicuspid showing apical foramen opening distally, well short of radiographic apex. **B,** Radiograph of mandibular molars with filled root canals shows similar situation in mesial roots.

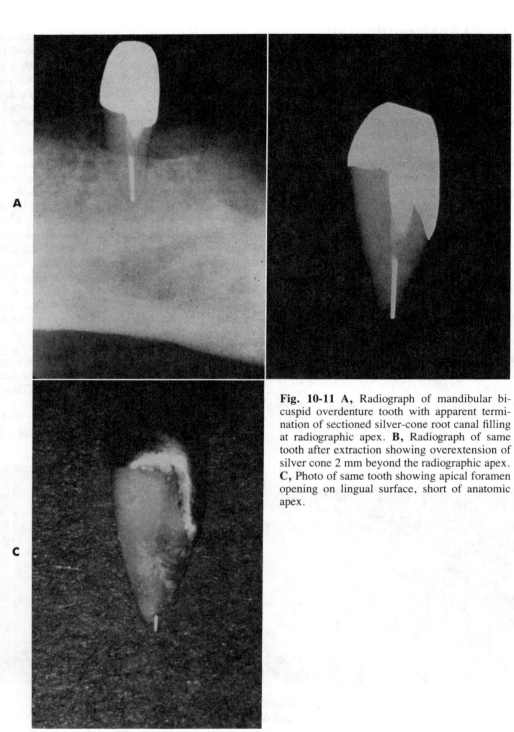

**Fig. 10-11 A,** Radiograph of mandibular bicuspid overdenture tooth with apparent termination of sectioned silver-cone root canal filling at radiographic apex. **B,** Radiograph of same tooth after extraction showing overextension of silver cone 2 mm beyond the radiographic apex. **C,** Photo of same tooth showing apical foramen opening on lingual surface, short of anatomic apex.

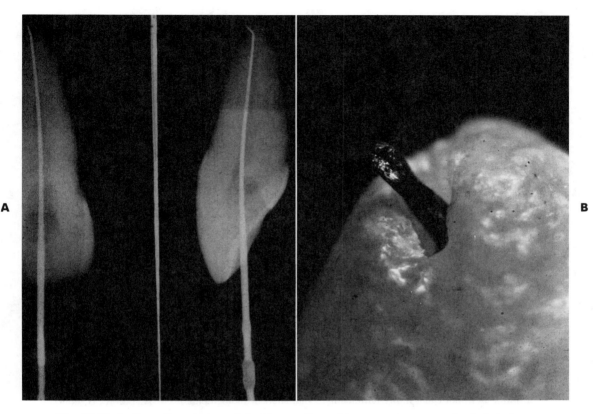

**Fig. 10-12 A,** Buccolingual view of the file at radiographic apex, whereas proximal view shows file exiting beyond apical foramen. **B,** Photo of same tooth with file extending beyond the apical foramen, which is well short of anatomic apex. (Courtesy Dr. John R. Grady, Lyndhurst, Ohio, and Dr. Howard Clausen, Newport, Rhode Island.)

result in overinstrumentation and overfilling a large percentage of the time.

The apical foramen can almost be obliterated by deposition of secondary dentin within the root canal and by deposition of cementum outside the root canal. Continuous dentin and cementum deposition throughout life will reduce the diameter of the apical foramen, but complete closure will not occur as long as the pulp remains vital. Aging, continuous cementum deposition, and mesial and occlusal drift will result in shifting of the apical foramen. Therefore the apical termination of root canal instrumentation and filling in the older adult may be shorter than the usual 0.5 to 1 mm from the radiographic apex (Fig. 10-13). Persistent attempts to

instrument and fill beyond this level may result in perforation, postoperative discomfort, and a greater chance of failure. The use of electronic measuring devices may be helpful in determining canal length in older adult teeth with cementum deposition, though inconsistency and inaccuracy have been reported with their use.[19] Provided that the canal is dry and no vital tissue is present, the patient who is not anesthetized for a root canal filling usually feels a mild sensation when the instrument or gutta-percha point passes beyond the apical foramen. Many patients prefer not to have an anesthetic during the root canal filling procedure once the rationale of not administering an anesthetic is explained to the patient. This is especially

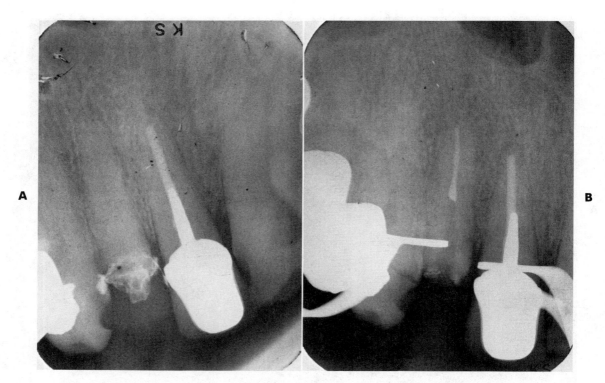

**Fig. 10-13** Cementum deposition at the apex of a maxillary lateral incisor in a 67-year-old patient resulting in a root canal filling terminating 2 mm short of radiographic apex. **A,** Before; **B,** after.

true in the older adult whose discomfort threshold is higher than the younger patient, probably because of less anxiety and fear.

Single-visit root canal therapy should be considered for the older adult for teeth with vital pulps, especially in teeth that can be prepared and filled short of the radiographic apex. Small, negotiable canals are also prime candidates for single appointment therapy. In a recent study, Goldman and associates[15] found that in 255 patients who had one-visit prophylactic endodontic treatment, there were only three flare-ups. This may be the treatment of choice for elderly patients who find it exhausting to travel to the dental office for treatment and for whom certain procedures, even isolation of the tooth, may be difficult.

Condensation of gutta-percha with sealer is the root canal filling of choice for the aged patient. Lateral condensation is preferred by most dentists.

However, caution should be exercised because the possibility of cracked teeth may be present. Rather than use lateral condensation on a tooth suspected of being cracked, the operator should consider the use of the warm gutta-percha diffusion technique or the use of injected thermoplasticized gutta-percha for filling root canals (Fig. 10-14). For teeth with pulp chamber access and calcified nonnegotiable canals, pulpotomy should be a consideration rather than root end filling. Frequent recall should be a part of the treatment plan to observe radiographic changes, which may necessitate surgical intervention.

## SURGICAL PROCEDURES

The number of endodontic cases requiring periradicular surgery has decreased dramatically in the past 20 years. More sophisticated instruments and materials, greater knowledge of root canal mor-

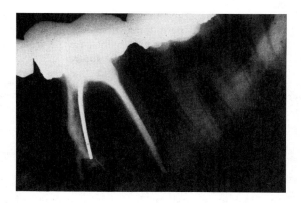

**Fig. 10-14** Lateral condensation of gutta-percha in mesiolingual canal resulting in fracture of a previously cracked mesial root. Procedural errors such as broken instrument in mesial root and overextension of gutta-percha in distal root are also evident.

phology, preparation and filling, and better endodontic teaching programs in our schools have contributed to this reduced need for surgical endodontics. However, the need still exists in certain situations, and it is expected to increase in the future especially in older patients. Nonsurgical endodontic therapy will continue to be the treatment of choice. However, there will be indications for surgical endodontics rather than extraction.

Certainly an increase in nonnegotiable calcified canals, pulp stones, and dystrophic calcifications will influence the need for periapical surgery (Fig. 10-15). Endodontic surgery will be indicated for retreatment of teeth with post and core crowns and for some teeth that cannot be retreated successfully nonsurgically, such as those with paste filling materials and irretrievable root canal fillings. Surgical procedures associated with periodontal disease

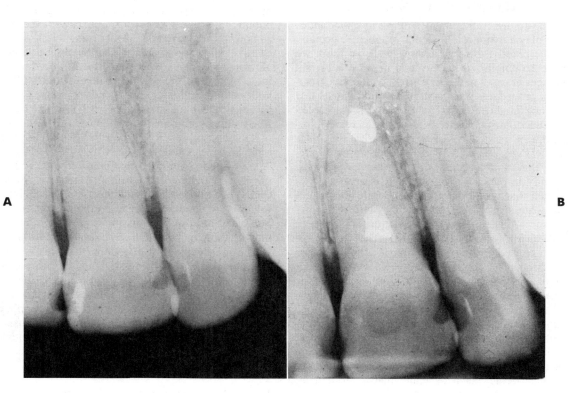

**Fig. 10-15 A,** Pretreatment radiograph of symptomatic central incisor with calcified canal. **B,** After futile attempt to find canal orifice, apex was sealed with amalgam, cement placed in apex, and tooth bleached and restored with composite.

will also increase in the older adult. The retention of strategic teeth may depend on root amputations and hemisections after the remaining roots are endodontically treated.

Furcation involvements, periodontal maintenance problems, deep interproximal root caries, fractures, and resorptions, many of which can be corrected by surgical procedures, are seen more frequently. However, remember that the contraindications and complications for endodontic surgery in the younger patient are accentuated in the older adult. There may be more conditions that complicate the surgical procedure and postoperative healing. However, with the proper precautions and more attention to the desires of the patient, endodontic surgery for selected cases may be less traumatic physically and mentally than tooth extraction.

## RETREATMENT PROCEDURES

In the future, retreatment therapy in endodontics will play a major role in dental practice, especially in the elderly. No matter how well we think we have accomplished our original therapy, a certain number of cases will fail. Current endodontic treatment procedures practiced by general dentists that are not taught in dental schools and not accepted by endodontists have resulted in an increase in retreatment procedures, especially with the older adult (Figs. 10-16 to 10-19). There are many factors that may account for failures. Most exist equally in patients of all ages. It is generally accepted that the primary cause of failure is an inadequate seal of the root canal system either because of inadequate instrumentation or failure to find all the canals (Fig. 10-17). The criteria for success used by most endodontists is the presence or absence of symptoms and evaluation of radiographs. When one is evaluating radiographs of the treated tooth, a case is considered a failure in need of retreatment if a lesion is present when none existed at the time of endodontic therapy or a preexisting lesion increases in size or does not appear to be decreasing in size after a reasonable length of time (Fig. 10-18). Some causes of failure are "dentistogenic" such as inadequate débridement, separated instruments, perforations, and overextended or underfilled root canal fillings resulting in a poor apical seal (Fig. 10-19). Morphologic variations may also contribute to failures as well as root fractures and periodontal disease. These entities account for most retreatment cases, a trend that will probably continue in the future.

There are some causes of failure that are more prevalent in the elderly. The presence of systemic disease such as diabetes, renal disease, blood dyscrasias, hepatic dysfunction, osteoporosis, and adrenal and hormonal disturbances may prevent or delay osseous regeneration and healing. The importance of obtaining an adequate medical history cannot be overemphasized, even when one allows for modifications in treatment, because it will aid the clinician in attaining a higher percentage of success thus keeping retreatments to a minimum.

A true failure in endodontics occurs only when the tooth is extracted. Most cases are potential failures. If we can determine the cause of the failure and treat the case accordingly, success is the usual result. Diagnosis and treatment planning of endodontic failures can be a frustrating experience and somewhat controversial.[8] Once diagnosed, most cases should be retreated nonsurgically, but there are some situations where a surgical procedure is indicated. With the use of a solvent, teeth filled with gutta-percha and sealer lend themselves well to nonsurgical treatment (Fig. 10-17, A). Teeth filled with a hard paste may require the careful use of solvents and rotary instruments. If teeth are not removable, endodontic surgery may be necessary. A well-fitted silver cone that is not visible within the pulp chamber is often difficult to retrieve. Some cannot be removed even with the use of specialized forceps, trephining drills, and tubular extractors. Sonic and ultrasonic devices may be helpful in removing these metallic and paste root canal fillings.

The management of endodontic failures is further complicated by the wide range of successful retreatment (53% to 91%).[14] This success rate is affected by variables as differences in technique, operator's ability and difficulty of the case, number of cases included with periradicular pathosis, length of observation period, and different interpretation of the criteria for success and failure.

## HEALING IN THE OLDER ADULT

Irreversible damage to the dental pulp results in a necrotic pulp and subsequent pathologic changes in the periradicular tissues. Normal healing of these

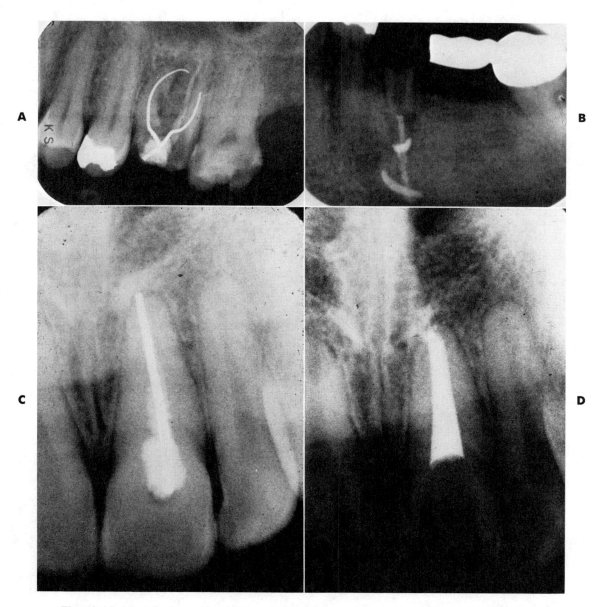

**Fig. 10-16 A** and **B,** Examples of unacceptable endodontic treatment procedures. **C,** Poor access and inadequate silver-cone root canal filling in this symptomatic discolored incisor. **D,** Retreatment with lateral condensation of gutta-percha.

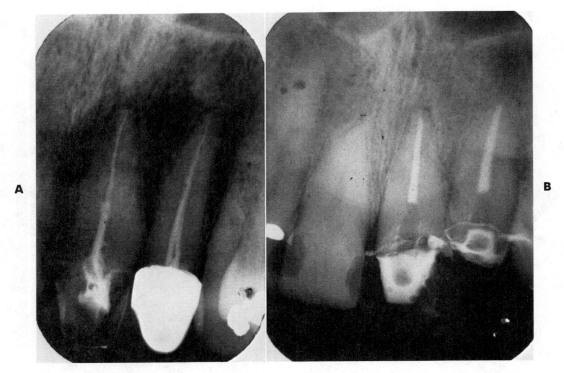

**Fig. 10-17 A,** Inadequate, poorly sealed gutta-percha root canal fillings. **B,** Retreatment with lateral condensation of gutta-percha.

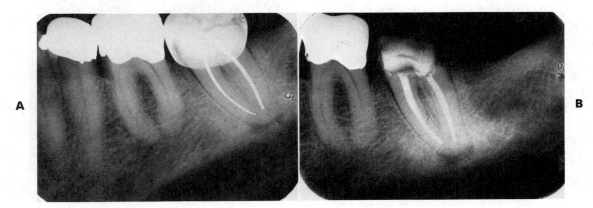

**Fig. 10-18 A,** Silver-cone root canal fillings with new periapical radiolucency. **B,** Retreatment with lateral condensation of gutta-percha.

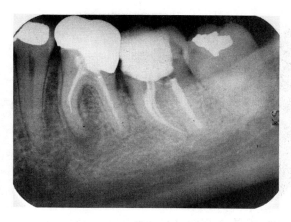

**Fig. 10-19** Endodontic failure in first molar because of inadequate instrumentation and separated instrument. Apparently successful root canal filling in second molar.

tissues depends on the complete removal of the irritant from the pulp spaces and the complete filling of the root canal system. This is the rationale of root canal therapy.

However, if all endodontic lesions healed completely, there would be no need for retreatment. Success depends on the repair of periradicular tissues injured either by the endodontic treatment, by the disease process itself, or by a combination of these elements. Both local and systemic factors influence the healing process. There is a direct relationship between the systemic factors influencing repair and the success of endodontic treatment.

According to Seltzer,[36] local factors influencing repair include infection, hemorrhage, and the physical injury to the periradicular tissues caused by instrumentation beyond the apex, decreased vascularization (as seen in older adults), and the presence of foreign bodies in the periradicular tissues. Root canal filling materials and sealers are the most common irritants found in the periradicular area, though separated instruments, amalgam fillings, cotton fibers, and paper points pushed beyond the apical foramen can also act as foreign bodies.

It has been shown that the percentage of clinical success is greater in teeth that have been prepared and filled short of the apex.[36] Sinai[42] has supplied histologic evidence to support these claims. The clinician should attempt to confine all preparation

and filling procedures within the confines of the root canal system and treat the periradicular tissues with tender loving care. Irritants, especially microorganisms, pushed beyond the apical foramen may cause acute flare-ups resulting in pain and discomfort and delayed healing especially where deceased host resistance and virulence of the organisms are contributing factors. Patients who are more likely to be susceptible to infectious agents and healing may be hindered by a reduction of nutritional factors necessary for healing. It is strongly recommended that root canals be prepared and filled at the dentinocemental junction or 0.5 to 1 mm from the radiographic apex in young teeth and probably more than 1 mm in older teeth because of cementum formation.

In the elderly, repair of tissues injured may be delayed but will occur in most endodontic cases (Fig. 10-20). In certain systemic conditions, endodontic therapy is preferable to extraction because of the greater risk of transient bacteremia.[1] Systemic diseases, such as tuberculosis and diabetes, if uncontrolled, will also interfere with the healing process. A controlled diabetic who is in need of endodontic therapy requires medical consultation and may require supplemental medications and antibiotic therapy. Blood dyscrasias such as anemia interferes with the healing of periradicular tissues.

Osteoporosis, a disturbance of bone matrix formation, may account for incomplete resolution of endodontic lesions. Osteoporosis is seen most frequently in postmenopausal women[36] where estrogen depletion hinders osteoblastic activity. In the patient who has had radiation therapy, nonsurgical root canal therapy is preferable to extraction or surgical endodontics because of the possibility of osteoradionecrosis. Even then, healing may be delayed or nonexistent because of reduction in the vascularization and subsequent decrease in circulatory elements and fibroblasts necessary for repair. Again, the risk of infection can be reduced by confining all instrumentation and filling within the confines of the root canal system.

The effect of stress and its relationship to healing is especially worthy of consideration. Selye's[39] general adaptation syndrome, which postulates that stress causes a reaction in different areas of the body, can result in delayed or nonexistent healing in the older patient, where irritants forced into

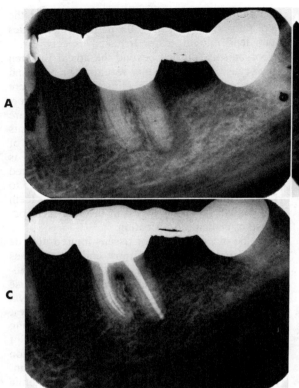

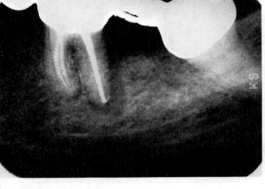

**Fig. 10-20 A,** Patient 81 years of age with lesion on molar abutment tooth. **B,** Root canal therapy completed. **C,** Recall radiograph 33 months later shows apparent healing.

## ENDODONTAL AND PERIODONTAL CONSIDERATIONS

Although periodontal disease can exist in both young and old patients, it is more prevalent in the elderly. Periodontics is closely associated with endodontics for many reasons. Biologically the tissues involved have a mesodermal derivation, and pulp tissue resembles periodontal ligament tissue in the apical area of the tooth. Retention of an endodontically treated tooth depends on the integrity of the periodontium. Cells in the periodontal ligament are intimately involved in periradicular repair. Communication between the pulpal spaces and periodontium exists via lateral and accessory canals and through the dentinal tubules.[46] Therefore the integrity of the pulp is of major concern in the treatment of advanced periodontal disease.[45]

Clinically it may be difficult to distinguish between pulp and periodontal disease, since the symptoms of mobility, swelling, and tenderness to percussion are common to both. The pulp test, which usually gives no response with a necrotic pulp, may also give no response with periodontal disease because of age changes. Although sinus tracts are usually of endodontic origin, they may also appear as a direct communication between the

the periradicular tissues can cause acute flare-ups. Comfort's[10] theory of aging known as the "wear-and-tear theory" could be likened to aging of the dental pulp where accumulation of irritants cause its death. Malamed[27] recommends a stress-reduction protocol for medically or emotionally compromised patients that if followed may help promote comfort and healing. This is especially pertinent to the repair of endodontic surgical cases, which are more stressful than nonsurgical ones.

The apical granuloma seen in many endodontic lesions is the body's first attempt at repair. The complete removal of the irritant found in the root canal system, through proper preparation and filling, will accelerate healing in most teeth in any patient, but in the elderly it may be necessary to provide additional therapy to promote the healing process because of medical complications.

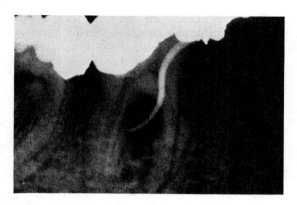

**Fig. 10-21** Primary endodontic lesion with secondary periodontal involvement. Tracing of sinus tract with gutta-percha point leads to lateral canal with furca bone loss.

apex and the gingival sulcus of a tooth with a necrotic pulp, thus indicating a combined endodontal-periodontal lesion. Generalized bone loss as is seen frequently in older patients usually indicates a periodontal problem, whereas a single tooth with bone loss is suggestive of a lesion of endodontic origin (Fig. 10-21). History and duration of pain are also important in aiding the clinician in choosing the correct therapy.

Determining the cause of an endodontal-periodontal lesion is important in the treatment planning. Endodontic treatment for a primary endodontic lesion with secondary periodontal involvement usually results in rapid healing. The periodontal lesion may exist by way of a furcation or lateral canal, a condition referred to as "retrograde periodontitis"[41] (Fig. 10-21). If a primary periodontal lesion exists with secondary endodontic involvement, periodontal treatment is mandatory and endodontic treatment is indicated. Retrograde pulpitis, which has been well documented,[34,38,44] may be caused by the injudicious use of ultrasonic and rotary instruments, and irritating chemicals resulting in exposure of lateral or accessory canals may induce an irreversible pulpitis. Actual extension of a periodontal lesion along the root surface may also result in a communication with the apex of the tooth and pulpitis. After endodontic therapy, proper maintenance and successful periodontal therapy are essential.

The true combined lesion, which exists when there is irreversible pulp pathosis and a periodontally involved tooth, requires combined therapy. The prognosis depends on the success of both endodontic and periodontal treatment. In the older adult, a cracked tooth or one with a vertical fracture may present a clinical picture similar to that of a true combined lesion. Carefully angled radiographs may show a vertical root fracture, but often the diagnosis is more clinical. One may make a diagnosis of a cracked tooth by placing a cotton roll or orangewood stick on the cusps of the suspected tooth and having the patient close and open. Usually with release in pressure, pain occurs. Staining techniques with fiberoptic transillumination are also useful in the detection of a cracked tooth.

There may be an untreatable periodontal defect involving one root of a posterior tooth such as the distobuccal root of a maxillary molar. Often these pulps show no evidence of abnormality. Endodontic therapy and root amputation may be necessary for healing. It is generally accepted that the sequence of treatment is first root canal therapy and then root amputation or hemisection.

Determining the cause of endodontal-periodontal problems will aid the clinician in the proper diagnosis and treatment of these lesions, thus affording patients proper care and improving the retention period of these teeth.

## OVERDENTURES

Retaining roots beneath dentures preserves bone and increases denture stability, thus affording greater retention. As the population ages, the number of overdentures will increase with more teeth retained. Endodontic overdenture abutments must be carefully evaluated clinically and radiographically. Both single-rooted and multirooted teeth may be utilized. The latter are often treated by hemisection or root amputation. The status of peridontally involved teeth must be thoroughly evaluated before their use as abutments.

If there is a diminution of the root canal space to a level below the alveolar mucosa with no pulp exposure or significant sensitivity after tooth reduction, teeth with vital pulps may be retained and used as overdenture abutments. However, Ettinger[13] reported that in a study of the rate of subsequent periapical pathosis in overdenture abutments, 14 of 82 teeth with vital pulps failed for a percentage of 17.1%. More than half were the result of pulp necrosis in previously vital pulps. Only three were viewed as purely endodontic failures—one unidentified second canal and two vertical root fractures. Although there was no detectable pulp exposure when the teeth were reduced, he suggested that there may have been a microexposure into the pulp canal eventually causing pulp necrosis.

At the time of endodontic treatment, reducing the crown-root ratio of an intended overdenture abutment to a level of 2 to 3 mm above the gingiva will help stabilize a mobile tooth while allowing for more expeditious treatment. Most teeth are restored with amalgam placed several millimeters into the root canal after being filled with gutta-percha and sealer (Fig. 10-22). Gold copings and attachments are also used for increased stability of the overdenture prosthesis.

In another report of 254 patients over a 12-year period, Ettinger[12] found that 28 of 679 overdenture abutment teeth were lost. Periodontal disease and caries accounted for 85% or all but four teeth lost. This study further emphasizes the importance of the integrity of the periodontium in the retention of endodontically treated teeth.

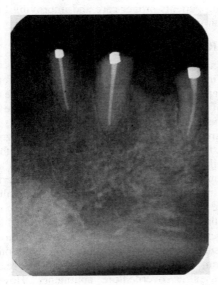

**Fig. 10-22** Root canal–filled teeth with amalgam restorations for overdenture case.

The overdenture with endodontically treated teeth is a valuable treatment procedure for someone missing many natural teeth. Tooth loss in the elderly is more traumatic than that in a younger patient. There is generalized patient acceptance of overdentures because older patients feel that they still retain some teeth thus reducing the emotional impact of tooth loss.

## FEAR AND ANXIETY IN THE ELDERLY

No chapter considering endodontic treatment in the elderly would be complete without a discussion of fear and anxiety. Forty-one percent of adults admit to delaying routine dental care because of fear.[26] Because of severe anxiety an estimated 12% to 15% avoid all dental care.[43] In a recent survey conducted on behalf of the American Association of Endodontists,[31] individuals who have received root canal therapy are four to five times more likely to feel that root canal therapy is painless than those who have never been treated. Three fourths of the respondents felt that root canal therapy was painful, yet only one fourth of the total number of respondents had received endodontic therapy. Older respondents, who were more likely to have endodontic therapy, were less likely to find the treatment painful. Kent[21] found that the more anxious a patient is, the higher the level of pain that may be anticipated, regardless of the planned procedure. The anxious patient is more likely to report a more painful experience during and after dental procedures.[22] Therefore efficient pain control and sedation procedures are especially useful in reducing the patient's anxiety in endodontic therapy.

Older patients appear to have a higher pain threshold than younger ones,[2] and so dental anxiety decreases with age.[35] The reason may be that more anxious patients usually experience greater pain during treatment than less anxious patients.[33] Milgram[28] found that the nature of the dentist-patient interaction and not the specific procedure may be the most significant factor when one is treating older adults. In a study by Bernstein,[6] the most negative aspect mentioned by patients was pain during an appointment, whereas the absence of pain ranked third among 17 positive aspects. In Rankin's[32] study of dentists' behavior and patients' attitudes, over 97% of patients wanted the dentist to fully explain the treatment procedures, and 89%

liked having the dentist to be truthful about the amount of anticipated pain.

Patient education plays a significant role in decreasing a patient's fear and anxiety. The importance of stress reduction, especially in the older adult, who may be medically compromised, has previously been discussed. Fear of the unknown is always a source of stress in our lives.[20] Since endodontic procedures effectively limit verbal communication, it is important to allow sufficient opportunity for this before one begins treatment.[24] Every patient deserves an explanation of the rationale of endodontic therapy. Patient information booklets are helpful, but direct, caring communication between dentist and patient explaining the endodontic therapy and the postoperative procedures to be followed, if discomfort occurs, is preferable and will reinforce what the patient has read. A sympathetic and concerned approach will help relieve the patient's fears and anxieties. When anxiety is high during treatment, the patient's pain threshold and pain tolerance are lowered.[11]

In promoting a good doctor-patient relationship, postoperative discomfort and sequelae are reduced and patients require less medication.[33] Failure to establish rapport and trust may complicate the endodontic procedure and decrease the chances of success.

## REFERENCES

1. Baumgartner JC and Harrison JW: The incidence of bacteremia related to endodontic procedures. I. Nonsurgical endodontics, J Endodont 2:135, 1976.
2. Bennett CR: Conscious sedation in dental practice, ed 2, St. Louis, 1978, The CV Mosby Co.
3. Bernick S: Age changes in the blood supply to human teeth, J Dent Res 46:544, 1967a.
4. Bernick S and Nedelman C: Effect of aging on the human pulp, J Endodont 3:88, 1975.
5. Bern-Klug M: AADS geriatric dentistry curriculum project, J Dent Educ 52(10):574, 1988.
6. Bernstein DA, Kleinknecht RA, and Alexander LD: Antecedents to dental fear, J Public Health Dent 39:113, 1979.
7. Bhussry BR: Modification of the dental pulp organ during development and aging. In Finn SB, editor: Biology of the dental pulp organ, University, Ala, 1968, University of Alabama Press.
8. Block RM and Lewis RD: Surgical treatment of iatrogenic canal blockages, Oral Surg 63:722, 1987.
9. Burch JG and Hulen S: The relationship of the apical foramen to the anatomic apex of the tooth root, Oral Surg 34:262, 1972.
10. Comfort A: The biology of senescence, London, 1956, Routledge.
11. Dworkin SF, Frence TP, and Giddon DB: Behavioral science and dental practice, St. Louis, 1978, The CV Mosby Co.
12. Ettinger RL: Tooth loss in an overdenture population, J Prosthet Dent 60:459, 1988.
13. Ettinger RL and Krell K: Endodontic problems in an overdenture population, J Prosthet Dent 59:459, 1988.
14. Friedman S and Stabholz A: Endodontic retreatment—case selection and technique. 1. Criteria for case selection, J Endodont 12:28, 1986.
15. Goldman M, Rankin C, Mehlman R, and Santa C: Immunological implications and clinical management of prophylactic endodontic treatment, Compendium 10(8):462, 1989.
16. Grady JR and Clausen H: Establishing your point, Clin Am Assoc Endodont, Apr 28, 1975.
17. Green D: Stereomicroscopic study of 700 root apices of maxillary and mandibular posterior teeth, Oral Surg 9:728, 1960.
18. Ingle JI: Geriatric endodontics, Alpha Omegan 79(4):47, 1986.
19. Ingle JI and Taintor JF: Endodontics, ed 3, Philadelphia, 1985, Lea & Febiger.
20. Katz CA: Stress factors operating in the dental office work environment, Dent Clin North Am 30:529, 1986.
21. Kent G: Anxiety, pain and type of dental procedure, Behav Res Ther 22:456, 1984.
22. Klepac RK, McDonald M, Hauge G, et al: Reactions to pain among subjects high and low in dental fear, J Behav Med 3:373, 1980.
23. Kuttler Y: Microscopic investigation of root apexes, J Am Dent Assoc 50:544, 1956.
24. Kuhn CC: Pain and helplessness in the anxious dental patient, J Can Dent Assoc 54:263, 1988.
25. Levy AB and Glatt L: Deviation of the apical foramen from the radiographic apex, J NJ Dent Soc 41:12, 1970.
26. Lindsay SJE, Wege P, and Yates J: Expectations of sensations, discomfort and fear in dental treatment, Behav Res Ther 22:99, 1984.
27. Malamed SF: Handbook of medical emergencies in the dental office, ed 3, St. Louis, 1986, The CV Mosby Co.
28. Milgram P, Weinstein P, and Getz T: Fear and anxiety reduction in the geriatric dental patient, Gerodontics 1:14, 1985.
29. Osetek EM: Case selection and treatment planning. In Cohen S and Burns RC, editors: Pathways of the pulp, St. Louis, 1987, The CV Mosby Co.
30. Philippas GG and Applebaum E: Age changes in the permanent upper canine teeth, J Dent Res 47:411, 1968.
31. Public knowledge and opinion about endodontics, Chicago, 1987, Public Communications, Inc.
32. Rankin JA and Harris MB: Patients' preferences for dentists' behaviors, J Am Dent Assoc 110:323, 1985.
33. Rossetti P: Dental anxiety, Boston, 1988. (Unpublished data.)
34. Rubach WC and Mitchell DF: Periodontal disease: accessary canals and pulp pathosis, J Periodontol 36:34, 1965.
35. Schuurs A, Duivenvoorden H, et al: Dental anxiety, the parental family and regularity of dental attendance, Community Dent Oral Epidemiol 12:89, 1984.

36. Seltzer S: Endodontology: biologic considerations in endodontic procedures, ed 2, Philadelphia, 1988, Lea & Febiger.
37. Seltzer S and Bender IB: The dental pulp, ed 3, Philadelphia, 1984, JB Lippincott Co.
38. Seltzer S, Bender IB, and Ziontz M: The interrelationship of pulp and periodontal disease, Oral Surg 16:1474, 1963.
39. Selye H: The general adaptation syndrome and diseases of adaptation, J Clin Endocrinol 6:217, 1946.
40. Sicher H: Orban's oral histology and embryology, ed 7, St. Louis, 1972, The CV Mosby Co.
41. Simon JH, Glick DH, and Frank AL: The relationship of endodontic-periodontic lesions, J Periodontol 43:202, 1972.
42. Sinai I, Seltzer S, Soltanoff W, et al: Biologic aspects of endodontics, II. Periapical tissue reactions to pulp extirpations, Oral Surg 23:664, 1967.
43. Sokol DJ, Sokol S, and Sokol CK: A review of non-intrusive therapies used to deal with anxiety and pain in the dental office, J Am Dent Assoc 110:217, 1985.
44. Staffileno H: Furcation treatment in periodontics, Dent Radiogr Photogr 38:85, 1965.
45. Staffileno H: Periodontal factors—endodontic considerations. In Controversies in dentistry, Chicago, 1987, The American Association of Endodontists and the AAE Endowment and Memorial Foundation.
46. Stahl SS et al: Speculations about gingival repair, J Periodontol 43:395, 1972.
47. Stanley HR and Ranney RR: Age changes in the human dental pulp. 1. The quantity of collagen, Oral Surg 15:1396, 1962.
48. Wescott WB: Current and future considerations for a geriatric population, J Prosthet Dent 49(1):113, 1983.
49. White R: Endodontics laboratory manual, Boston, 1988, Tufts University School of Dental Medicine. (Unpublished data.)

# 11

# Periodontal Diseases in the Older Adult

*Jon B. Suzuki*
*Linda C. Niessen*
*Denise J. Fedele*

The need for periodontal services for elders will continue to escalate because of the decrease in edentulism and the increase in the retention of natural teeth in the population. In addition, an enhanced awareness of oral facial esthetics and self-esteem and the desire to maintain a high quality of life serve as strong motivating factors for periodontal care. The purpose of this chapter is to discuss the diagnosis, treatment and prevention of periodontal diseases in the older adult.

## ETIOLOGY OF PERIODONTAL DISEASE IN THE ELDERLY

The significance of bacterial plaque and other local irritants in the cause of the various periodontal diseases has been well established.[29,32,56] Until recently, the nonspecific plaque hypothesis in the cause of the periodontal diseases was well accepted.[56] However, periodontitis is now recognized to be caused by specific bacteria.[15] The specificity of microorganisms appears to be related to clinical and radiographic entities of periodontitis patients.[49,55] Certain types of bacteria are involved, and, apparently, specific species or combination of species may be associated with different diseases.

Recent developments have been published since Page and Schroeder's concept of the pathogenesis of the periodontal lesion.[52] The four states of the periodontal lesion (initial, early, established, and advanced) are histopathologic designations of an increasingly complex inflammatory infiltrate into the connective tissue of the marginal gingiva concomitant with increasing plaque formation. The complex inflammatory infiltrate of the marginal gingiva includes neutrophils (polymorphonuclear leukocytes), lymphocytes, plasma cells, and mast cells.[52] Table 11-1 summarizes the four stages of periodontal lesions, histologically and by clinical diagnosis. Types of periodontal disease that occur in younger persons such as rapidly progressive periodontitis, juvenile periodontitis, postjuvenile periodontitis, and prepubertal periodontitis are associated with altered cell function. These diseases possibly have genetic implications with a familial tendency, whereas periodontal disease in the older adult at this time does not appear to have the same type of genetic implications and immune dysfunction.

## ADULT PERIODONTAL DISEASES
## GINGIVITIS

Gingivitis is an inflammatory process affecting the soft tissues surrounding the teeth. The inflammatory process does not extend into the alveolar bone, periodontal ligament, or cementum. The primary etiologic agent of gingivitis is bacterial plaque. The first three states (initial, early, and established) are consistent with the clinical diagnosis of gingivitis.

Plaque-associated gingivitis is the most common form of gingivitis and probably the most common form of all periodontal diseases. Plaque-associated gingivitis has clinical features including some or all of the following: inflammation, edema, bleeding upon probing, spontaneous gingival sensitivity, and itching. However, by definition, no loss of

**Table 11-1** Review of pathogenesis of the periodontal lesion

| Stage | Primary cell type | Clinical diagnosis |
|---|---|---|
| Initial | PMN (polymorphonuclear leukocytes) | Gingivitis, early |
| Early | PMN, lymphocytes | Gingivitis, moderate |
| Established | PMN, lymphocytes, plasma cells | Gingivitis, advanced |
| Advanced | PMN, lymphocytes, plasma cells | Periodontitis |

Adapted from Page RC and Schroeder HE: Lab Invest 33:235, 1976.

attachment or radiographic loss of bone is associated with gingivitis in young and old patients.

Other factors modify the course and clinical presentation of gingivitis. These factors permit a classification (see box) of gingivitis based upon secondary etiologic factors.[52] The primary agent for most if not all forms of gingivitis is bacterial plaque. Steroid hormone–influenced gingivitis may be seen in older female patients who are on postmenopausal steroid therapy. Acute necrotizing ulcerative gingivitis (ANUG, Vincent's infection, trench mouth) is not discussed in this chapter because it occurs primarily in younger adults.

Medication-influenced gingival overgrowth (such as gingival "hyperplasia" secondary to phenytoin) frequently results in pseudopockets (that is, junctional epithelium at the level of the cementoenamel junction with no loss of attachment). Medications having this potential include phenytoin (Dilantin) used for the control of seizures,[4,59] cyclosporin A used for immunosuppressive therapy of renal transplant patients,[51] and calcium-channel blockers (nifedipine) used for treatment of cardiovascular disease. The new immunosuppressive drug FK-506, used for organ transplantation patients, may also have oral implications but has not been investigated yet. Since neurologic and cardiovascular diseases increase with age, dental professionals can expect to see many more older adults with some or all of their natural dentition taking these medications.

Fibroblasts in the connective tissue of the periodontium respond with abnormal rates of mitosis in the presence of these medications resulting in apparently normal cells and a fiber and matrix composition. Bacterial plaque is a significant etiologic factor in medication-influenced hyperplastic gingivitis. Other forms of gingivitis may be influenced

---

**FORMS OF GINGIVITIS**

Plaque-associated gingivitis
ANUG (acute necrotizing ulcerative gingivitis)
Steroid hormone-influenced gingivitis
Medication-influenced gingival overgrowth
Other forms of gingivitis

From Suzuki JB: Dent Clin North Am 32(2):195, 1988.

---

by nutritional deprivation states. Although little is known regarding the impact of nutrition on periodontal status, indirect evidence on impaired protein intake,[50] folic acid,[62] zinc,[38] and vitamin C[2] indicates probable alteration of the periodontal tissues. Older adult patients may experience a variety of nutrition-deprivation states. (See Chapter 15.)

The progression from plaque-associated gingivitis to periodontitis has been investigated[3,21,39] and represents a conversion from the established stage to the advanced stage of the periodontal lesion. Understanding the functional roles of immunocompetent cells observed histopathologically in periodontal lesions may provide clues regarding the progression of disease.

One study has shown that when bacterial plaque accumulates, the periodontal tissues of older adults become inflamed sooner and more severely than the tissues of younger adults.[22] However, when oral hygiene procedures were reinstated, gingivitis decreased and there was no difference in the rate of healing between the young and old patient groups. One hypothesis for greater plaque retention in older adults is that as a result of gingival recession there is a larger surface area on which plaque can accumulate. Also, the two tooth surfaces, cementum and enamel, may differentially affect the rate at which plaque may accumulate.

Altered host response with increasing age may also affect the increased rate at which plaque accumulates in older adults manifesting in a more pronounced inflammatory reaction in marginal gingivae. However differences between young and old patients in the rate of progression of periodontitis has not been clearly demonstrated.

## Periodontitis

Periodontitis is defined as inflammation involving the gingival unit (gingiva and alveolar mucosa) and extends to the periodontal ligament, alveolar bone, and cementum. Periodontitis involves loss of clinical attachment and radiographic loss of bone. The reasons for the progression from gingivitis to periodontitis remain unclear but may reflect aberrations of host-cell responsiveness to plaque infection or may represent colonization and infection by highly pathogenic plaque bacteria.

Fig. 11-1 schematically presents three plausible hypotheses for periodontal destruction: (1) direct tissue destruction caused by bacterial plaque and metabolic products, (2) immune hyperresponsiveness precipitated by immune complexes, lymphocyte blastogenesis, or activation of complement pathways, or (3) immune deficiencies involving neutrophil function (chemotaxis, phagocytosis), neutropenia, or the autologous mixed lymphocyte response (AMLR).

## Chronic adult periodontitis

Chronic adult periodontitis usually occurs in adults over 35 years of age, and there appears to be no predilection for either gender. This form of periodontitis is directly related to accumulations of tooth-associated materials (plaque and calculus). The features of adult periodontitis are listed in the box on the next page. The rate of pathogenesis of chronic adult periodontitis commonly takes years and even decades to progress. The extent and distribution of bone loss and loss of attachment are variable and often are related to plaque-related areas. Based on statistical models,[18,29] there may be cyclic patterns of exacerbations and remission (periods of quiescence and disease activity).

Radiographically, deposits of calculus may be seen in patients with gross neglect. Middle-aged to older patients with adult periodontitis may have dentitions with missing teeth, large and numerous restorations (amalgams, composites, crowns, and fixed prostheses), medical, nutritional and genetic factors, along with malposed teeth and food-impaction areas, may enhance plaque retention and therefore result in furthering loss of clinical at-

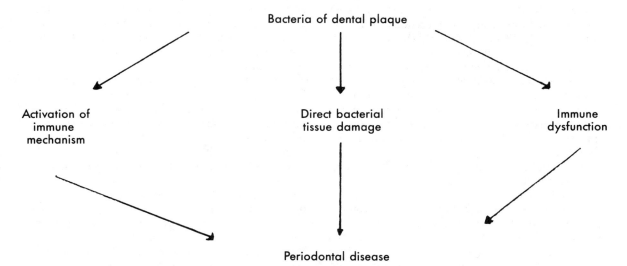

Fig. 11-1 Current concepts of pathogenesis of periodontitis.

---

### FEATURES OF ADULT PERIODONTITIS

Patients over 35 years of age
Approximately equal sex distribution
Variable lesions
Plaque and calculus present
Caries rate variable but usually high
Host-response apparently normal
Genetic implications unknown

---

From Suzuki JB: Dent Clin North Am 32(2):195, 1988.

tachment. Host-response factors, including neutrophil and lymphocyte function, are apparently normal.

Lymphocyte function studies historically implicate enhanced blastogenesis (transformation) when challenged by components of bacterial plaque.[5,23,25] In addition, patients with advanced periodontitis were reported[25] to have a significantly depressed lymphocyte blastogenic response to selected preparations of plaque mitogen and antigens. More recent evidence[60,61] indicates that lymphocyte blastogenic responsiveness to a battery of preparations of putative periodontal pathogens may be within expected ranges of age- and gender-matched healthy subjects. In controlling laboratory tissue culture conditions using incorporations of $^3$H-thymidine into the DNA of lymphocytes, investigators have demonstrated an intact cell-mediated immunity in adult patients with periodontitis.[53-54,60]

Because age of onset of the disease, age of the patient, medical and dental histories, bacterial composition of dental plaque, plaque-retentive areas, level of oral hygiene, and other variables are extremely difficult to control, genetic studies of adult periodontitis have not been pursued. Therefore genetic implications of this form of periodontitis are not known.

Periodontal disease in the elderly does not appear to be a specific disease but the result of a chronic adult periodontitis since adulthood. Although age-related changes have been documented in the periodontium of elders,[49] these changes do not appear to be the cause of periodontal disease in the elderly.

Immunologic alterations in T-cell function occur in the elderly, but periodontal disease may be a disease more related to B-cell and plasma cells.

Changes in selected serum hormone levels and increased susceptibility to microbial inflammation have also been suspected etiologic agents.[49] The increased prevalence and severity of periodontal disease in older adults does not appear to be the result of increased susceptibility because of aging but, rather, the more likely result of increased additive influence of sequential lesions over time.

### RISK ASSESSMENT IN THE ELDERLY

The history and physical examination are most important to the assessment of treatment risk and prognosis in the elderly. The elderly have increased morbidity and mortality, not because of age itself, but because of underlying disease and disability.[37] Although consultation with the patient's physician is frequently indicated, a careful and detailed history can elicit valuable clues to the patient's overall medical status, and this assists in the determination of surgical risk or treatment prognosis.

Signs and symptoms of acute or chronic systemic disease can often be detected by an astute clinician during a careful history. Cardiovascular and pulmonary diseases, hypertension, diabetes, mental status, and nutritional status affect the ability of the elderly to successfully tolerate and recover from invasive dental therapy. Over-the-counter (OTC) and prescription medications provide clues to the extent and severity of an individual's chronic disease. An individual's functional status will assist the dental practitioner in formulating a prognosis for the patient.

A useful tool to predict surgical mortality has been established by the American Society of Anesthesiologists (ASA). Table 11-2 provides the ASA classification system. This system stratifies patients into five categories while adjusting for age by not allowing an elderly person to be assigned class I.[37] This classification system has been validated in patients over 80 years of age.[37] Although this system was originally designed to assess surgical risk under general anesthesia, it currently is used to assess risk before diagnostic testing and outpatient surgery. Thus it serves as a useful tool to allow assessment of invasive dental therapy such as periodontal surgery, for the elderly.

**Table 11-2** American Society of Anesthesiologists physical status scale

| Class | Physical status |
| --- | --- |
| I | Normal healthy person |
| II | Patient with mild systemic disease |
| III | Patient with severe systemic disease that is not incapacitating |
| IV | Patient with incapacitating systemic disease that is a constant threat to life |
| V | Moribund patient who is not expected to survive 24 hours with or without operation |
| E | Added to any class patient undergoing emergency surgery |

Data from Meneilly GS, Rowe JW, and Minaker KL: Anesthesia and surgery in the elderly. In Rowe JW and Besdine RW: Geriatric medicine, Boston 1988, Little, Brown & Co.

## PERIODONTAL TREATMENT IN THE ELDERLY

Longitudinal clinical trials evaluating the effect of various modalities of periodontal treatment have shown that the progression of periodontal disease can be slowed in both young and old patients with meticulous oral hygiene.[30-31] Thus a primary variable in the periodontal disease equation is oral hygiene, not necessarily age. The extent to which age alone influences oral hygiene care has not been studied extensively. In healthy community-dwelling older adults, oral hygiene does not appear to decline with age.

The approach to periodontal disease treatment differs from that of younger adults. Several factors must be considered during treatment planning for older dental patients. Generally, periodontal disease in the elderly is not a quickly progressive disease. The onset of adult periodontal disease often occurs in young to middle adulthood. By older adulthood, periodontal disease presents as a long-standing chronic disease.

Recent studies indicate that advanced periodontal disease in the elderly may be less prevalent than moderate disease.[24,43,49] The cohort effect of this current group of elders could account for this finding, with current elders having already lost teeth to advanced periodontal disease during their middle age. Since periodontal disease has periods of ex-

acerbation and remission, understanding and documenting periods of active disease versus quiescent periods will be essential to the formulation of the treatment plan and prognosis.

The dental practitioner should consider the disease prognosis for both surgical and nonsurgical therapy. The patient's health status including the risks and benefits of both surgical and nonsurgical therapy should be considered. The patient's periodontal disease severity, medical diagnosis, OTC and prescription medications, ambulation, ability to perform adequate oral hygiene procedures, and ability to tolerate treatment are factors the practitioner should evaluate during treatment planning.

Depending on the nature of the periodontal defect, surgical periodontal therapy may be indicated in elderly persons. The elderly responding best to surgical intervention are those who are able to maintain the surgical result. The elderly who are frail or medically compromised can often be managed by aggressive nonsurgical therapy including meticulous oral hygiene home care, scaling, root planing, and closed curettage. Recall appointments may need to be scheduled more frequently to coincide with patients' needs (every 2 to 3 months) rather than the dental office's standard operating procedure (usually every 6 months).

## PERIODONTAL DISEASE PREVENTION AND MAINTENANCE OF ORAL HEALTH

Since periodontal diseases are bacterially mediated diseases, controlling oral bacteria can prevent them. Poor oral hygiene is a risk factor for periodontal diseases. The ability to remove oral debris and plaque is directly related to a person's manual dexterity as well as to one's physical and cognitive abilities.

Although a person's oral hygiene capabilities do not change with age, certain physical conditions, if they occur, can alter a person's ability to perform routine oral hygiene. Visual impairment often increases with age; approximately 12% of the elderly have some type of visual impairment.[42] Such impairment can alter a person's ability to see oral debris, and this indirectly affects oral hygiene. Chronic diseases, such as arthritis, or stroke resulting in paralysis, will alter a person's ability to use a toothbrush or dental floss.

Xerostomia is the most common adverse side

effect of many medications. Without the buffering and antibacterial properties of saliva, people are at increased risk for bacterial plaque adherence and colonization and therefore for periodontal disease. In addition, oral dryness can impair or limit chewing and speaking.

Medications that induce xerostomia include antidepressants, antihistamines, antineoplastics, antipsychotics, antispasmodics, decongestants, diuretics, and tranquilizers. As part of the medical history, the dentist should record the medications a patient is taking and must comprehend the effect of those medications on the oral cavity. For patients who complain about oral dryness and are not taking medication, appropriate referral and diagnostic tests for primary salivary gland disease are indicated.

### Mechanical plaque control

Toothbrushing is the most common form of mechanical plaque control in the United States.[14] Although the majority of the population will state that they brush their teeth once or twice a day, they often do not remove plaque satisfactorily. Flossing is the recommended method for cleaning the interproximal surfaces of the teeth. However, persons floss much less frequently than they use a toothbrush. Over 80% of people report that they either do not floss or floss only sporadically. The proportion of people who report that they floss their teeth decreases with age after 40 years of age.

There is no evidence of changes in adults' brushing habits resulting from age alone. However, older adults with disabilities, those who are hemiplegic as a result of a cerebrovascular accident (CVA) and can no longer use their dominant hand, those with visual problems, or those with dementia, who may not remember when or how to brush their teeth, may have difficulty practicing oral hygiene.[45] Persons with these disabling conditions will need assistance with daily oral hygiene. In addition, persons with disabilities may need assistance inserting, removing, and cleaning prostheses.

The problems nursing home residents have practicing oral hygiene have been documented.[10,41] Because of their medical problems, nursing home residents are often unable to practice daily oral hygiene and must rely on the nursing staff to assist them. Unfortunately, nurses receive minimal training in oral health and disease as part of their nursing education. As a result, nurses may feel uncomfortable cleaning a patient's denture or brushing a patient's teeth.

As part of the initial dental examination, the patient should be evaluated for the ability to perform oral hygiene. McLeran categorized older adults into four categories (Table 11-3) based on their abilities to practice oral hygiene.[36] The oral hygiene needs of older adults in category I do not differ from those of young or middle-aged adults. Category II patients will need some assistance with daily oral hygiene depending on the disability. Category III patients will need assistance brushing but

**Table 11-3** Patient oral hygiene categories

| Category | Criteria |
|---|---|
| I | Patient is completely self-sufficient and able to perform all oral hygiene techniques possible except for flossing and other skills requiring fine motor ability. |
| | Mentally alert and able to comprehend and demonstrate motivation to perform hygiene procedures. |
| II | Patient is self-sufficient but unable to perform techniques adequately because of arthritis, limited range of motion, and limited use of hands. Needs some assistance. |
| | Mentally alert but may exhibit depression, forgetfulness, or little interest in self-care. |
| III | Patient unable to care for daily needs; dependent on others to perform oral hygiene procedures but can cooperate with caregiver. |
| | Mentally unable to comprehend or communicate but cooperative or noncombative. |
| IV | Comatose patient, completely dependent on others for self-care, or noncooperative patient. |

Adapted from McLeran H: Oral hygiene care of the elderly, Module 13, Geriatric curriculum series, Iowa City, 1982, University of Iowa College of Dentistry.

will be able to cooperate by opening their mouths for the person providing care. Category IV patients, unable to assist, will require a caregiver to provide oral hygiene care. These categories can be applied to patients with natural dentition, complete dentures, or a combination of natural dentition and prosthesis.

People with upper-extremity disabilities may require modifications to toothbrushes or floss holders. For people needing toothbrush-grip modifications, a Styrofoam ball, tennis ball, or customized acrylic handle can be added to the toothbrush handle.[36] Similarly, floss-holding devices have been manufactured to assist people with upper-extremity disability.[40] Some older adults and nurses in nursing homes have found electric toothbrushes or the new rotary electric toothbrushes very helpful for mechanical plaque control.

In category III, brush-on fluoride gels may be easier for caregivers to control and apply than fluoride mouthrinses, since the patient may not be able to swish and then expectorate the rinse. Mouthrinses are contraindicated for patients in category IV, since they are likely to aspirate the mouthrinse because of their comatose condition.

### Chemotherapeutic agents

*Fluorides.* Fluoride works in a variety of ways.[11,63] First, it reduces the enamel solubility by both systemic and topical action. Second the topical effect of fluoride promotes remineralization in the early stages of caries development.[44] Third, fluoride appears to affect the metabolic processes of bacterial plaque.[12,64] Studies have shown fluoride to have a bactericidal effect on those bacteria that cause caries and periodontal disease.[28,35,64] However, as recently as 1983, a survey of dentists, dental researchers, and the public found that only dental researchers considered fluorides as the most important factor in preventing caries.[47] Practitioners and the public ranked oral hygiene measures above fluoride.

Topical fluorides are recommended as antiplaque agents because of their antibacterial properties, particularly stannous fluoride. Stannous fluoride, sodium fluoride, or acidulated phosphate fluoride (APF) are the most common forms of self-applied topical fluorides.

Self-applied fluorides can be in the form of rinses or gels. Table 11-4 lists some currently available fluoride rinses and gels and their fluoride concentrations. The choice of a rinse or a gel should be made by the dentist in consultation with the patient. Gels are often easier to use and may adhere to the teeth longer than rinses. As happens with children, gels can be applied for adults in preformed or customized trays or with a toothbrush (brush-on gels). Mouthrinsing requires people to hold the rinse in the mouth for a certain period of time and then expectorate it. Adults with neurologic diseases, particularly dementia, often do not have the ability to rinse.[46] For these persons, brush-on gels are the best approach when they use a topical fluoride. In addition, for persons who depend on caregivers to provide oral hygiene care, such as residents of nursing homes who depend on nurses to provide oral hygiene, brush-on gels may be easier for the caregivers to apply.

*Antiplaque agents.* Many patients are unable to remove plaque thoroughly. Lack of motivation, poor mechanical ability, or lack of knowledge are some of the reasons contributing to poor plaque control. The idea of a mouthrinse that removes plaque or kills the pathogenic bacteria is very appealing. Over the years a variety of agents have been tested with limited success. Antibiotics have had some success. However, the development of resistant organisms is a concern with long-term antibiotic use.[1,33] Enzymes that affect the metabolism of the bacterial plaque also have been considered and tested and used in Europe since the 1970s. Recently the American Dental Association (ADA) has approved two agents, chlorhexidine and Listerine, to help "prevent and reduce supragingival plaque and gingivitis."[7-8]

Chlorhexidine is a cationic bis-biguanide that has been used as a broad-spectrum antiseptic in clinical medicine since the 1950s. Chlorhexidine had been used as a preventive and therapeutic dental agent in Europe for more than 20 years. It is rapidly adsorbed to the negatively charged bacterial surface. The positively charged chlorhexidine molecule most likely attaches to the phosphate groups in the lipopolysaccharide and carboxyl groups in proteins.[26]

In an earlier trial that used the experimental gingivitis model, a twice-daily rinse with 0.2% chlorhexidine gluconate prevented the accumulation of plaque and gingivitis.[34] Other studies have found that brushing with chlorhexidine dentifrices effec-

**Table 11-4** Topical fluoride rinses and gels

| Brand name | Type | Concentration of compound (%) | Concentration of fluoride ion (%) | pH |
|---|---|---|---|---|
| **Topical fluoride rinses** | | | | |
| ACT | NaF | 0.05 | 0.02 | Neutral |
| Florigard | NaF | 0.05 | 0.02 | Neutral |
| Fluorinse | NaF | 0.05 | 0.02 | Neutral |
| NafRinse | APF | 0.05* | 0.02 | Acidic |
| Phos-Flur (Rx) | APF | 0.05* | 0.02 | Acidic |
| StanCare | SnF$_2$ | 0.10 | 0.025 | Neutral |
| NafRinse (Rx)† | NaF | 0.2* | 0.1 | Neutral |
| Point-Two (Rx)† | NaF | 0.2 | 0.1 | Neutral |
| **Topical fluoride brush-on gels** | | | | |
| Easy Gel | SnF$_2$ | 0.4 | 0.1 | Acidic |
| Flo-Gel | SnF$_2$ | 0.4 | 0.1 | Acidic |
| Gel-Kam | SnF$_2$ | 0.4 | 0.1 | Acidic |
| Gel-Tin | SnF$_2$ | 0.4 | 0.1 | Acidic |
| Iradicav Gel | SnF$_2$ | 0.4 | 0.1 | Acidic |
| Omni-Gel | SnF$_2$ | 0.4 | 0.1 | Acidic |
| Previstan | SnF$_2$ | 0.4 | 0.1 | Acidic |
| Stop Gel | SnF$_2$ | 0.4 | 0.1 | Acidic |
| Ultra-Gel | SnF$_2$ | 0.4 | 0.1 | Acidic |
| Gel II (Rx) | SnF$_2$ | 0.4 | 0.1 | Acidic |
| Karigel (Rx) | APF | 1.1 | 0.5 | Acidic |
| Thera-Flur (Rx) | APR | 1.1 | 0.5 | Acidic |
| Prevident (Rx) | NaF | 1.1 | 0.5 | Neutral |
| Thera-Flur-N (Rx) | NaF | 1.1 | 0.5 | Neutral |

* Approximate.
† Weekly usage.

tively reduces plaque and gingivitis.[6,16]

A recent study by Grossman et al. found that 0.12% chlorhexidine gluconate mouthrinse used twice daily reduced plaque accumulation, gingivitis, and gingival bleeding in an adult population.[20] This was one of the few studies that included middle-aged adults. Although the age range of the population was 18 to 60 years, the mean age of the population studied was 33 years. Side effects of chlorhexidine include an increase in calculus accumulation, staining of the teeth, and a bitter taste.

The Council on Dental Therapeutics of the American Dental Association recently accepted Peridex (Procter & Gamble Co.), a 0.12% chlorhexidine gluconate mouthrinse, to help prevent and reduce supragingival plaque and gingivitis.[8] Al-though chlorhexidine has not been studied in older adults (over 65 years of age), the results in younger populations indicate its efficacy for older adults. It may be particularly useful for adults who have difficulty with mechanical plaque control. Adults taking phenytoin or calcium-channel blockers are at risk for a medication-induced gingivitis and may benefit from daily chlorhexidine use.

Diabetic patients undergoing oral or periodontal surgery may benefit from a chlorhexidine mouthrinse after surgery. Chlorhexidine has been suggested for use with patients wearing provisional restorations to promote gingival healing before placement of the final fixed prothesis. Chlorhexidine appears to be most useful on a short-term basis—6 months or less. Its use on a long-term basis (over 6 months) has not been extensively studied. Chlorhexidine is available by prescription only. Its recommended use is to rinse twice daily, in the morning and before bedtime, with 15 ml for 30 seconds.

Listerine antiseptic is a hydroalcohol solution that recently has been accepted by the Council on Dental Therapeutics of the American Dental Association to help prevent and reduce supragingival plaque and gingivitis.[7] Three clinical studies of 6 months or more showed Listerine to be effective in reducing plaque and gingivitis when compared to placebo rinses.[9,19,27] These studies, like those for chlorhexidine, were conducted among primarily young, healthy adult populations. Although Listerine's effectiveness has not been investigated in older adults or medically compromised populations, Listerine should be considered for plaque control in persons who have difficulty with mechanical plaque control. Side effects of Listerine are minimal. However, it contains 26.9% alcohol and may be contraindicated in patients who cannot tolerate the high alcohol content (such as patients taking Antabuse), patients who are alcoholics or recovering alcoholics, or patients with severe oral mucositis. The use of Listerine should be considered if patients cannot tolerate the taste or staining that may result from using chlorhexidine. In addition, Listerine is a nonprescription mouthrinse and is less expensive and easier for patients to obtain than chlorhexidine.

## Saliva substitutes

Saliva plays an essential role in maintaining oral health. Xerostomia, or dry mouth, can result from primary salivary gland disease, such as Sjögren's syndrome, radiation to the head and neck area, or the anticholinergic activities of medications, that is, medication-induced xerostomia.[13,17,57] Older adults with multiple chronic diseases may be taking a variety of medications that can induce xerostomia.[13,17,57] This can compromise chewing, speaking, or swallowing abilities. In addition, without the antibacterial properties of saliva, the person can be at increased risk for periodontal disease. (See Chapter 17 for more information on xerostomia.)

Saliva substitutes are currently available on the market that can help relieve the symptoms of dry mouth.[58] Several saliva substitutes and their manufacturers are listed in Table 11-5. Commercially

**Table 11-5** Saliva substitutes

| Product | Manufacturer |
|---|---|
| Glandosane | Fresenius AG<br>Distributed by:<br>Universal International Corp.<br>Boynton Beach, Florida |
| Moi-stir | Kingswood Canada, Inc.<br>Toronto, Canada |
| Oral Balance | Laclede Professional Products<br>15011 Staff Court<br>Gardena, CA 90248 |
| Orex | Ing's Dental Specialties<br>Fort Wayne, Indiana |
| Saliment | Richmond Pharmaceuticals<br>Richmond Hill, Ontario, Canada |
| Sali-synt | Remeda Pharmaceuticals<br>Finland |
| Salivart | Westport Pharmaceuticals<br>1 Turkey Hill South<br>Westport, CT 06880 |
| Xero-lube | Colgate-Palmolive Company<br>Medical Products<br>300 Park Ave.<br>New York, NY 10022 |

available saliva substitutes contain salt ions; a lubricant-sweetener, usually glycerin or sorbitol; and a flavoring agent. Several saliva substitutes contain fluoride. Most saliva substitutes can be used *ad libitum* by patients. Some come in a spray dispenser and can be misted into the mouth when needed. Others come in a bottle and can be rinsed or swished in the mouth. Saliva substitutes are available by prescription or over the counter depending on the regulations of each state.

## Periodontal assessment

A complete and accurate periodontal assessment, using a full-mouth radiograph, probing depths of each tooth, defining gingival architecture, and so on is an integral component of the dental record. The standard of care will require that dental professionals document periodontal health and disease as well as we currently document dental caries. This assessment will allow the dental professional and patient to monitor periodontal status over time and

PATIENT_____ DATE _____

Periodontal Case Classification (AAP): I   II   III   IV

Medical Health Status        (ASA): I   II   III   IV

1) SIGNIFICANT FINDINGS (C.C. Medical History, General Comments)_____

_____

2) PERIODONTAL DIAGNOSIS

    1. Gingivitis    ☐ generalized    ☐ localized    (Specify)_____

    2. Periodontitis    ☐ generalized    ☐ localized    (Specify)_____

    3. Occlusal Trauma    ☐ Primary    ☐ Secondary

    4. Emergency    ☐ Periodontal/Gingival Abscess    ☐ ANUG    ☐ TMJ

3) PROGNOSIS    Poor _____

                  Fair _____

                  Good _____

4) ETIOLOGICAL FACTORS

  ☐ Plaque _____

  ☐ Calculus _____

  ☐ Defective Restorations _____

  ☐ Occlusal Factors and Habits _____

  ☐ Systemic Factors _____

6) ORAL HYGIENE

  ☐ Frequency _____

  ☐ Brush Type _____

  ☐ Floss (waxed/unwaxed) _____

  ☐ Interdental Stimulation _____

  ☐ Irrigation _____

  ☐ Recommended Changes _____

  ☐ Last Preventive Dentistry Appointment _____

5) PERIODONTAL TREATMENT PLAN

  ☐ Initial Therapy (S/RP, polish, Fl, OHI)

  ☐ Occlusal Control (Adjustment/Appliance)

  ☐ Surgeries _____

  ☐ Maintenance (Frequency) _____

Form 125982 Colwell Systems. Inc., Champaign, IL

**Fig. 11-2** Sample diagnosis assessment form. Forms are available from Colwell Systems, Inc., Champaign, Illinois.

| PROBE | | | | | | | | | | | | | | | | |
|---|---|---|---|---|---|---|---|---|---|---|---|---|---|---|---|---|
| RECESSION | | | | | | | | | | | | | | | | |
| ATTACHMENT LOSS | | | | | | | | | | | | | | | | |

| PROBE | | | | | | | | | | | | | | | | |
|---|---|---|---|---|---|---|---|---|---|---|---|---|---|---|---|---|
| RECESSION | | | | | | | | | | | | | | | | |
| ATTACHMENT LOSS | | | | | | | | | | | | | | | | |

| PROBE | | | | | | | | | | | | | | | | |
|---|---|---|---|---|---|---|---|---|---|---|---|---|---|---|---|---|
| RECESSION | | | | | | | | | | | | | | | | |
| ATTACHMENT LOSS | | | | | | | | | | | | | | | | |

| PROBE | | | | | | | | | | | | | | | | |
|---|---|---|---|---|---|---|---|---|---|---|---|---|---|---|---|---|
| RECESSION | | | | | | | | | | | | | | | | |
| ATTACHMENT LOSS | | | | | | | | | | | | | | | | |

## OCCLUSAL ANALYSIS

| CENTRIC RELATION | 1 2 3 4 5 6 7 8 | 9 10 11 12 13 14 15 16 |
|---|---|---|
| | 32 31 30 29 28 27 26 25 | 24 23 22 21 20 19 18 17 |
| RT. LATERAL | 1 2 3 4 5 6 7 8 | 9 10 11 12 13 14 15 16 |
| | 32 31 30 29 28 27 26 25 | 24 23 22 21 20 19 18 17 |
| LT. LATERAL | 1 2 3 4 5 6 7 8 | 9 10 11 12 13 14 15 16 |
| | 32 31 30 29 28 27 26 25 | 24 23 22 21 20 19 18 17 |
| PROTRUSIVE | 1 2 3 4 5 6 7 8 | 9 10 11 12 13 14 15 16 |
| | 32 31 30 29 28 27 26 25 | 24 23 22 21 20 19 18 17 |

Form 125862 Colwell Systems, Inc., Champaign, IL

**Fig. 11-2, cont'd.** For legend see opposite page.

thus plan optimal patient care. A sample diagnostic assessment form is shown in Fig. 11-2.

## SUMMARY

Periodontal diseases can and do affect older adults. Gingivitis and chronic periodontitis are the most common types of periodontal diseases seen in older adults. Research has shown that periodontal diseases can be treated successfully in adults. However successful treatment first depends on accurate, adequate diagnosis and assessment. Dentists must document signs and symptoms of periodontal diseases as carefully and completely as they chart for dental caries. In addition, prevention of periodontal diseases plays a major role in dental care for older adults.

## REFERENCES

1. Ainamo J: Control of plaque by chemical agents, J Clin Periodont 4:23, 1977.
2. Alvares O et al: The effect of subclinical ascorbate deficiency on periodontal health in non-human primates, J Periodont Res 16:628, 1981.
3. Ammons WF, Schectman LR, and Page RC: Host tissue response in chronic periodontal disease. I. The normal periodontium and clinical manifestations and periodontal disease in the marmoset, J Periodont Res 7:131, 1972.
4. Babcock FR: Incidence of gingival hyperplasia associated with Dilantin therapy in a hospital population, J Am Dent Assoc 71:1447, 1965.
5. Baker JJ, Chan SP, Socransky SS, et al: Importance of *Actinomyces* and certain gram-negative anaerobic organisms in the transformation of lymphocytes from patients with periodontal disease, Infect Immun 13:1363, 1976.
6. Bay LM: Effect of toothbrushing with different concentrations of chlorhexidine on the development of dental plaque and gingivitis, J Dent Res 57(2):181, 1978.
7. Council on Dental Therapeutics: Council on Dental Therapeutics accepts Listerine, J Am Dent Assoc 117:515, 1988.
8. Council on Dental Therapeutics: Council on Dental Therapeutics accepts Peridex, J Am Dent Assoc 117:516, 1988.
9. DePaola LG, Overholser CD, Meiller TF, et al: Chemotherapeutic inhibition of supragingivits dental plaque and gingivitis development, J Clin Periodontol 16:467, 1989.
10. Duncan JL: Incorporating oral hygiene procedures in geriatric nursing homes, Dent Hygiene 53:519, 1979.
11. Ericsson SY: Cariostatic mechanisms of actions of fluorides: clinical observations, Caries Res 11(suppl 1): 2, 1977.
12. Fejerskov O, Tylstrup A, and Larsen MJ: Rational use of fluorides in caries prevention: a concept based on possible cariostatic mechanisms, Acta Odontol Scand 39:241, 1981.
13. Fox PC, van der Ven PF, Sonies BC, et al: Xerostomia: evaluation of a symptom with increasing significance, J Am Dent Assoc 110:519, 1985.
14. Frandsen A: Mechanical oral hygiene practices: state of the science review. In Löe H and Kleinman DV, editors: Dental plaque control measures and oral hygiene practice, Washington, DC, 1986, IRL Press.
15. Genco RJ, Zambon JJ, and Christersson LA: Use and interpretation of microbiological assays in periodontal diseases, Oral Microbiol Immunol 1:73, 1986.
16. Gjermo P and Rolla G: Plaque inhibition by antibacterial dentifrices, Scand J Dent Res 78(6):464, 1970.
17. Glass BJ, Van Dis M, Langlais RP, and Miles DA: Xerostomia: diagnosis and treatment planning considerations, J Oral Maxillofac Surg 58:248, 1984.
18. Goodson J, Tanner AC, Haffajee AD, et al: Patterns of progression and regression of advanced destructive periodontal disease, J Clin Periodontol 9:472, 1982.
19. Gordon JM, Lamster IB, and Sieger MC: Efficacy of Listerine antiseptic in inhibiting the development of plaque and gingivitis, J Clin Periodontol 12:697, 1985.
20. Grossman E, Reiter G, Sturzenberger O, et al: Six month study of the effects of a chlorhexidine mouthrinse, J Periodont Res 21(suppl 16):33, 1986.
21. Heijl LC, Rifkin BR, and Zander HA: Conversion of chronic gingivitis to periodontitis in squirrel monkeys, J Periodontol 47:710, 1976.
22. Holm-Pederson P, Agerbaek NM, and Theilade E: Experimental gingivitis in young and elderly individuals, J Clin Periodontol 2:14, 1975.
23. Horton, JE, Leiken S, and Oppenheim, J: Human lymphoproliferative reaction to saliva and dental plaque-deposits: an in vitro correlation with periodontal disease, J Periodontol 43:522, 1972.
24. Hunt RJ, Levy SM, and Beck JD: The prevalence of periodontal attachment loss in an Iowa population aged 70 and older, J Public Health Dent 50(4):251, 1990.
25. Ivanyi I and Lehner T: Lymphocyte transformation by sonicates of dental plaque in human periodontal diseases, Arch Oral Biol 16:1117, 1971.
26. Kornman KS: Antimicrobial agents: state of the science review. In Löe H and Kleinman DV, editors: Dental plaque control measures and oral hygiene practices, Washington, DC, 1986, IRL Press.
27. Lamster IB: The effect of Listerine antiseptic on reduction of existing plaque and gingivitis, Clin Prevent Dent 5(6):12, 1983.
28. Lilienthal B: The effect of fluoride on acid formulation by salivary sediment, J Dent Res 35:197, 1956.
29. Lindhe J, Haffajee A, and Socransky S: Progression of periodontal disease in adult subjects in the absence of periodontal therapy, J Clin Periodontol 10:433, 1983.
30. Lindhe J and Nyman S: The effect of plaque control and surgical pocket elimination on the establishment and maintenance of periodontal therapy in cases of advanced disease, J Clin Periodontol 2:67, 1975.
31. Lindhe J, Socransky SS, Nyman S, et al: Effect of age on healing following periodontal therapy, J Clin Periodontol 12:774, 1985.
32. Listgarten M: Structure of the microbial flora associated with periodontal health and disease in man, J Periodontol 47:1, 1976.
33. Lobene RR: Chemotherapeutics for the prevention of dental plaque, J Prevent Dent 3:32, 1976.

34. Löe H and Schiött CR: The effect of mouthrinse and topical complication of chlorhexidine on the development of dental plaque and gingivitis in man, J Periodont Res 5:79, 1970.
35. Loesche WJ: Topical fluoride as an antibacterial agent, J Prevent Dent 4:21, 1977.
36. McLeran H: Oral hygiene care for the elderly, Module 13, Geriatric curriculum series, Iowa City, 1982, University of Iowa College of Dentistry.
37. Meneilly GS, Rowe JW, and Minaker KL: Anesthesia and surgery in the elderly. In Rowe JW and Besdine RW: Geriatric medicine, Boston, 1988, Little, Brown & Co.
38. Miles DA: Functions of zinc: a literature résumé, J Oral Med 37:95, 1963.
39. Moulton R, Ewen S, and Thieman W: Emotional factors in periodontal disease, Oral Surg 5:833, 1952.
40. Mulligan R and Wilson S: Design characteristics of floss-holding devices for persons with upper extremity disabilities, Spec Care Dentist 4:168, 1984.
41. Napierski GE and Danner MA: Oral hygiene for the dentulous total care patient, Spec Care Dentist 2:257, 1982.
42. National Center for Health Statistics: Current estimates from the National Health Interview Surveys: United States, 1979, Series 10, No. 136, Public Health Service pub no. 81-1564, 1981.
43. National Institute of Health, National Institute of Dental Research: Oral Health of United States Adults: the national survey of oral health in U.S. employed adults and seniors: 1985-86: national findings, Public Health Service publ no. 87-2868, 1987, US Dept of Health and Human Services.
44. Newbrun E: Cariology, Baltimore, 1978, Williams & Wilkins.
45. Niessen LC and Jones JA: Alzheimer's disease: a guide for dental professionals, Spec Care Dentist 6(1):6, 1986.
46. Niessen LC, Jones JA, Zocchi M, and Gurian B: Dental care for the Alzheimer's patient, J Am Dent Assoc 110:207, 1985.
47. Opinion Research Corporation: Dental caries: what people know: surveying the "knowledge gap," Princeton, NJ, 1983.
48. Page RC: Periodontal disease in the elderly: a critical evaluation of current information, Gerodontology 3(1):63, 1984.
49. Page RC and Schroeder H: Periodontitis in man and other animals, Basel, 1982, S Karger, AG.
50. Pinborg JJ et al: Oral changes in South Indian children with severe protein deficiency, J Periodontol 38:218, 1967.
51. Rateitschak-Pluss E et al: Initial observation that cyclosporin-A induces gingival enlargement in man, J Clin Periodontol 10:237, 1983.
52. Schluger S, Page RC, and Yuodelis R: Periodontal disease: basic phenomena, clinical management and occlusal and restorative interrelationships, Philadelphia, 1977, Lea & Febiger.
53. Sims T, Clagett JA, and Page RC: Effects of cell concentration and exogenous prostaglandin on the interaction and responsiveness of human peripheral blood lymphocytes, Clin Immunol Immunopathol 12:150, 1978.
54. Sims T and Page RC: Effects of endogenous and exogenous inhibitors on the incorporation of labeled precursors into DNA by human mononuclear cells, Infect Immunol 38:502, 1982.
55. Slots J, Hafström C, Rosling B, et al: Detection of *Actinobacillus actinomycetemcomitans* and *Bacteroides gingivalis* in subgingival smears by the indirect fluorescent-antibody technique, J Periodont Res 20:613, 1985.
56. Socransky SS: Microbiology of periodontal disease: present status and future considerations, J Periodontol 48:497, 1977.
57. Spielman A, Ben-Aryeh H, Gutman D, et al: Xerostomia: diagnoses and treatment, J Oral Surg 51(2):144, 1981.
58. Sreebny LM and Schwarz SS: A reference guide to drugs and dry mouth, Gerodontology 5(2):75, 1986.
59. Steinbert SC and Steinberg AD: Phenytoin-induced gingival overgrowth control in severely retarded children, J Periodontol 53:429, 1982.
60. Suzuki JB, Sims T, and Page RC: Effects of factors other than pathologic status on responsiveness of peripheral mononuclear cells from patients with chronic periodontitis, J Periodontol 54:408, 1983.
61. Tew JB, Ranney RR, and Donaldson SL: Blastogenic responsiveness in periodontally healthy subjects: evidence for mitogenic activity in oral bacteria, J Periodontol Res 17:466, 1982.
62. Vogel RI et al: The effect of folic acid on gingival health, J Periodontol 47:677, 1976.
63. Wei S, editor: Clinical uses of fluoride, Philadelphia, 1985, Lea & Febiger.
64. Yoon N and Berry CW: An in vivo study of the effects of fluorides (SnF 0.4%, APR 1.23% and neutral NaF 0.05%) on levels of organisms resembling actinomyces, gingival inflammation and plaque accumulation, J Dent Res 58:535, 1979.

# 12

# Prosthodontic Treatment with Implants for Geriatric Edentulous Patients

*George A. Zarb*
*Adrianne Schmitt*

Many international reports indicate a global trend in the increasing survival of the elderly.[23] Quite understandably governments and health professionals are seeking to predict the influence of the aging factor on the growth of health expenditure. These concerns also seek an improvement and preferably an enhancement in the quality of life of a country's senior citizens. In recent years the dental profession has made considerable progress in fulfilling a comparable remittence for elderly dental patients by prescribing preventive and restorative measures. As a result, patients with advanced oral diseases and several missing teeth are routinely treated successfully irrespective of their age. Furthermore the introduction of controlled maintenance programs for these patients can virtually guarantee the longevity of even the most severely depleted dentitions.[9,20] A similar claim cannot be made vis-à-vis the edentulous geriatric population. Regrettably, a significant number of elderly patients are already edentulous and wear complete dentures, whereas others may not be able to avail themselves of current methods for retention of their partial dentitions. Over the years texts and published articles have extolled the virtues of the mechanical principles of partial complete denture therapy. Such correctly applied principles are purported to virtually guarantee a happy coexistence between dentures and their host tissues. As a result, dentists have been remarkably successful in convincing themselves, if not always their patients, that technically well-made removable dentures can be worn satisfactorily and perhaps even indefinitely. Strangely enough this notion has persisted, despite the very obvious fact that 45 $cm^2$ of a superbly evolved tooth attachment and support mechanism has been replaced by a qualitatively and quantitatively compromised area of support for a prosthetic dentition[32] (Fig. 12-1). Published evidence reveals that although it is difficult to define denture satisfaction a significant number of patients in all age groups are dissatisfied with their dentures.[2,24] Furthermore, many elderly patients experience difficulty in attaining comfortable and efficient oral function with removable dentures.[18] Both this textbook and other recent references[27] emphasize the important relationship between adequate oral function (and by implication good prosthetic function) and proper digestion and nutrition. The greater life expectancy of edentulous patients is very likely to increase or prolong the risk of denture dissatisfaction and its functional implications. This risk is particularly compelling in the context of the denture-supporting tissues' well-documented vulnerability to adverse changes as a result of long-term denture wearing.[14]

It is not surprising therefore that therapeutic initiatives in this area have included many attempts at providing patients with analogs for tooth roots, or dental implants that will ensure the provision of stable functional prostheses. The objective of this chapter is an analysis of the impact of the use of implants to support and retain dental prostheses in geriatric edentulous patients.

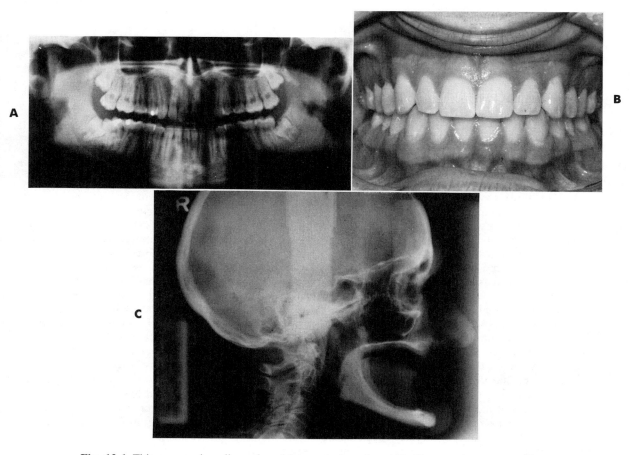

**Fig. 12-1** This panoramic radiograph and intraoral view, **A** and **B**, illustrate the amount of bone, tooth, and periodontal tooth attachment present in the intact natural dentition. This is in sharp contrast to the amount available in the edentulous mouth, **C**.

## EDENTULOUS PREDICAMENT AND PROMISE OFFERED BY DENTAL IMPLANT RESEARCH

Despite well-documented and anecdotal claims for the success of complete denture therapy, dentists and patients do not always agree as to what constitutes a successful denture experience. Although criteria for technically adequate dentures exist, they do not give sufficient recognition to patient-mediated factors such as ability to handle dentures, patient opinion about treatment, or screening for potential emotional problems. In fact, research attempts at establishing valid and responsive out-

come measures of prosthetic effectiveness have proved unreliable because of difficulties in establishing quantifiable and reproducible parameters. Most of these attempts have included assessments of patient attitude, systemic health status, classifications of ridge morphology, mucosal health status, tongue position, quality and quantity of saliva, bite-force levels, functional assessments of the masticatory system, subjective reports and evaluations of dietary choices and chewing ability, as well as overall satisfaction.[6,10,15,26] A few recent reports have also sought to assess the possible contributory roles of physical, emotional, and psychologic components.[11] A synthesis of these items may reveal anticipated treatment difficulties and even indicate a possible level of treatment outcome to be achieved. However this information will not help the patient who simply cannot wear a complete denture.

Diverse reasons have been proposed to account for the cause and frequency of gradual or chronic inability to wear complete dentures. Most dentists identify anatomic, physiologic, and psychologic reasons as causing the edentulous predicament. They normally attempt to cope with the problem by patient counseling, by modifying and improving the denture fabrication technique, and occasionally by resorting to a preprosthetic surgical intervention. Regrettably these efforts may still prove to be inadequate, and these patients end up by being diagnosed as maladaptive.

Traditional preprosthetic surgical endeavors (sulcus deepenings and vestibuloplasties) have largely sought to provide a comfortable enlargement of the potential denture-bearing area. Although such an approach may appear sensible in the context of traditional associations of better prosthetic prognoses with favorable ridge morphology, longitudinal documentation favoring minimal morbidity and clinical effectiveness for the surgical methods has not been compelling.[33]

Current research indicates that the provision of a stable prosthesis may very well be the single most important determinant of success in complete denture therapy along with the fulfillment of a patient's esthetic expectations.[35] This compelling conclusion has resulted from the fact that osseointegrated dental implants have been shown to reliably and safely provide long-term prosthetic stability for edentulous patients of all age groups.[35] This statement contrasts sharply with the profession's traditional attitude toward dental implant therapy.

The search for an implant system or systems that provide dentists and patients with alloplastic tooth roots or their equivalent for prosthesis support and with scientific documentation for their longitudinal survival has until recently been remarkable mainly for its anecdotal value. Several implant systems have indeed been commercially available for several decades, but the lack of scientific justification for both their prescription and long-term clinical efficacy have underscored their lack of routine acceptance in clinical academia or practice. None-

theless several patients have benefited from the work of pioneering colleagues such as Bodine and particularly Small, at least in the short term. The lingering conviction is, however, that subperiosteal implants and variations such as ramus frames fail slowly, creating an illusion of relative longevity. Furthermore these techniques are not easily retrievable and certainly limited in clinical application. As a result the teaching of implant prosthodontics has not featured prominently in most dental schools' prosthodontic curricula.

The seminal work of Brånemark, published in 1977,[7] introduced the technique of osseointegration. This is based upon a demonstrated, mechanical, and perhaps even structural interlocking of functional implant and loaded bone such that optimal force or stress distribution occurs from implant to surrounding bone. His basic science and clinical research indicated the use of a versatile and predictable attachment mechanism for tooth root analogs. This was in striking distinction to a concept of implant-retention efficacy based on three-dimensional stabilization such as the subperiosteal or the blade implant.

The Brånemark work ushered in a new era of research endeavor in the treatment of edentulous patients with implants. It also introduced a standard of quality, predictability, and longevity that qualifies for the interim or current yardstick against which other implant systems must be measured. This status is predicated on the following three considerations:

1. The dentist now has a compelling biologic rationale for implant host-tissue support that can safely and predictably reduce the burden of illness associated with routine implant prescription for edentulous patients.
2. The clinical application of this rationale survives longitudinal scientific scrutiny.
3. The biologic rationale for osseointegration appears to be reconcilable with diverse prosthodontic applications.

## OSSEOINTEGRATED IMPLANTS: METHODOLOGY, INDICATIONS, AND CONTRAINDICATIONS

The clinical techniques for achieving and maintaining osseointegration are well described in the literature.[8] Fig. 12-2 identifies the salient stages of

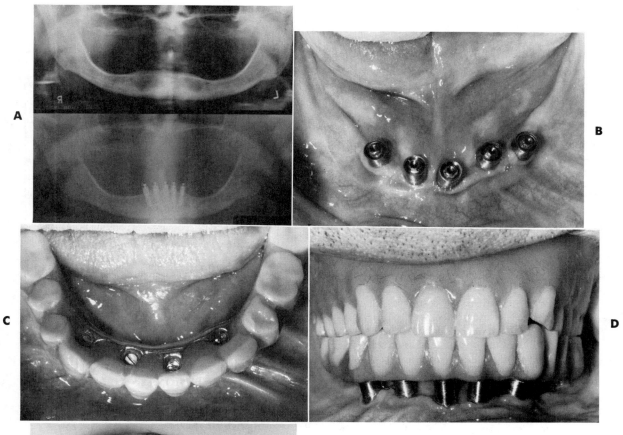

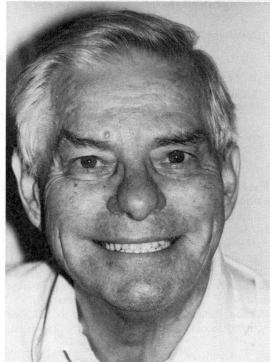

**Fig. 12-2** Five implants were surgically inserted into this edentulous arch, **A** and **B**. They are used to support an electively removable prosthesis that is retained by five gold screws, **C** and **D**. The bridge has a cast frame to provide support and retention for the acrylic teeth and base. **B** to **E** were taken 8 years after completion of prosthodontic treatment, and this patient continues to enjoy the stability of his implant-support bridge.

the procedure. The basic objective of osseointegration is the provision of an attachment mechanism for the man-made root analog, which is somewhat analogous to a periodontal ligament. It therefore aims at a host bone response that is highly differentiated and biomechanically adequate to resist occlusal stresses. Such an achievement appears to depend on the following clinical protocol:

1. Careful surgery that does not compromise the predictability of a favorable healing response as manifested by subsequent, well-differentiated host-tissue response.
2. Use of a commercially pure unalloyed titanium material. This means that the oxide layer that builds up over the metallic surface prevents an actual contact between bone and metal. This layer is purported to beneficially affect the host-tissue response, albeit in an imperfectly understood way.
3. Design of a root analog that allows immediate stability of the implant and an excellent scope for eventual stress distribution.
4. Unloaded healing phase for the implant to ensure a predictable optimal healing response.
5. An impeccable fit of the prosthetic superstructure and correct occlusal relationships as well. These are standard objectives in prosthodontics, but the absence of a resilient periodontal ligament support in tissue-integrated prostheses indicates a need for technical prosthodontic accuracy that may very well exceed what is required for tooth abutments.[2]

The original inclusion criteria in studies with the osseointegration technique were limited to maladaptive edentulous patients. Exclusion criteria were also clearly delineated (see boxes). Given the virtual absence of morbidity that has been reported, it is therefore tempting to suggest that any edentulous patient whose systemic health does not preclude a minor oral surgical procedure may be considered a candidate for osseointegration. Preliminary studies indicate that osteoporosis is not a contraindication for treatment.

## TORONTO OSSEOINTEGRATION GERIATRIC STUDY

The literature documenting the longitudinal efficacy of osseointegrated implants in geriatric pa-

---

**CLINICAL CONSIDERATIONS THAT SINGLY OR COLLECTIVELY PRECLUDED COMFORTABLE WEAR OF A COMPLETE DENTURE**

Severe morphologic compromise of denture-bearing area accompanied by nonretentive prosthesis

Parafunctional oral activity associated with recurrent soreness of supporting tissues and virtual absence of denture stability

Apparent lack of oromuscular coordination

Hyperactive gag reflex elicited by removable prosthesis

Patient-reported inability to adapt to wearing denture(s)

---

**CLINICAL CONSIDERATIONS AS EXCLUSION CRITERIA**

Patient inability to undergo a minor oral surgical procedure for systemic health or personal reasons

Edentulous jaw with bony dimensions that could not accommodate Brånemark implant dimensions available at the time

History of drug abuse

Unrealistic expectations regarding cosmetic improvement of previously achieved cosmetic results

---

tients specifically is limited.[17] However there exists extrapolated evidence that confirms the beneficial results of this method.[1,34] In our original prospective Toronto study, which sought to test the veracity of the Brånemark claims, our patient treatment group consisted of 46 edentulous patients with 49 implant-supported prostheses.[34] Eleven of these patients were over 60 years of age when their treatment was completed between 1979 and 1983. In addition, nine patients over the age of 60 were included in our second ongoing study into the diverse applications of osseointegration. Their treatment was completed between 1984 and the spring of 1987. The combined population numbered 20 (six males and 14 females) with an age range for male subjects of 60 to 76, with a mean age of 66.92 years, and 60 to 75 for the female subjects, with a mean age of 69.29 years. All 20 patients presented for treatment with a chronic history of inability to tolerate a mandibular denture.

All the patients met our criteria of adequate systemic health to allow for a minor oral surgical procedure, and the mandibular treatment comprised 15 fixed prostheses and 5 overdentures. The males were treated with 24 implants, and the females with 65 implants, for a total of 89 implants. At each annual recall appointment and at the most recent examination (1989), that is, 6 to 10 years after treatment for the first study patients and 2 to 5 years for the second study patients, all reported and demonstrated evidence of complete resolution of their original prosthetic problem. Eighty-four (94%) out of the originally placed 89 implants demonstrated evidence of osseointegration as judged by our proposed success criteria. Five of the 84 implants were not in functional use because their location precluded a simple maintenance type of prosthetic design. The 79 implants (87%) in functional use accounted for a 100% continuous-use functional success of the prescribed prostheses. Furthermore all 20 patients reported satisfaction with the esthetic result achieved, along with their completely restored functional status. We therefore regard Brånemark's original results[1] and the Toronto replication study[34] as quite compelling in terms of their extrapolated therapeutic implications for geriatric patients.

## SALIENT FEATURES OF THE OSSEOINTEGRATION PROCEDURE

Multicenter studies carried out on large, diverse, and consecutive population groups have endorsed the treatment efficacy of the osseointegration technique.[13,19,22,30,34-35] It is therefore understandable that most prosthodontists who have so frequently come up short in their efforts to deal with the predicament of the elderly edentulous, now regard the osseointegration method as a profound therapeutic breakthrough. Although clinical and scientific discretion may indicate that moving this information laterally into the geriatric field may be premature,

we would argue that published documentation warrants such an initiative. This argument becomes very compelling when stock is taken of the salient feature of osseointegration.

1. Almost all eligible edentulous sites are qualitatively and quantitatively suitable for osseointegration. Infrequent loss of individual implants is accompanied by rapid healing of the failed bone site, and secondary reimplantation can usually be readily undertaken. Both this observation and the design of the components allow for maximum scope for retrievability of the entire system. Reported implant failure is very low and virtually innocuous to the patient.[1,31,36]

2. Success of individual implants is over 85% in 10-year observation periods. Virtual 100% prosthetic success has been reported even when an abbreviated number of implants osseointegrate.[1,13,17,19,22,30,34,36] This success reflects the versatility of the system, since either a fixed prosthesis or an overdenture type may be prescribed depending on morphologic, financial, and other considerations.

3. Patients' problems of function, pain, and compromised life quality are dramatically reduced.[5] Patient reports on increased or enhanced masticatory efficiency, comfort, biting force, and tactile sensation were matched by measurable objective assessments.[12,16,22]

4. Bone loss around implants, even in patients with advanced residual ridge resorption, appears to be minimal and significantly less than bone loss under removable prostheses.[1,38] Furthermore the longitudinal soft-tissue response to osseointegrated implants appears to be uneventful even in the frequent absence of attached gingival tissue. The latter condition had traditionally be regarded as a prerequisite for implant success. As a result of our Toronto prospective study, we concluded that conventional clinical periodontal parameters appear to be of limited value or perhaps even irrelevant in predicting the longevity of osseointegration. The presence of plaque around osseointegrated titanium implants does not appear to render the attachment mechanism vulnerable in the way plaque on natural teeth may, at least within

the limits of the reported one- to two-decade-long documented observation and analysis. This does not mean that implant oral hygiene aspects should be ignored entirely. It does appear to mean, however, that elderly patients whose oral hygiene maintenance motivation or digital skills may be impaired are unlikely to have to devote the same obsessive hygienic maintenance of their implant abutments, as necessitated by teeth acting as abutments for extensive fixed bridges[21] or for overdentures.[29] Furthermore most prosthesis designs (especially in the mandible) lend themselves to easy home care procedures, such as rinsing with antiplaque mouth washes and use of Water Pik.* The periodontal ligament surrounding a natural tooth is regarded embryologically, histologically, and functionally as unique connective tissue. The interfacial response elicited by the osseointegration process is quite different from the periodontal ligament and as such cannot be expected to respond to the oral environment in a similar manner. Clearly a great deal more research has to be done to clarify the nature and specifics of this difference. In the meantime clinical descriptive reports underscore the longitudinal viability of osseointegrated implants even when far less than optimal oral hygiene is present.

5. A new set of success and efficacy criteria has evolved.[3] These criteria are a yardstick against which other systems claiming osseointegration must be measured. It would be unrealistic to suggest that the demonstrated biomechanical efficacy of osseointegration is exclusively limited to the Brånemark system. However only preliminary scientific documentation is available from other systems and their claim for longevity can be regarded only as provisional at this stage. The recommended conditions for application of the criteria and the criteria themselves[25] are shown in the box.

6. Although the therapeutic breakthrough in the treatment of edentulous patients has occurred, prosthodontists should be careful to

---

*Teledyne Water Pik, 1730 East Prospect St., Fort Collins, CO 80521.

---

## CONDITIONS FOR APPLICATION OF SUCCESS AND EFFICACY CRITERIA

1. Only osseointegrated implants should be evaluated with these criteria.
2. They apply to individual endosseous implants.
3. At the time of testing the implants must have been under a functional load and in occlusion.
4. Implants that are beneath the mucosa and in a state of health in relation to the surrounding bone should not be included in the evaluations but may be reported as complications.
5. Complications of an iatrogenic nature that are not attributable to a problem with material or design should be considered separately when one is computing the percentage of success. This includes such problems as impingement on the mandibular canal and intrusion into the sinus and nasal cavity.

## CRITERIA FOR SUCCESS

1. The individual unattached implant is immobile when tested clinically.
2. There is no evidence of peri-implant radiolucency as assessed on distorted radiographs.
3. The mean vertical bone loss should be less than 0.2 mm annually after the first year of service.
4. There should be no persistent pain or discomfort attributable to the implant.
5. The implant design should not preclude placement of a crown or prosthesis with an appearance satisfactory to the patient and dentist.
6. In the context of the above, a success rate of 85% at the end of a 5-year observation period and 80% at the end of a 10-year period should be regarded as minimum levels for success.

---

not get carried away and prescribe the technique indiscriminately. The reported edentulous successes need not automatically translate to partially dentate patients whose edentulous segments do not coincide with the host zones selected for edentulous patients.

Here again the temptation to extrapolate data is a very strong one, and here again we would argue in favor of discretion and prudence until results from long-term clinical trials are available. Until then we cannot yet subsume the versatility and routine application of the technique. See second box on p. 206.

Implicit in this list of salient features underscoring the argument favoring osseointegration for elderly edentulous patients is the risk the profession runs of losing sight of even better science and its application that is published up to now. The profession and prosthodontists in particular must resist such a temptation.

It should also be possible to produce an implant system that does all the things the Brånemark one does but at a fee that does not deny it to those who need it most. The majority of elderly patients are on fixed incomes, a fiscal predicament that is likely to preclude "state-of-science" prosthetic dentistry. The hallmark of a health service is not only the intelligence and ingenuity that reflects its therapeutic innovations, but also the universality of its application. Anything short of such an objective usurps the notion of a health profession.

## CONCLUSION

The predicament of being elderly and edentulous has taken a fair toll in undermined life quality for patient and dentist alike. The former suffered because of their morphologic and functional compromise, the latter because of a dearth of safe and predictably successful clinical modalities to prescribe. The advent of osseointegration appears to have profoundly changed this predicament. The biologic anchorage of tooth-root analogs in elderly edentulous jaws is finally tenable. Prosthodontic treatment has entered a new scientific era of restorative therapy. Our elderly patients are bound to benefit from this breakthrough.

## REFERENCES

1. Adell R, Leckholm U, Rockler B, and Brånemark P-I: A 15-year study of osseointegrated implants in the treatment of the edentulous jaw, Int J Oral Surg 10:387, 1981.
2. Agerberg G and Carlsson GE: Chewing ability in relation to dental and general health: analysis of data obtained from a questionnaire, Acta Odontol Scand 39:147, 1981.
3. Albrektsson T, Zarb GA, Worthington P, and Eriksson AR: The long-term efficacy of currently used dental implants: a review and proposed criteria of success, Int J Oral Maxillofac Implants 1(1):11, 1986.
4. Bergen E, Johnsen TB, and Ingerbretsen R: Patient motives and fulfillment of motives in renewal of complete dentures, Acta Odontol Scand 42:235, 1984.
5. Blomberg S and Lindquist LW: Psychological reactions to edentulousness and treatment with jawbone-anchored bridges, Acta Psychiatr Scand 68:251, 1983.
6. Bolender CL, Swoope CC, and Smith DE: The Cornell Medical Index as a prognostic aid for complete denture patients, J Prosthet Dent 22:20, 1969.
7. Brånemark P-I, Hansson BO, Adel R, Breine U, et al: Osseointegrated implants in the treatment of the edentulous jaw: experience from a ten-year period, monograph, Stockholm, 1977, Almquist & Wiksell.
8. Brånemark P-I, Zarb GA, and Albrektsson T: Tissue integrated prostheses osseointegration in clinical dentistry, Chicago, 1985, Quintessence Int Co.
9. Budtz-Jørgensen E: Prosthetic considerations in geriatric dentistry. In Holm-Pederson P and Löe H, editors: Geriatric dentistry, Copenhagen, 1986, Munksgaard.
10. Friedman JW: A guide for the evaluation of dental care, Los Angeles, 1972, School of Public Health, University of California.
11. Friedman N, Landesman HM, and Wexler M: The influence of fear, anxiety, and depression on the patient's adaptive response to complete dentures, Part 2, J Prosthet Dent 59:45, 1988.
12. Haraldson T: Functional evaluation of bridges on osseointegrated implants in the edentulous jaw, thesis, Göteborg, Sweden, 1979, University of Göteborg.
13. Henry PJ: Osseointegrated dental implants: two-year follow-up replication study. 24th Australian Dental Congress, Aust Dent J 31(4):247, 1986.
14. Hickey JC, Zarb GA. and Bolender C: Prosthodontic treatment for edentulous patients, ed 9, St. Louis, 1985, The CV Mosby Co.
15. Ismail Y, Zullo T, and Kruper D: The use of the psychological screening inventory as a predictor of problem patients, J Dent Res 54:L513, 1974 (abstract).
16. Jemt T: Masticatory mandibular movements, doctoral thesis, Göteborg, Sweden, 1984, University of Göteborg.
17. Köndell PA, Nordenram A, and Landt H: Titanium implants in the treatment of edentulousness: the influence of patient's age on prognosis, Gerodontics 4(6):280, 1988.
18. Landt H and Hedegard B: Patientgruppen, bei denen Adaptationsschwierigkeiten vorkommen. In Haunfelder D, Hupfauf L, Ketterl W, and Schmuth G, editors: Die Praxis der Zahnheilkunde, München-Wien-Baltimore, 1983, Urban und Schwarzenberg.
19. Laney WR, Tolman DE, Keller EE, et al: Dental implants: tissue-integrated prosthesis utilizing the osseointegration concept, Mayo Clin Proc 61:91, 1986.
20. Lang NP and Weber HP: Fixed prosthodontics in geriatric dentistry. In Holm-Pederson P and Löe H, editors: Geriatric dentistry, Copenhagen, 1986, Munksgaard.
21. Lindhe J and Nyman S: Scaling and granulation tissue removal in periodontal therapy, J Clin Periodontol 12(5):374, 1985.
22. Lindquist LW: Prosthetic rehabilitation of the edentulous mandible, doctoral thesis, Göteborg, Sweden, 1987, University of Göteborg.

23. Matthiessen PC: Demography: impact of an expanding elderly population. In Holm-Pederson P and Löe H, editors: Geriatric dentistry, Copenhagen, 1986, Munksgaard.
24. Osterberg T: Odontologic studies in 70 year old people, thesis, Göteborg, Sweden, 1981, University of Göteborg.
25. Smith D and Zarb GA: Criteria for success of osseointegrated endosseous implants, J Prosthet Dent 62(5):567, 1989.
26. Sobolovik CF and Larson HJ: Predicting denture acceptance through psychotechnics, J Dent Educ 32:67, 1968.
27. Steen B: Nutrition in the elderly: implications for oral health care. In Holm-Pederson P and Löe H, editors: Geriatric dentistry, Copenhagen, 1986, Munksgaard.
28. Swoope CC: Identification and management of emotional patients, J Prosthet Dent 27:437, 1972.
29. Toolson LB and Smith D: A five-year longitudinal study of patients treated with overdentures, J Prosthet Dent 49(16):749, 1983.
30. van Steenberghe D, Quirynen M, Calberson L, and Demanet M: A prospective evaluation of the fate of 697 consecutive intraoral fixtures modum Brånemark in the rehabiliation of edentulism, J Head Neck Pathol 6:53, 1987.
31. Worthington P, Bolender C, and Taylor T: The Swedish system of osseointegrated implants: problems and complications encountered during a four-year trial period, Int J Oral Maxillofac Implants 2(2):77, 1987.
32. Zarb GA: The edentulous milieu, Toronto Conference on Osseointegration in Clinical Dentistry, J Prosthet Dent 49(6):825, 1983.
33. Zarb GA: Impact of osseointegration on preprosthetic surgery. In Albrektsson T and Zarb GA, editors: The Brånemark Osseintegrated Implant, Chicago, 1989, Quintessence Int Co.
34. Zarb GA and Schmitt A: The longitudinal clinical effectiveness of osseointegrated dental implants: the Toronto Study, Part I, Surgical results, J Prosthet Dent 63(4):451, 1990.
35. Zarb GA and Schmitt A: The longitudinal clinical effectiveness of osseointegrated dental implants: the Toronto Study, Part II, The prosthetic results, J Prosthet Dent 64(1):53, 1990.
36. Zarb GA and Schmitt A: The longitudinal clinical effectiveness of osseointegrated dental implants: the Toronto Study, Part III, Problems and complications encountered, J Prosthet Dent 64(2):185, 1990.
37. Zarb GA, Schmitt A, and Apse P: Longitudinal effectiveness of osseointegrated dental implants: peri-implant mucosal response, IADR Abstr no 367, 1989.
38. Zarb GA, Schmitt A, and Chaytor D: Longitudinal effectiveness of osseointegrated dental implants: radiographic analysis, IADR Abstr no 362, 1989.

# 13

# Oral and Maxillofacial Surgery for the Geriatric Patient

*Lonnie H. Norris*

In the geriatric population, the need for preprosthetic surgery for the treatment of edentulous atrophic alveolar ridges and for pathology surgery to remove neoplastic lesions is greater than the need in younger age groups. There is less need for elective orthognathic surgery for correction of craniofacial skeletal anomalies. But overall, the types of oral and maxillofacial surgical procedures that can be performed for the geriatric patient is essentially the same for all adults. Individuals differ greatly in their aging process; therefore chronologic age is not always a reliable index of the ability to undergo surgical procedures. The need for special concern for oral and maxillofacial surgery in the geriatric patient is not related to the kinds of operations but rather to the greater incidence of complicating systemic diseases, to the increased use of medications to stabilize debilitating medical conditions, and to the differences in physiologic and psychologic responses to surgery.

Often major modifications in general patient management must be considered to compensate for compromising physiologic and psychologic differences. Each patient must be thoroughly individually assessed.

Management can be divided into preoperative, intraoperative and postoperative considerations.

## PREOPERATIVE CONSIDERATION

In the preoperative management of geriatric patients it is essential to:

1. Review the medical and psychologic stability of the patient to tolerate surgical procedures.

2. Review both prescribed and over-the-counter medications being taken for possible side effects or adverse drug interactions, which may alter management and surgical plans.
3. Establish surgical treatment plans at levels of intervention that coincide with the extent of surgery the elderly patient can physiologically and psychologically tolerate.
4. Select the appropriate anesthesia technique based on the patient's overall physiologic and psychologic status and on the surgical procedure planned.
5. Plan the number and length of surgical appointments required that will be the least stressful.
6. Select the most appropriate surgical environment for the patient, that is, outpatient versus hospital.

As a consequence of the physiologic changes associated with aging, there are high incidences of chronic diseases as well as effects of the use of medications. About 80% of the elderly suffer from at least one chronic disease; 40% may suffer from two or more chronic diseases.[34,62] Forty-two percent are limited in activity because of chronic conditions. Surveys reveal that in those elderly seeking dental treatment there is a high prevalence of arthritis (58%), hypertension (41%), disorders of vision, hearing, nose, and throat (28%), cardiac problems (25%), histories of benign or malignant tumors or cyst (25%), and allergies (20%). Gastrointestinal disorders, liver and gallbladder problems, kidney disorders, rashes and skin diseases, diabetes, and sinusitis were reported in 15% to 20%. In addition, slightly more than 7% reported mental and nervous disorders.[5,9,86]

A study involving 3,217 rural Iowans who were 65 years or older stated that 77% reported taking at least one medication that could significantly affect dental treatment or patient management. Fifty-one percent reported medications known to cause xerostomia, 39% reported medications possibly affecting hemostasis, 28% were at risk of drug-inducted soft-tissue reactions, 22% reported medications that could interact with drugs commonly prescribed in dentistry for pain and anxiety control, 20% reported medications requiring that vasoconstrictor use be minimized, and 16% reported medications indicating reduced stress tolerance.[5,47-48] Problems in surgical management can be associated either with the compromising systemic disease process or to the medications taken for treatment of the systemic disease.

Although preoperative history and clinical examination are important in all patients, they are more essential in the elderly because of the higher incidence for more advanced medically compromising diseases.[45] However, obtaining an accurate history may be more difficult because of poor memory, diminished comprehension, or hearing, speech, or vision problems. Infrequently, the past medical history may be too detailed about outdated coincidental episodes. Considerable time can be consumed trying to obtain significant data. A review of older patients of a dental school found 87% used multiple medications. Yet, 18% were unaware of the name of at least one of their prescriptions, and 8% did not know the name of the medications or why they were taking them.[64] Care must be taken in directing questions or providing information in simple language. Patience and sensitivity are essential in the management of older patients.

It is often necessary to rely on family members or friends to provide information, but frequently, more reliable information can be obtained from discharge summaries of hospital medical records or consultation with their current physician. However, because of potential problems in obtaining a reliable medical history or contacting reliable sources, there is greater dependence on clinical examination to reveal the signs of systemic diseases. A minimal clinical examination should in-

clude evaluation of blood pressure, pulse, and respiration and observation of the general apperance for assessment of coloration, stamina, chest configuration, distension of neck veins, or ankle edema. Based on clinical findings, laboratory evaluations may be indicated, including blood and urine analysis, chest radiograph, electrocardiogram, and reevaluation by their physician before surgical intervention. Often, in consultation with the patient's physician, medication regimens must be modified preoperatively to prevent unfavorable surgical sequelae, or preoperative antibiotics must be initiated as special precautions to prevent bacteremias or infections.

In patients with compromising systemic diseases, it is important to prevent stress.[44,45] The need for adequate pain control during treatment may be even more compelling than in other patients. Once a surgical procedure is planned, it is important to choose an appropriate anesthesia technique.

For oral and maxillofacial surgery procedures for the elderly, local anesthesia, nitrous oxide–oxygen inhalation sedation, parenteral sedation, and general anesthesia techniques are all available. Choice of which would be most appropriate is dependent on the surgical procedure required and the overall medical and emotional status of the patient. There are no specific contraindications to administration of local anesthesia agents to older patients. Local anesthesia agents are generally preferred and are less problematic in monitoring. However, carefully used sedation techniques or even general anesthesia may offer advantages dependent on the difficulty of the surgical procedure or the medical and emotional condition of the patient.

Using a local anesthesia agent containing a small concentration of epinephrine is usually not contraindicated provided that intravascular injection is avoided by a proper aspiration. However, in patients with organic heart disease and compromised cardiac function such as angina pectoris, congestive heart failure, history of myocardial infarction, and hypertension, it is recommended that the total amount of epinephrine be limited to 0.04 mg during an appointment.[8,35,47] This is equivalent to 4 ml or approximately two cartridges of 2% lidocaine solution containing 1:100,000 concentration of epinephrine. Mepivacaine 3%, without a vasoconstrictor, can be used effectively to provide a satisfactory level of anesthesia with sufficient duration. It is preferred whenever there is a question of myocardium sensitivity to vasoconstrictors. In addition, vasoconstrictors should be avoided in patients with hyperthyroidism or patients taking medications in that the vasoconstrictor may result in the potentiation of the vasopressor effect or a hypertensive crisis. Monoamine oxidase inhibitors, such as tranylcypromine (Parnate) or phenelzine sulfate (Nardil), adrenergic neuron-blocking agents, such as guanethidine or reserpine, or even tricyclic antidepressant agents, such as amitriptyline, are included in these medications.[56,90]

In the administration of local anesthetic agents, special caution must be taken not to cause a toxicity reaction from an inadvertent overdose. Total dosages of local anesthetic agents should be based on a recommended dose per unit of body weight, either milligrams per pound, or milligrams per kilogram. For lidocaine 2% with 1:100,000 epinephrine and for mepivacaine HCl (Carbocaine) 3% without a vasoconstrictor, the recommended maximum dose is calculated based on 2 mg/lb (4.4 mg/kg), with 300 mg being the absolute maximum dose. The Council on Dental Therapeutics of the American Dental Association revised the maximum recommended safe dosages for local anesthetics and no longer adjusts dosages for the inclusion of a vasoconstrictor.[51] Maximum calculated local anesthetic dosages should always be decreased for the medically compromised, debilitated, and elderly patients because of the unknown degree of hepatic and renal dysfunction. Decreased renal perfusion and hepatic dysfunction will produce increased plasma levels of drugs and therefore exaggerated clinical actions as well as prolonged duration. At each appointment a medically compromised 100-pound patient should be administered less than 5.5 cartridges of 2% lidocaine (36 mg/cartridge) or less than 3.5 cartridges of 3% mepivacaine (54 mg/cartridge).

*Nitrous oxide–oxygen inhalation sedation* is probably the most highly recommended sedation. It is easily administered in noninvasive techniques and is readily reversed. The major indication for the use of nitrous oxide–oxygen ($N_2O/O_2$) inhalation sedation is the management of fear and anxiety. However, $N_2O/O_2$ sedation has an important role in the management of medically compromised

patients. In elderly patients with cariovascular disease, $N_2O/O_2$ sedation has the advantage of producing both a reduction in anxiety and an elevation in the pain reaction threshold and of providing a minimum of 30% oxygen content. (Room air has only an 18% to 21% oxygen content). All these factors indirectly decrease the work load of the myocoradium and the potential for ischemia. In addition, in the presence of hepatic dysfunction, nitrous oxide does not undergo biotransformation in the liver and causes no additional toxicity risk.

Chronic obstructive pulmonary disease, for example, emphysema and chronic bronchitis, represents a relative contraindication to the use of $N_2O/O_2$ inhalation sedation because of the potential effect of an oxygen-enriched gas mixture to produce apnea during the procedure. The stimulus for breathing in a healthy person is an increase in the blood carbon dioxide level. However, patients with chronic obstructive pulmonary disease have lost their ability to respond to this stimulus because of already existing chronic elevated carbon dioxide levels. The stimulus in these patients is a lowered blood oxygen content. When the oxygen saturation of blood is raised during administration of $N_2O/O_2$, the stimulus for involuntary breathing is removed. Yet, in the conscious patient where voluntary control over breathing is still possible, prolonged apnea does not develop.[52]

*Parenteral (intravenous) sedation* is more profound in effect than $N_2O/O_2$ inhalation sedation and is recommended for patients with more intense anxiety or more involved surgical procedures. Caution must be employed in the administration of central nervous system–depressant drugs to patients over 65 because of a greater than usual incidence of overreaction to therapeutic dosages. In addition, a major limitation in the use of intravenous sedation techniques is the lack of integrity of veins. As people age, veins lose elasticity and become more brittle or fragile, causing increased difficulty when venipuncture is performed and higher incidents of hematoma, venospasms, and infiltrations. Yet the amnesia effect and the depth of sedation that can be titrated make parenteral sedation favorable as compared to $N_2O/O_2$ inhalation. Parenteral sedation techniques use hemodynamically safer agents for management than general anesthesia techniques do. In fact, many patients respond to parenteral sedation with conscious levels similar to general anesthesia but without the physiologically depressing side effects of general anesthesia.

The most used agents in parenteral sedation are the benzodiazepines *diazepam* and *midazolam*. However, because of midazolam's potency and its potential to cause severe respiratory depression, it should be used with extreme caution in the medically compromised and geriatric patient. The benzodiazepines undergo biotransformation in the liver and must be used with caution in patients with hepatic dysfunction. Overall, older patients have increased sensitivity to agents, and the dosages of benzodiazepines should be decreased as compared to other adults. The rate at which the drug undergoes biotransformation is decreased. There is decreased protein binding of drugs in the geriatric age group. This means that there will be more of the free, unbound drug available within the blood to cross the blood-brain barrier and produce central nervous system depression.

In all sedation techniques, whether inhalation or parenteral, local anesthesia must still be used to block the pain stimulus. Only with general anesthesia can there be a complete loss of response to pain.

*General anesthesia* is defined as a controlled state of depressed consciousness accompanied by partial or complete loss of protective reflexes, including the ability to independently maintain an airway and respond purposefully to physical stimulation or verbal command. The most common agent used in outpatient general anesthesia is methohexital, an ultrashort-acting barbiturate that offers the advantage of quick metabolism. Yet deep general anesthesia is not recommended for geriatric patients in outpatient clinics and should be used with discretion in medically compromised patients in the hospital. Because the aging process involves physiologic changes with gradual reduction in the functional capacity of most organs of the body, older patients are automatically considered an anesthesia risk, even without significant past medical histories. In cases in which extensive surgery is required, hospitalization with treatment as an inpatient is recommended. Generally, the morbidity risk/benefit ratio of the anesthesia should not be greater than the morbidity risk/benefit of the surgery. For example, for a geriatric patient with significant cardiac compromise, general anesthesia may be indicated to reduce and stabilize an edentulous atrophic bilateral mandible fracture, but it would not be indicated for the removal of mobile periodontally involved teeth. Further, in the anxious patient with a high cardiac risk the use of local anesthesia with $N_2O/O_2$ inhalation or intravenous diazepam sedation, to reduce stress and the myocardial work load, would be preferred over local anesthesia in performing minor oral surgery.

*Orally administered and intramuscularly administered sedation techniques* are also available. However, orally administered drugs cannot be titrated and can give unpredictable clinical responses. Intramuscular administered drugs are more traumatic in delivery to the fragile patient and also cannot be titrated for reliable responses. Diazepam and other benzodiazepines are popular oral premedications. If they are used for the geriatric patient, it is recommended to use smaller than recommended therapeutic dosages. It is not recommended to use intramuscular sedation because of the increased risk of exaggerated untitrated drug effect.

Most patients with associated medical problems tolerate surgery better both physiologically and psychologically when it is performed in the morning. An exception may be patients with chronic obstructive pulmonary disease because longer periods of ambulation enables them to improve pulmonary ventilation,[45] in which case early afternoon appointments would be preferred. The length of appointments and the amount of surgery performed per appointment should generally be decreased in the physiologically compromised. Thus, in preoperative treatment planning, multiple short appointments are usually preferred.[85] An exception would be if medications have to be altered preoperatively to decrease the risk of surgically related complications, but by alteration of the medications the overall risk for a medically related complication is increased. For example, with patients on anticoagulation therapy, with high risk of recurrent thromboembolistic episodes, it may be best to manage these patients with fewer appointments and with less interruptions of their anticoagulation therapy. Close monitoring in a hospital environment would be suggested.

## INTRAOPERATIVE CONSIDERATION

Physiologic changes associated with aging alter the geriatric patient's ability to respond to the trauma and stress of surgery. These changes include reduced protein turnover and conversion, reduction in tissue elastin, declines in cellular reproduction and metabolic rate, impaired cardiovascular function and peripheral microcirculation, and decreased calcium absorption.[10,16,26,45,72] Special care must be taken to minimize tissue damage and to limit the potential of infection. Important surgical considerations in the intraoperative management of geriatric patients include the following:

1. Sterile techniques
2. Gentle handling of tissues
3. Proper flap design to maintain adequate blood supply
4. Minimal stripping of the periosteum
5. Avoidance of dead space in the wound to prevent hematoma formation and infection

Thin and delicate tissue with reduced elasticity, hypertension, and increased capillary fragility contribute to the increased intraoperative bleeding problems and extensive postoperative ecchymosis.[45] Since many older patients are also borderline anemic, it is more essential to obtain proper hemostasis and minimize blood loss during surgery. Blood loss can be limited if one keeps the tissue reflected to the minimum to gain appropriate access, applies retraction forces with care to prevent unnecessary stripping of tissue or soft-tissue tears, and limits the amount of surgery done at any appointment. In addition, immediate suturing and pressure application to a surgical site, that is, one extraction quadrant, before one proceeds to another site is advantageous in controlling blood loss. One must constantly remember that the healing capabilities are far less forgiving to errors in surgical techniques and planning than those errors in young healthy persons.

Oral and maxillofacial surgical services most frequently provided for geriatric patients can be classified in the procedural areas of exodontia surgery, preprosthetic surgery, trauma surgery, and surgical management of pathologic lesions. The surgical techniques used in treatment are no different from those applicable to younger healthy persons. The armamentarium and techniques of oral and maxillofacial surgery procedures have been well documented.[43,66] Thus, in a discussion of oral and maxillofacial services, emphasis will be placed on the uniqueness in management of geriatric patients rather than on established techniques.

## EXODONTIA SURGERY

The combination of genetic predisposition, life style and socioeconomic environment, exposure to fluorides, oral hygiene at home, and dental visit behaviors throughout a person's lifetime contributes to the state of oral health or lack of it in later years. Indications for the removal of teeth increase with age. This does not result solely from enhanced susceptibility but also reflects the accumulation of insults over time.[29] Oral and maxillofacial surgeons agree with other dental health providers that all possible efforts should be made to maintain natural dentition, yet there are still many indications for removal of teeth. Following are the most common indications for removal of teeth:

1. Nonrestorable teeth secondary to advanced caries or unfavorable fracture
2. Severe periodontal disease with excesive bone loss and irreversible tooth mobility
3. Impacted teeth with associated pathologic lesions
4. Preradiation with or without chemotherapy extraction of compromised dentition
5. Severely compromised teeth in line with a jaw fracture
6. Medical and economic limitations in a restorative treatment plan

Before extraction, teeth must be examined carefully for assessment of the difficulty of the extraction. It is essential to take proper radiographs. In general, periapical radiographs provide the most accurate and detailed view of the tooth roots and the surrounding bony tissue. Panoramic radiographs are most useful for views of impacted teeth and in the management of compromised patients limited to tolerate multiple intraoral radiographs. When one is reviewing radiographs to assess the difficulty of extraction, the root portion of the radiograph is most important. The configuration of the roots, the status of the periodontal ligament, the density of the surrounding bone, the relation-

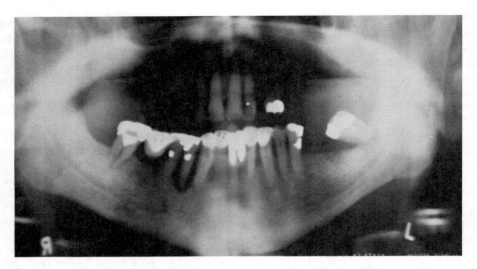

**Fig. 13-1** Panoramic radiograph showing root caries and severe periodontal disease. Clinical mobility of teeth facilitates in uncomplicated extractions.

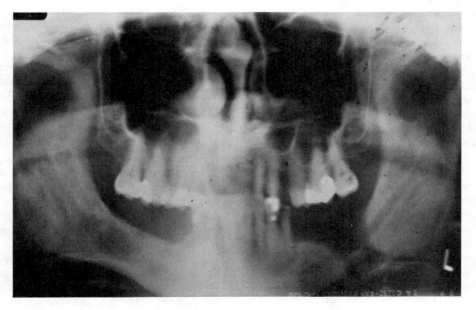

**Fig. 13-2** Pneumatized left maxillary sinus in association with roots of teeth. Great chance of sinus exposure if molars are extracted. Chronic osteomyelitis with pathologic fracture from recently exfoliated infected tooth from left mandible.

ship of the roots to associated vital structures, and possible periapical lesions influence the surgical trauma the patient must undergo, as well as the required armamentarium and anesthesia technique (Figs. 13-1 and 13-2).

Clinical evaluation can be made of the condition of the tooth's crown, the access into the oral cavity, the cooperation of the patient, and the mobility of the tooth.

Devitalized teeth and teeth with large restorations have a high probability of fracture on removal. Long roots with excessive curvature, bulbous roots with hypercementosis, or wide divergence of roots indicate surgical extraction and splitting of teeth. Short conical roots usually make the extractions easier. It is important to assess the level of bone loss as well as the density of bone, the status of the periodontal ligament space, and the clinical mobility of teeth. With equal levels of vertical bone loss, differences in difficulties of removal of teeth have been encountered because the surrounding bone often becomes sclerotic. If the bone appears more dense than normal with evidence of condensing osteosis or chronic diffuse

sclerosing osteomyelitis and there is no clinical tooth mobility, conservative endodontic or periodontic therapy would be preferable to extraction. Often, these teeth cannot be extracted with forceps but must be surgically drilled out and often result in complications attributable to long delayed healing with multiple acute exacerbations. Sclerotic bone is relatively avascular and responds poorly to any trauma or bacterial infection[73] (Fig. 13-3).

When performing extraction of isolated maxillary molars in partially edentulous patients, one must make special consideration to the fact that there is a likelihood of only a thin layer of bone between the pneumatized maxillary sinus and the roots of these teeth. The potential for perforation of the sinus during routine forceps extraction is high. Therefore, if preoperative radiographs indicate the likelihood of accidental sinus exposure, the adjacent buccal alveolar bone should be removed and the tooth sectioned to limit the forces exerted on the sinus wall during tooth removal.

If a small perforation (1 to 3 mm) occurs into the sinus and the sinus is disease free, additional soft-tissue flap closure is not required.[53,66] Efforts

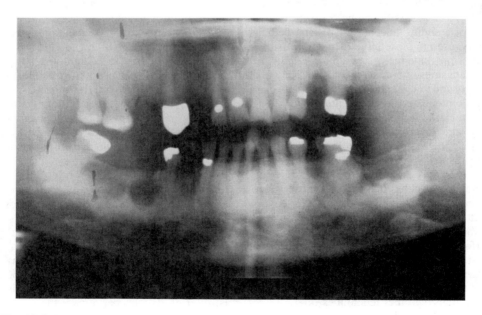

**Fig. 13-3** Chronic sclerosing osteomyelitis with dense avascular bone. Endodontic and periodontic treatment preferred over extractions in order to prevent long-term postoperative nonhealing complications.

are made to establish a clot in the site by gentle insertion of a piece of absorbable gelatin sponge into the socket and by pressure over the extraction site for 1 to 2 hours. Soft tissues displaced during the extraction should be repositioned and sutured. The patient is instructed to avoid nose blowing, inhaling cigarettes, or sucking straws and to avoid any other situation that may produce pressure changes between the nasal passages and oral cavity. The patient is given an antibiotic. Usually penicillin is the antibiotic of choice, since the perforation was of odontogenic origin. It is noted that in maxillary sinusitis of nonodontogenic cause ampicillin or amoxicillin are commonly used as the antibiotic of choice because of the prevalence of *Haemophilus influenzae* in the sinus. Regardless of the antibiotic choice, the patient is also placed on nasal spray decongestant and an oral systemic decongestant for 7 to 10 days to shrink mucous membranes and to lessen nasal secretions.

Surgical closure is indicated if large perforations occur or if chronic oroantral communications develops. Varied surgical techniques are used for closure of oroantral fistulas that require mobilization and rotation of soft-tissue flaps to cover the defects.[15,46,53,76,91-93] A small opening is readily sealed by means of a sliding buccal flap. Palatal pedicle flaps can be used to close large fistulas, or fistulas that recur or preclude the use of a buccal flap. The mucosal flaps must be designed to have a good blood supply and to least alter the surrounding anatomy to accommodate use of a denture.

Various metallic foil plates have been advocated for the closure of oroantral fistulas. Twenty-four carat, 36-gauge gold plate has been used with encouraging results.[19,27] The foil is placed over the bony defect and is positioned beneath overlying buccal and palatal flaps. It provides a more stable base to support mucosal flaps and directly covers the defect. This technique offers particular advantages to the edentulous geriatric patient with large sinus perforations, in that it requires less reflection and repositioning of large soft-tissue flaps, shorter convalescent period, and less reduction of vestibule depth that interefere with denture retention on atrophic ridges than the other techniques do.

In young healthy patients, as a general rule, all impacted teeth should be removed as soon as they can be determined to be nonfunctional, unless removal is otherwise contraindicated. This decision is usually made during the late teenage years between 16 and 18 years of age, when the roots are between one third to two thirds formed. This is the preventive philosophy of dentistry extended to the removal of impacted teeth to circumvent the necessity of removal later in life when the surgery is more likely to be complicated by the bone being denser and less vascular and the patient being more medically compromised. Younger patients physiologically and psychologically tolerate surgical procedures better and heal more quickly.

In the geriatric patient, impacted teeth are removed only if associated pathosis indicates the necessity of removal. If the impacted tooth has been retained for many years without periodontal exposure, caries, or cystic enlargement, it is unlikely any pathosis will begin in the later years. Therefore in the elderly patient with an asymptomatic impacted tooth found on routine radiographic examination that has no associated disease and has a reasonably thick layer of overlying bone, the impacted tooth should not be removed. Periodic radiographic examination of the area is advised every 1 or 2 years to ensure that favorable conditions for retention remain stable.

All too frequently, the patient presents with pericoronitis or caries involving a previously impacted tooth in an otherwise edentulous, atrophic mandible. The alveolar process gradually undergoes resorption with age. Thus the impacted tooth finally comes to the surface, as if erupting. In addition, dentures may compress bone to increase the resorption rate, or compress soft tissue over the underlying tooth to result in soft-tissue perforation and subsequent infection. If cystic lesions occur, the presenting complaint is often the inability to retain the denture over the expanding alveolar ridge or notice of a soft area on the ridge (Figs. 13-4 to 13-7).

Caution must be taken in the surgical management of older patients in the removal of impacted teeth. The risk of systemic complications is higher because of their compromised physiologic status. In addition, the risk of local complications—that is, inferior alveolar nerve paresthesia and fracture of the mandible or of the maxillary tuberosity—is higher. The changes in bone elasticity and density of the atrophic ridge, the possible occurrence of

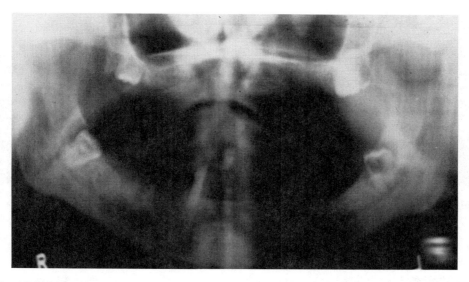

**Fig. 13-4** Advanced caries in impacted third molars of medically compromised geriatric patient with severe angina pectoris and scheduled for coronary bypass surgery.

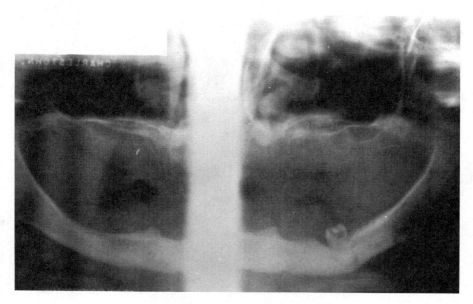

**Fig. 13-5** Impacted molar with exposure into oral cavity after long-term denture wear. High risk of mandible fracture. Autogenous bone grafting and immobilization of mandible indicated if tooth is removed.

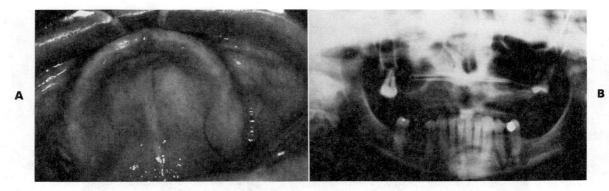

**Fig. 13-6 A,** Maxillary right third molar exposed into oral cavity after long-term denture wear. **B,** Panoramic radiograph reveals impacted maxillary left third molar not clinically exposed yet, with maxillary right third molar seen clinically.

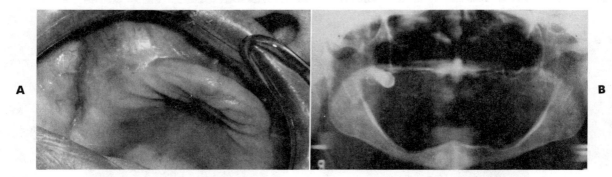

**Fig. 13-7 A,** Buccal expansion with acute symptoms at edentulous maxillary ridge. **B,** Radiograph reveals impacted maxillary third molar with cystic lesion.

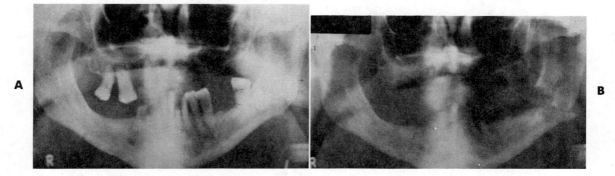

**Fig. 13-8 A,** Impacted ankylosed third molar in geriatric patient. Bone density is the same as tooth structure. **B,** Fractured mandible from fall 1 week after removal of teeth.

ankylosis with long-retained impacted teeth, and frequent inability to clinically distinguish the difference between tooth and bone coloration or hardness can make the removal of impacted teeth an extremely difficult surgical procedure. Special care must be taken not to exert excessive force. Thus bone must be removed and teeth sectioned to give the least amount of resistance on removal (Fig. 13-8).

In the geriatric patient, indications for removal of bony impacted teeth must be overwhelmingly convincing to justify a good ratio of benefit to risk of complication.

## PREPROSTHETIC SURGERY

Preprosthetic surgery is surgical preparation and recontouring of the remaining soft tissue and bony alveolar ridges after removal of teeth to better accommodate the use of a prosthesis. Many oral and maxillofacial surgery procedures including maxillary tuberosity reduction, palatal or mandibular torus removal, frenectomy, and alveoloplasty are in this category of surgery (Fig. 13-9). However, in the older population one of the most challenging areas of preprosthetic surgery is the management of the atrophic ridge.

Improvements in oral health status and the considerable decrease in the incidence of caries attributable to fluoridation have caused a gradual reduction in the percentage of completely edentulous Americans.[29,63] Yet, based on National Health In-terview Survey (NIHIS) data in 1983, 45% of persons over 74 years of age and 34% of persons in the age group 65 to 74 are edentulous.

Although fluoride traditionally has been associated with prevention of decay in children, a study in Canada showed that the occurrence of root decay in adults with lifelong histories of fluoridated water consumption was approximately 60% less than it was in nonfluoridated areas.[29,89] This finding is particularly important to the geriatric population in which the high incidence of nonrestorable root and cervical caries often leads to edentulism. In the National Survey of Oral Health in U.S. Employed Adults and Seniors, 1985-1986, 67% of the males and 61% of the females in the geriatric population had root surface lesions, with almost 66% unrestored in males and 38% unrestored in females.[63]

Despite progress in preserving dentition, there is a significant number of patients in need of preprosthetic surgery to modify edentulous ridges for better denture retention. While teeth are present, alveolar bone responds to physiologic stress by aligning the trabeculas appropriately. There are several interpretations that explain edentulous bone loss after the teeth have been removed. First, disuse atrophy undoubtedly plays a role in a low turnover type of remodeling. Second, excessive loading in the pressure-resorption phenomenon may contribute to a higher turnover type of remodeling.[1,25]

As teeth are removed, the corresponding alveolar bone undergoes osteoclastic activity. Of all the lo-

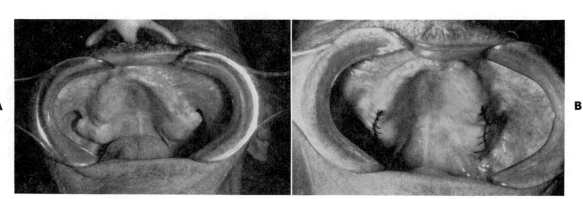

**A** **B**

**Fig. 13-9** **A**, Bilateral tuberosity enlargements with buccal exostosis. **B**, Postoperative tuberosity reductions and alveoloplasties.

cal and systemic factors involved in ridge resorption, years of denture wear appears to be the most important.[58-60,81] The edentulous ridge that has accommodated a denture for many years frequently exhibits extensive resorption to the basal bone by the geriatric years. Resorption of the alveolar residual ridge is a chronic progressive and irreversible process that occurs slowly. The average rate of loss of the residual anterior ridge height is 5 to 8 mm per 10-year period.[65a]

The principle objectives of preprosthetic surgical treatment of severely atrophic alveolar ridges should include:[25]

1. Creation of a broad ridge form
2. Adequate fixed tissue over the denture-bearing area
3. Adequate vestibular depth for prosthesis extension
4. Proper interarch relationship
5. Added strength where mandible fracture may occur
6. Protection of the neurovascular bundle
7. Adequate palatal vault form
8. Proper posterior tuberosity notching

Some preprosthetic surgical procedures used to accomplish ideal reconstruction objectives are more surgically invasive than others. They require the harvesting of autogenous soft tissue or bone grafts from donor sites and significant reflection of soft-tissue flaps at recipient sites. Each patient's medical status and restorative expectations must be assessed before a surgical treatment plan is established. The frail, severely medically compromised patient may not be able to tolerate many of the advanced preprosthetic surgery procedures. Expectations of both the patient and the dental care providers may have to be modified. Only conservative surgical approaches of improvement may be allowable for the severely compromised geriatric patient.

In the development of an appropriate preprosthetic surgical treatment plan for the edentulous atrophic ridge, panoramic and cephalometric radiographs are helpful in determining ridge configuration, vertical height, and relationships. In severely atrophic ridges, computerized tomography (CT) scans provide more accurate definition of ridge configuration and the specific location of the

associated anatomy, such as inferior alveolar nerve and maxillary sinus.

Clinically the soft-tissue denture-bearing area should be examined for adequate surface area of nonmobile keratinized mucosa, for high mucosal and muscular attachments that limit vestibular depth and interfere with denture retention, and for possible hyperplastic tissue.

When adequate bone of at least 12 to 15 mm in height is available and yet soft-tissue attachments are close to the superior crest of the ridge or if there is a lack of keratinized mucosa, a vestibuloplasty technique can be performed to reposition soft-tissue attachments from the crest of ridges to inferior positions. Many vestibuloplasty techniques have been documented, including vestibuloplasty with secondary epithelialization, vestibuloplasty with soft-tissue graft, transpositional flap vestibuloplasty (lip switch), and submucosal vestibuloplasty.[17,32,36-37,54-55,65,68] Regardless of which technique is employed, the goal of vestibuloplasty ridge extension is to uncover existing basal bone of the atrophic ridge by surgically repositioning the overlying mucosa, muscle attachments, and muscle to create a deeper sulcus for increase extension of the denture flange to improve retention.

In secondary epithelialization vestibuloplasty techniques, in which overlying mucosa is repositioned to create a deeper sulcus and the underlying exposed periosteum is allowed to granulate and reepithelialize, 50% of maxillary cases relapse in 3 years. This relapse incidence can reach 80% to 95% in mandibular surgeries.[30] Submucosal vestibuloplasty with secondary epithelialization techniques have been shown to result in excessive failure, especially in the mandible, and are considered unacceptable.

Vestibuloplasty with soft-tissue grafts placed to cover the denuded periosteum are preferable in the mandible. The grafts limit scar contraction with concurrent migration of vestibular soft tissue, the combination of which obliterates the created sulcus. Various soft tissues have been used as grafts in vestibuloplasty techniques. Autogenous skin, dermis, buccal mucosa, and palatal mucosa are most commonly used tissues.[32,55,79,80]

Skin and dermis donor sites allow for more available grafting tissue for transfer to extensive intraoral recipient sites and are preferred in major

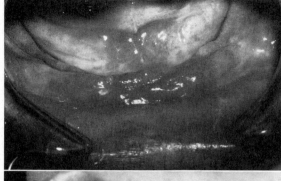
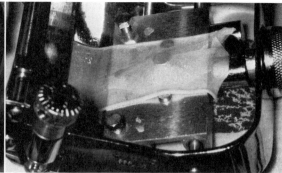
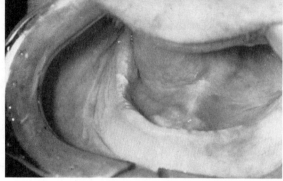

**Fig. 13-10 A,** Edentulous mandibular ridge with high muscle attachments. **B,** Dermatome used to harvest skin graft from the hip area. **C,** Vestibuloplasty with skin graft.

reconstruction cases (Fig. 13-10). The disadvantages of using skin or dermis include:

1. The need for two different surgical areas.
2. The use of general anesthesia being preferred to harvesting of the graft.
3. Body scars, even though the thigh and buttocks are the chosen donor sites, which are usually covered by clothes.
4. Grafts retain the coloration and character of the donor sites. Thus skin pigmentation and occasionally hair growth may be seen at the vestibuloplasty with skin grafts.

Mucosa from the hard palate offers the potential graft advantages of providing a firm, resilient, keratinized tissue with minimal contraction of the grafted area. Palatal tissue is relatively easy to obtain, but there is the possibility of bleeding secondary to the greater palatine vessels and only a limited amount of tissue is available. Also discomfort is associated with the postoperative healing

phase of palatal-graft donor sites. Surgical packs, dentures, or palatal splints can be used to protect the areas to lessen the discomfort.

Buccal mucosa grafts from the inner aspect of the cheek have the advantage of accessibility of graft-harvest site and more tissue availability as compared to the hard palate. However, buccal mucosa does not become keratinized, and its general mobility could result in inadequate denture-bearing surface. As with all graft donor sites of the oral cavity, in comparison to skin or dermis donor sites, concerns in management of postoperative healing can be limited to one general area.

In the medically compromised patient, if functionally possible, it is preferable to limit the vestibuloplasty extension to the anterior region of the edentulous ridge and to use soft-tissue grafts from the oral cavity. Only one surgical site (oral cavity) is required, and the surgery could be performed under local anesthesia alone or in combination with a conscious sedation technique. Thus shorter surgery time is possible with less risk of surgical or anesthetic complications.

When ridge resorption is too advanced for effective soft-tissue reposition for creation of an adequate sulcus depth in a vestibuloplasty technique, or mandibular resorption has progressed to the level that the mental foramen is exposed at the crest of the ridge causing neurosensory disturbances, ridge augmentation of the atrophic ridge may be indicated. Augmentation grafting improves the height and contour of the available denture-bearing area, adds strength to an extremely deficient mandible, and protectively covers related anatomy from trauma. Sources of graft material include autogenous rib and iliac crest, allogeneic rib, iliac crest and mandible, and alloplastic hydroxyapatite synthetic bone.

Autogenous bone has been the most biologically acceptable material used in augmentation and has the advantage of having osteogenic potential. Disadvantages in the use of autogenous bone include the need for stable health status to undergo significant donor site surgery, morbidity associated with harvesting the graft, extensive unpredictable postoperative resorption of the bone graft, and the necessity of not wearing dentures for 6 to 8 months after surgery. At least 40% to 60% of grafted bone may be resorbed during the first 1 to 2 years and 60% to 100% by the end of 3 to 5 years.[4,24,88] Various autogenous bone grafting techniques have been employed in an attempt to minimize limitations in reconstruction and to resolve some of the resorption problems. Superior border augmentation, onlay grafts, inferior border augmentation, interpositional grafts, and sagittal (visor) osteotomy with pedicled grafts have all been used with limited success in preprosthetic surgery application.[6,20,33,67,71,84] Most techniques result in better denture retention because of increased ridge bulk. However, most undergo extensive loss of ridge vertical height and require a secondary soft-tissue procedure, and possible neurosensory deficit can occur in some techniques. In the medically compromised patient, the risk of morbidity in autogenous bone graft procedures must be considered before elective preprosthetic surgery.

The use of freeze-dried allogeneic bone in preprosthetic surgery eliminates the morbidity associated with harvesting autogenous bone at a second surgical site. However, it has resorption rates similar to those of autogenous bone and does not have the osteogenic potential of autogenous bone to strengthen weak recipient areas. Also, dehiscence of overlying soft tissue has been reported with augmentation using freeze-dried bone. The combination of freeze-dried rib being used as a vertical strut on the lingual of the mandible and autogenous iliac crest bone for bulk and contour on the buccal has offered advantages of supporting the ridge height during placement of medullary bone for osteogenic potential (Fig. 13-11).

Hydroxyapatite, a dense ceramic alloplastic material, has become popular for use in preprosthetic ridge augmentation because it is readily available and has long-term dimension stability. It solves many problems related to autogenous bone grafting techniques including donor-site morbidity and excessive postoperative resorption. In addition, selected cases with moderate ridge resorption may be recontoured with use of local anesthesia. Hydroxyapatite used as synthetic bone is placed subperiosteally adjacent to bone and binds physically and chemically to the bone. Particles not directly adjacent to bone are primarily surrounded in a fibrous tissue capsule with infiltration of vascular tissue throughout the graft material. Except for the severely atrophic mandible, hydroxyapatite can be used alone as an outpatient procedure with use of local anesthesia possibly combined with a conscious sedation technique to fill undercuts and concavities, change ridge configuration, increase ridge width, and make limited increases in ridge height (Fig. 13-12).

Based on a classification of the anatomy of alveolar ridge deficiency, appropriate treatment protocols in the use of hydroxyapatite have been recommended.[25,39-40] Since hydroxyapatite does not have osteogenic potential, in the reconstruction of the severely atrophic pencil-thin flat ridge, autogenous cancellous iliac bone is mixed with it to add bone strength and to improve its capability to be contoured to desirable vertical height. Hydroxyapatite is nonresorbable and postoperative graft resorption is negligible. In addition, since it allows vascular tissue in growth around the particles, adequate vascularity is available for secondary vestibuloplasty with soft-tissue grafts. The disadvantages of hydroxyapatite in preprosthetic surgery are related to the difficulty in containing the particle

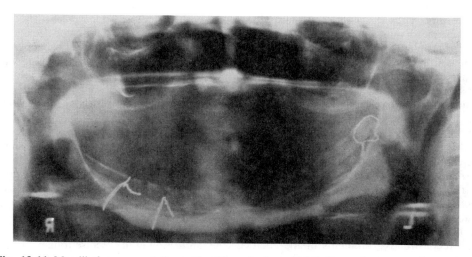

**Fig. 13-11** Mandibular augmentation with allogeneic freeze-dried rib used as a strut for vertical height and autogenous iliac crest bone packed on anterior surface for osteogenic potential and contour.

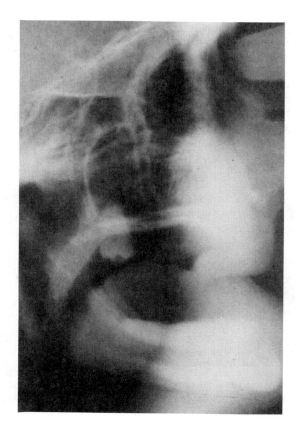

**Fig. 13-12** Lateral radiographic view of edentulous mandible with hydroxyapatite alloplastic graph. Retained maxillary third molar without any pathologic condition.

material within a confined subperiosteal tunnel and achieving adequate augmentation height. The particles tend to spread to increase width rather than consolidate vertically, a tendency that is often desirable for correction of ridge relationships and for denture retention. Various soft-tissue flap designs, tissue expanders, and splinting techniqes have been used in efforts to control particle position. Hydroxyapatite in solid block form establishes the necessary vertical height but is associated with soft-tissue dehiscence over the grafts.

Although hydroxyapatite has provided significant advancement in augmentation alternatives with overall less morbidity, it has limitations in preprosthetic surgery. In the preprosthetic reconstruction of the patient with severely atrophic ridges, autogenous cancellous iliac bone graft should be mixed with hydroxyapatite for best augmentation results. Thus the associated morbidity risk of harvesting an autogenous graft and the requirement for hospitalization and general anesthesia must be considered.

In conclusion, advanced preprosthetic reconstruction surgery procedures using autogenous bone grafting to restore prosthetic function may be too surgically invasive for the medically compromised patient. Emphasis should be placed on prevention rather than corrective treatment. Health education and prevention should be promoted early in life to maintain dentition and maximum basal bone in efforts to avoid the surgery required to reconstruct severely atrophic ridges.

With advancements in modern dental implantology, signicant interest has been generated in resolving the reconstructive problems of the edentulous patient using implantology techniques. Implantology is of special interest in the management of patients because maximum prosthetic retention can be gained with overall less surgical intervention as compared to augmentation procedures for the severely atrophic ridge. As implantology applications increase, the use of preprosthetic augmentation procedures, whether using autogenous, allogeneic, or alloplastic grafts, is less indicated.

Modern dental implantology became popular in prosthetic reconstruction in the1960s. During this period, the subperiosteal implant, a metal-alloy lat-ticework frame was placed beneath periosteum onto bone. They are fabricated from direct bone impressions of the surgically exposed alveolar ridge and are designed with transgingival posts to support a removable prosthesis.[31,74] Subperiosteal implants have the advantage of being able to be fabricated for severely atrophic ridges with minimal bone height because they are adapted on the cortical surface of the superior portion of the existing ridge. They had acceptable application in mandibular reconstruction. However, since they are large frameworks not anchored firmly into bone, they are not as acceptably functional to resist the constant forces of gravity downward against the upward forces of mastication in maxillary reconstruction. In addition, any new resorption changes in the ridge after the fabrication of the precise framework could alter the subperiosteal implant's adaptation to the ridge. The probability of implant mobility with significant gingival pocket formation around the posts and failure of the implant would drastically increase (Fig. 13-13).

Endosteal blade implants, consisting of a thin wedge-shaped or rectangular base submerged into bone for anchorage and a post that extends through the mucosa into the oral cavity to support prosthetic appliances, were used by the early 1970s.[2,25,49] Immediate rigid prosthetic fixation was required so that the implant remained firm during the bone-

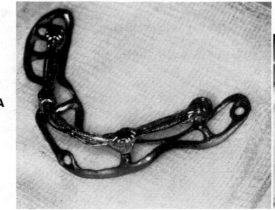
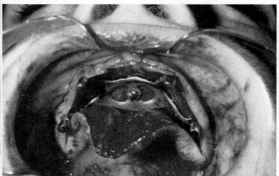

**Fig. 13-13 A,** Subperiosteal implant framework designed to sit on top of bone with post extending through soft tissue into oral cavity. **B,** Maxillary subperiosteal implant must resist gravity forces downward and occlusal forces upward for long-term success rate.

remodeling phase of healing. Subepithelial gingival fiber insertion into cementum, which is crucial to the periodontal health of the natural teeth, does not exist around the neck of dental implants. Instead there is a tight cuff of fibrous connective tissue fibers parallel to the implant surface, which supports the epithelial seal and provides a barrier to pocket formation.[57] Mobility during bone remodeling results in a widened peri-implant capsule, gingival inflammation with progressive pocket formation, and interface bone loss, which leads to short-term failure of the implant.

The mandibular frame implant is designed as an anterior endosteal blade with bilateral bar extensions that fit into surgically prepared ramus slots. The design of the implant took advantage of the areas of most available bone in the edentulous atrophic mandible and gained immobility through its tripod effect. This design of implants had similar implant-to-bone interface problems common with the endosteal blades.

During the mid-1970s, staple transosteal implants were introduced for use in the edentulous atrophic mandible in an attempt to resolve implant mobility problems that lead to early failure. It is composed of a submandibular stabilizing bone plate with multiple short retaining posts and two long posts that pass from the inferior border of the mandible through the entire vertical height of bone to enter the oral cavity in the canine region of the alveolar ridge[25,61,77-78] (Fig. 13-14). Significant implant stability is provided for mandibular overdenture retention. However, insertion of this type of implant requires a submental skin incision in an extraoral procedure performed under general anesthesia. In the rare incidence of transosteal implant failure, which necessitates its removal, the risk of mandibular fracture during its removal from the severely atrophic mandible may be significant. Favorable results are achieved with proper case selection.

Finally, in the early 1980s endosteal osseointegrated cylinder implants with two-stage implantation procedures were introduced with widespread use. The clinical insertion of cylinder implants had been initiated as early as 1965, and by 1980 substantial statistical data were available to support their excellent long-term success rate. Because of

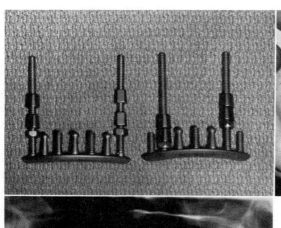

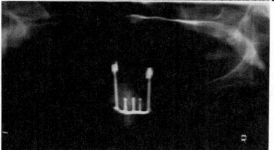

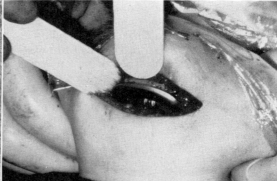

**Fig. 13-14** Staple transosteal implants of various designs inserted through the inferior border of the mandible in the symphysis area. Long posts extend into the oral cavity for prosthesis support; short posts are used for retention in base of mandible.

the advancements in methodology and in design of osseointegrated implants, improved application in the reconstruction of edentulous atrophic ridges and increased implant success rates have been realized. Osseointegration is defined as a direct contact between living haversian bone and the implant without any intervening fibrous tissue layers.

The cylindric design, two-stage surgery, and precise system of insertion appear to be crucial to the development and maintenance of a direct bone-implant interface, osseointegration.[3,12-14,42] In stage I, a precision set of internally and externally irrigated drills were designed for atraumatic preparation of the implant receptor site on the ridge to allow a precision fit between the bone and implant cylinder. One important factor that governs the outcome of an implantation procedure is the control of surgical trauma. When the implant site is prepared and the implant is inserted, a necrotic border zone is inevitably established around the foreign device caused by the frictional energy generated in drilling. This border zone must heal with new bone instead of fibrous tissue if osseointegration is to occur. The use of well-sharpened drills, careful cooling during drilling, and the avoidance of excessive drill speeds are important factors to be controlled to minimize bone trauma.

It has been reported that temperatures in excess of 43°C can produce protein coagulation with subsequent formation of necrotic bone and soft-tissue encapsulation of the implant.[22,23] In order to reduce initial bone trauma and promote healing, drill sets have been designed to operate at low rotary speeds from 10 to 20 rpm for preparation and insertion of various component parts of the system up to 1600 rpm with irrigation for bone receptor site preparation. Light and electron microscopic studies have demonstrated that bone undergoing atraumatic drilling procedures will heal directly against the titanium implant surface with a glycoprotein interface of only 20 nm.

After insertion, the implant top is covered on the crest of the ridge by the previously reflected soft-tissue flap and allowed to heal stress free for 3 to 6 months. Osseointegration with stabilization of the implant occurs during this period, and early loading is avoided to ensure optimal healing.

Stage II involves exposure of the implant, placement of a second-phase healing screw to extend the implant into the oral environment, and impressions for fabrication of the prosthesis. Either a fixed-bridge prosthesis or a full-removal denture prosthesis with clip bar can be constructed dependent on presurgical planning. The availability of bone, the number of implants inserted, and the overall medical and economic status and expectations of the patient all influence the prosthetic design decision (Figs. 13-15 and 13-16).

Bone loss is reported to be 1.5 mm in the first year and then only 0.1 mm per year on average thereafter. This is a lesser bone loss rate than that in edentulous patients without implants. Similar results with high success rates have been reported with one-stage osseointegrated cylinder implants. However, more long-term statistical data on success rates are available for two-stage osseointegrated implants, and currently one-stage osseointegrated implant systems are less commonly used.

Osseointegrated implants have generated special interest in the reconstruction of the problematic atrophic ridge of the geriatric patient because they offer:

1. Less surgical intervention as compared to autogenous bone graft techniques used in preprosthetic surgery and the capacity to be inserted with use of local anesthesia or conscious sedation techniques
2. Minimal additional bone loss after insertion in the already atrophic ridge
3. Maximum prosthesis retention with minimal available bone and more predictable prosthesis retention as compared to soft-tissue ridge-extension techniques
4. Options of full-arch fixed prosthesis versus full-removal prosthesis with clip bars
5. Less area of bony destruction associated with implant failure and easy in retrieving implants if osseointegration does not occur, as compared to other implant designs

In healthy older patients with severely atrophic ridges, the use of osseointegrated implants have been combined with autogenous, allogeneic, and alloplastic graft procedures and with mental nerve repositioning and maxillary sinus lift techniques, if indicated, to make the associated anatomy more accommodating for successful implantation.[11,38,82]

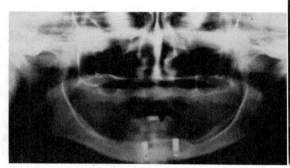
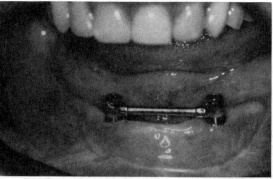

**Fig. 13-15 A,** Radiographic view of osseointegrated cylinder implants placed in application for removal clip denture—Stage I. **B,** Clinical view of clip bar attached to osseointegrated implants— Stage II.

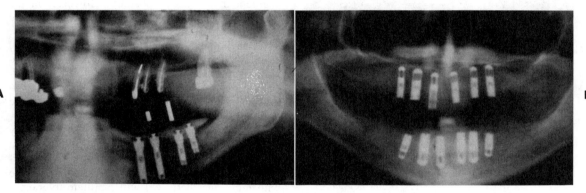

**Fig. 13-16** Radiographic views of osseointegrated cylinder implants placed in application for fixed bridge prosthesis.

Overall, the use of implantology in prosthetic reconstruction can provide a more functional prosthesis, less surgical morbidity, and improved long-term success rates as compared to other modalities of advanced preprosthetic surgery. Yet, each patient's appropriateness for the use of implantology must be evaluated individually.

In the evaluation of the geriatric patient, along with parameters on systemic health, the criteria of the motivation and dexterity to maintain oral hygiene standards must be met for implantology acceptability.

## TRAUMA SURGERY

As in the general population, the older patient may substain multiple trauma from various causes, including motor vehicle accidents, assaults, and accidental falls. However, because of the aging process, bones in the older population are less vascular and more atrophic with less elasticity. Thus overall less force is required to cause fractures and longer periods of immobilization are required for bone healing.

As in the management of any multiple trauma

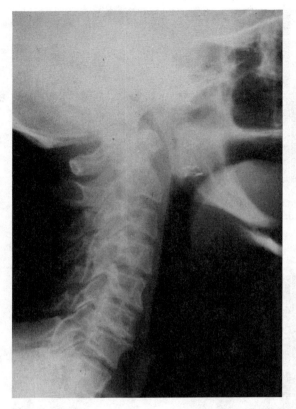

**Fig. 13-17** Bilateral parasymphysis fractures of atrophic edentulous mandible causing posterior displacement of the tongue.

management, methods of fracture stabilization, and lack of sufficient vascularity and of medullary bone to promote healing (Fig. 13-17).

Trauma to the edentulous severely atrophic mandible readily results in grossly displaced bilateral mandibular fractures. Because of the superior position maintained by the mandibular angle-and-ramus segment caused by the pull of the muscles of mastication and the inferior and backward displacement of the anterior symphysis segment and tongue by the suprahyoid muscles, acute airway obstruction can occur. As in the administration of cardiac pulmonary resusitation to the unconscious patient, manual traction of the chin is necessary to maintain the airway.

In a patient with dentition, loop wires can be placed around adjacent teeth on each side of the fracture lines to temporarily maintain the anterior segment in a reduced position. However, in the edentulous patient there is not a quick, atraumatic way to temporarily stabilize the bony segments. Thus, in the establishment of an emergency airway, emphasis is placed on repositioning of the associated soft tissues.

Placement of nasopharyngeal or an oropharyngeal airway tube may be sufficient to displace the tongue slightly forward and maintain the airway. In the conscious patient, a deeply inserted airway tube will not be tolerated well and could initiate gagging and vomiting. Spraying of the nasopharynx with local anesthetic and lubrication of the tube with local anesthetic gel will facilitate tolerance. If insertion of the airway tube is tolerated, its mere presence does not necessarily imply that satisfactory passage of air is ensured because the tube may become kinked or blocked by blood and mucus. It is essential that the patency of these tubes be maintained by frequent aspiration with fine suction catheters, which must be passed beyond the pharyngeal end, and that constant airway monitoring be maintained.[70] Beware not to cause hypoxia when suctioning.

Another option to maintain the airway in the conscious edentulous patient, if nasopharyngeal or oropharyngeal airway tubes cannot be used effectively, is to suture the tongue forward to the extraoral chin area to relieve the obstruction until more definitive treatment can be initiated.

If the airway is considerably compromised or its

patient, the first priorities for managing the patient with multiple trauma are to ensure a patent airway with adequate ventilation, assess cardiopulmonary stability by monitoring of vital signs, and control excessive bleeding. Definitive treatment of facial injuries generally can be deferred until the patient's overall status is stabilized. Since fractures of the facial bones have the potential to severely compromise the ability to maintain a patent airway, temporary repositioning facial fractures with their attached soft tissue may be of the highest priority.

Of all possible facial fractures to manage, bilateral fractures of the edentulous atrophic mandible may be one of the most challenging. The unique problems encountered in the management of these maxillofacial fractures include airway integrity is deteriorating as a result of hematoma formation or soft-tissue swelling, intubation is the satisfactory way of maintaining a clear airway. In a conscious patient an endotracheal tube is an extremely stimulating foreign body. The options are either to keep the patient's reflexes profoundly depressed pharmacologically or to perform a tracheotomy because a tracheostomy is better tolerated than an endotracheal tube. If sedation is used to tolerate the tube, the possibilities of respiratory depression and central nervous system depression may obscure the ability to accurately monitor conscious levels in neurologic evaluation.

In oral and maxillofacial trauma, regardless of the age group, airway management is of primary concern to prevent obstruction by blood clots, vomit, saliva, avulsed teeth, parts of dentures, or displaced fractures with their attached soft tissues. In the older patient with fracture of an atrophic pencil-thin mandible, the probability of airway obstruction, as well as the difficulty in its management, is more problematic. With vertical height loss, the mandible overcloses and rotates to a protruded position. Thus, because of the forward position of the mandible and the character and atrophic size of the mandibular bone, bilateral fractures of the thin mandible readily occur with trauma. Since the bone is so thin, significant backward displacement can occur from muscle pulls because of lack of interference from opposing segments to impede displacement. Once obstruction exists from displacement of the fractured edentulous mandible, the ability to temporarily stabilize the fracture to alleviate the obstruction is difficult. Finally, the incidence of compromised cardiac or pulmonary function is higher than that in the general population, and the establishment of effective ventilation is even more critical for survival with already tenuous cardiopulmonary systems.

In mandibular or maxillary fractures within stable dentition areas, with minimal displacement, and with muscle pulls in a direction to assist in reduction of the fracture, closed reductions can be performed by intermaxillary fixation. The dentition is used to establish a proper occlusal relationship and to maintain immobility of the fracture. A common technique consists in using prefabricated arch bars that are adapted to each arch and wired to the teeth. Then heavy elastics or wires are used be-

tween the two arch bars to hold the jaws together in an immobilized position, thus reducing and stabilizing the fracture.[43,70]

In grossly displaced fractures with muscle pulls that distract the fractures or in fractures behind areas of dentition or denture contact—that is, angle fractures—surgical opening of overlying soft tissue and placement of wires or plates directly into the fractured segments to reduce and stabilize them are indicated. This procedure is termed an "open reduction."

In the edentulous patient, existing dentures or newly fabricated cold-cure acrylic splints stabilized by skeletal wire fixation can be used to achieve closed reduction with intermaxillary fixation. Circummandibular wires in the mandible and circumzygomatic, anterior nasal spine, infraorbital, piriform aperture, frontal, zygomatic buttress, and perialveolar wires in the maxillae have all been used for skeletal wire fixation. Because of the surgery involved with possible associated complicationns, general anesthesia is preferred for the placement of skeletal wire fixation (Fig. 13-18).

In the medically compromised patient who cannot tolerate having their jaws wired together in intermaxillary fixation—that is, those with chronic obstructive pulmonary disease or nutritional problems—open reduction with direct bone plating or external skeletal fixation may be indicated (Fig. 13-19). The most commonly used external skeletal fixation used for stabilization of mandibular fractures is external biphasic pin fixation.[41,70] In this technique, specifically designed bone screws are placed through small skin incisions into bone on each side of major fractured segments. The fracture is reduced and held into place temporarily with a mechanical metal splint set until a cold cure acrylic bar can be appllied to the extraoral screw heads to maintain the fracture stable during the healing phases (Fig. 13-20).

In the geriatric patient, healing of bone is delayed, in many cases, because of diminished circulation, less active periosteal osteogenesis, reduced area of bone contact because of atrophy, and decreased systemic calcium absorption. Thus, in this older age group, a 9- to 10-week period of immobilization is recommended to healing as compared to a 5- to 6- week healing phase in the general adult population.

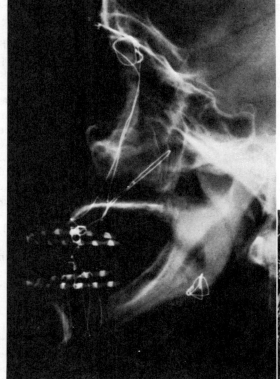

A

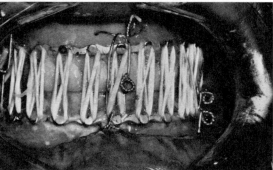

B

**Fig. 13-18 A,** Radiographic view of open reduction right angle and of left zygomatic complex fractures. Closed reduction using left frontal, right circumzygomatic, anterior nasal spine, and three circummandibular skeletal fixation wires to stabilize full dentures. **B,** Clinical view of closed reduction by use of skeletal fixation wires to full dentures with attached arch bars. Elastics used for intermaxillary fixation.

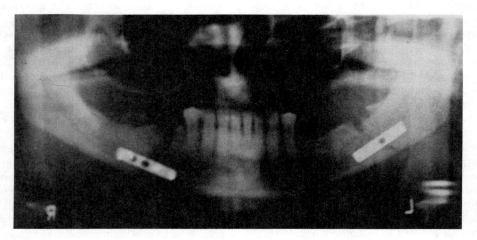

**Fig. 13-19** Use of bone plates to stabilize bilateral mandibular body fractures in patient with chronic obstructive pulmonary disease.

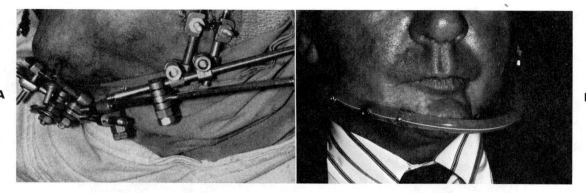

**Fig. 13-20 A,** Intraoperative reduction and stabilization of fractures with temporary metal splint set to gain surgical access to infected fracture site. **B,** Placement of acrylic bar to pin heads at end of surgery for stability during healing phase.

External skeletal biphasic pin fixation has played an important role in the management of fractures in the edentulous geriatric patient because of the following:

1. More rigid stability can be achieved as compared to techniques of wiring dentures into place for closed reduction.
2. Fractures not in the denture-bearing area, that is, unfavorable angle fractures, can be managed, and significant periosteal reflection can be avoided at the fracture site as compared to open reduction techniques. Thereby maximum periosteal blood supply is maintained to the relatively reduced vascularity of the atrophic mandible.
3. Intermaxillary fixation can be avoided because immobilization can be maintained in one jaw.
4. Direct wiring or bone plating into infected fracture sites can be avoided, since the acrylic bar can achieve stabilization with the screws being spaced farther from the fracture line.

The major disadvantages of extraoral skeletal biphasic pin fixation are the following:

1. External pins with an acrylic bar extending externally around the mandibular area are too conspicuous in daily activities and may interfere with head positions during sleep.
2. Difficulty in facial washing or shaving

3. Small soft-tissue scars are caused by the pin holes

In the management of the severely atrophic pencil-thin mandible consisting of only cortical bone with very limited medullary bone, closed reductions using dentures wired in for stabilization are associated with a high incidence of malunion of the fracture sties.[21,69,70] In addition, in these cases, open reductions with stripping of the periosteal blood supply for placement of direct transosseous wires or bone plates are associated with a high incidence of osteomyelitis (Fig. 13-21). Autogenous bone graft to the fracture sites are recommended to add strength and osteogenic potential for healing. Although efforts are being directed to advance technology in preprosthetic surgery to avoid the necessity of autogenous bone grafts except in extreme cases, in trauma surgery, autogenous bone grafts are still advocated to prevent postoperative long-term healing complications. Two commonly used autogenous bone graft techniques for management of severely atrophic mandibular fractures are the following:

1. Autogenous rib split and wired into place on the buccal and lingual aspects of the mandible to sandwich the reduced fracture site. External skeletal biphasic pin fixation is used to immobilize the fracture.
2. Autogenous iliac crest bone placed into freezed dried allogeneic bone struts or into a

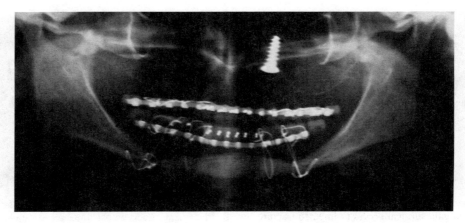

**Fig. 13-21** Bilateral open reductions and closed reduction of severely atrophic mandible. Acute osteomyelitis developed because of limited bone contact, poor vascularity, and circummandibular wires in proximity to fracture sites.

titanium mesh tray used to sandwich the mandible in the buccal and lingual aspects of the reduced fracture.

Because of complicating medical problems and altered physiologic capabilities in healing, the overall goal in management is to be conservative in elective surgical intervention. However, in the management of the geriatric patient who has sustained oral and maxillofacial trauma, often because of difficulties in stabilization and healing of fractures, more surgical intervention is required to achieve effective results as compared to that in younger patients.

## SURGICAL MANAGEMENT OF ORAL LESIONS

Neoplasms are new uncoordinated growth of abnormal tissue that is potentially capable of unlimited proliferation and does not regress after removal of the stimulus that produced the lesion. Neoplasms may be classified as benign or malignant, depending on their behavior pattern and cellular structure. A benign tumor grows slowly and is usually encapsulated. It enlarges by peripheral expansion, pushes away adjoining structures, and manifests no metastasis. A malignant tumor endangers the life of its host by its rapid infiltrating extension into surrounding vital structures and the phenomenon

of metastasis, which creates secondary growth in distant parts of the body, usually through the lymphatic system and bloodstream.[43] Although oral neoplasms constitute only a small minority of the pathologic conditions, they are of great significance, since they have the potential to jeopardize the overall health and longevity of patients.

The progressive effects of smoking, drinking, the use of smokeless tobacco, and chronic trauma from denture irritation in the development of soft-tissue neoplasms, especially oral cancer, is more apparent in the older population. The average age of onset of oral malignancies is 60 years of age. Thus, in the oral and maxillofacial surgery management of the older patient with higher risk of neoplasms as compared to the younger age groups, the importance of thorough oral examinations and of expedient biopsies for histopathologic evaluation is emphasized.

If the lesion is small, less than 1 cm, and appears clinically benign in nature, one can remove it in toto using an excisional biopsy technique. Larger lesions or lesions with malignant characteristics can be evaluated by tissue samples from the margin of the lesion using incisional biopsy techniques. If larger lesions change in clinical appearance at various areas, multiple incisional biopsy specimens can be taken from the lesion.

In a diagnostic survey of 9000 biopsies from

three age groups, under 60 years, 60 to 69 years, and over 70 years of age, it was found that neoplastic lesions were found 44% more often in the 60 to 69 age group and 90% more frequently in the over-70 age group than in the under-60 group.[75] Lesions that were significantly decreased in the older groups included mucocele, apical periodontal cyst, and periapical granuloma. Lesions that were at least twice as frequent in the older age groups as compared to the general population included epidermoid carcinoma, ulcer, hyperkeratosis, chronic inflammatory hyperplasia, and lichen planus. Biopsy specimens taken from persons less than 60 years old resulted in the diagnosis of malignancy for about 1 in every 133 biopsies, whereas 1 in every 12 biopsy specimens was diagnosed as malignant in persons 70 and over. Squamous cell carcinoma accounted for most intraoral malignancies (Figs. 13-22 and 13-23).

Surgical treatment of neoplasms consists essentially in removal of the entire mass if it is confined to an operable area. Surgery has been confined with radiation or chemotherapy based on the location, extent, and nature of the neoplasm. Basically, the earlier the neoplasm is detected before extensive expansion if benign or before metastasis if malignant, the less surgical intervention is required and the better long-term prognosis is achieved. In addition, the overall health status of the geriatric patient may not allow toleration of extensive surgical and medical treatment of metastatic lesions.

Malignant lesions are generally asymptomatic and frequently are dismissed as inconsequential by the elderly patient. Unfortunately the lesions are generally discovered as a neck mass secondary to cervical lymph node involvement when the prognosis is poor. Therefore it is essential in the high-risk older population to perform meticulous periodic oral examinations for possible early detection of neoplasms in order to improve the prognosis of survival (Fig. 13-24).

## POSTOPERATIVE CONSIDERATIONS

Because of physiologic changes normally associated with the aging process, the older patient generally has greater susceptibility to infection and delayed healing. For these reasons, the patient usually requires more time postoperatively to adjust to the physical stress of surgery and to compensate for further alterations in already compromised physiologic function.[45]

Immediately postoperatively, cold applications and pressure dressings to minimize swelling and ecchymosis are most essential. Thin, delicate skin, loose connective tissue with reduced elasticity, and increased capillary fragility often lead to exaggerated tissue responses to surgical trauma. Although in most cases swelling and ecchymosis are only mild postoperative sequelae, occasionally their appearance can be quite psychologically alarming. Efforts must be made to minimize both the physical and mental stress related to them (Fig. 13-25).

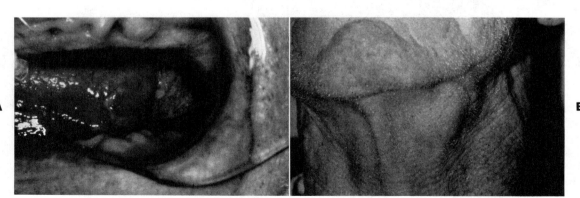

**A**

**B**

**Fig. 13-22  A,** Malignant lesions of the oral cavity are often located in difficult-to-view areas. Epidermoid carcinoma at the posterior border of the tongue. **B,** Cervical lymph node enlargement with posterior border of tongue epidermoid carcinoma.

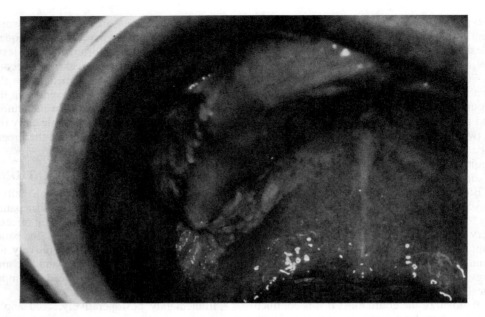

**Fig. 13-23** Leukoplakia-appearing squamous cell carcinoma located under denture area of posterior area of maxilla.

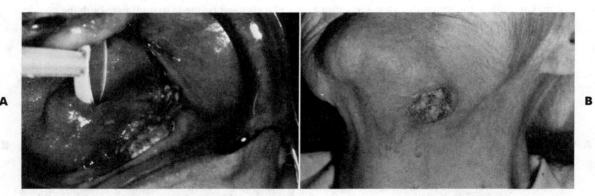

A                                                                                          B

**Fig. 13-24 A,** Extensive squamous cell carcinoma in floor of the mouth. **B,** Submandibular skin ulceration by invasion from squamous cell carcinoma in floor of the mouth.

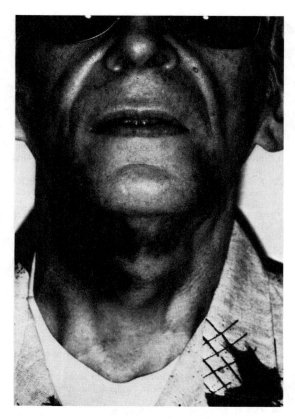

**Fig. 13-25** Ecchymosis extending into the neck region after extractions and alveoloplasty on a geriatric patient.

Secondary to the overall compromised vascularity and circulation, antibiotics are used to control the increased risk of infection. In addition, analgesics are used to reduce the harmful effects of stress on systemic function caused by postoperative pain. However, since it is necessary to be concerned about anesthesia types and dosage in preoperative considerations, caution must be also taken in the postoperative administration of drugs. The absorption, metabolism, and excretion of drugs diminish with age, particularly when there are changes in liver and kidney function.[7,28,45] In addition, the incidence of adverse drug reactions increase with age as well as with the number of drugs being taken.[87] Thus it is advisable to use the guidelines for minimal, recommended adult dosage in prescribing medications for geriatric patients and to make adjustments in dosage after the response to treatment is observed.

Patients often become discouraged and unmotivated after surgical procedures and must be encouraged both in nutrition and hydration and in ambulation. As compared to surgical procedures performed on other parts of the body, oral and maxillofacial surgery procedures also physically make eating properly difficult. Thus increased attention must be taken in the maintenance of proper dietary intake to recuperate. Prolonged bed rest can result in venous thrombosis, pulmonary embolism, pneumonia, urinary retention, and generalized decreased morale and physical strength. Early ambulation should be encouraged. If the patient must remain in bed, it is recommended to:[45]

1. Use support stockings and leg movements to increase circulation.
2. Encourage deep breaths and coughing to remove secretions and decreased risk of atelectasis and pneumonia.
3. Make frequent changes in lying positions to prevent stasis ulceration.

Since the patient will not be hospitalized throughout his or her postoperative healing phase, it is essential that the responsible person to care for him or her be fully advised and understand postoperative home care procedures. Both verbal and written instructions should be given in simple, logical language.

Finally, frequent postoperative observations are necessary until healing is completed, so that possible complications can be recognized early and treatment measures taken expeditiously to limit their severity.

## CONCLUSION

The best surgical outcome in the management of the older patient is based on the following:

1. Thorough preoperative treatment planning to prepare the patient medically and psychologically for surgery
2. Selection of the appropriate surgical intervention to agree with the health status, economics, and functional expectations of the patient
3. Careful intraoperative surgery to handle tis-

sue with less trauma and minimize intra-operative blood loss

4. The prevention of postoperative pain and infection while encouraging nutrition and mental and physical activity

These factors are important in the management of all surgical patients regardless of the age group but are more important in the older population because existing compromising systemic diseases and differencies in physiologic responses to surgery reduces the margin to recuperate from the stress of surgery. Yet, with proper planning and appropriate modifications in approaches when indicated to meet individual limitations, oral and maxillofacial surgery in older geriatric patients can be managed successfully.

## REFERENCES

1. Atwood D.,: Bone loss of edentulous alveolar ridges, J Periodontol 50(4):11, 1979.
2. Babbush C.: Endosteal blade-vent implants, Dent Clin North Am 30:97, 1986.
3. Babbush C, Kirsch A, Mentag P, and Hill B: Intramobile Cylinder (IMZ) two stage osseointegrated implant system with the Intramobile Element (IME): Part I. Its rationale and procedure for use, Int J Oral Maxillofac Implants 4(2):203, 1987.
4. Baker R, Terry B, Davis H, and Connole P: Long-term results of alveolar ridge augmentation, J Oral Surg 37:486, 1979.
5. Barnes G and Parker W: Gerontology: its increasing role and relevance to dentistry, Dentistry 8(2):21, 1988.
6. Bell W, Buche W, Kennedy J, and Ampel J: Surgical correction of the atrophic alveolar ridge: a preliminary report on a new concept of treatment, Oral Surg 43:485, 1977.
7. Bender D: Pharmacologic aspects of aging: a survey of the effects of increasing age on drug activity in adults, J Am Geriatr Soc 12:116, 1964.
8. Bennett C: Monheim's local anesthesia and pain control in dental practice, ed 7, St. Louis, 1984, The CV Mosby Co.
9. Berkey D: Clinical decision-making for the geriatric dental patient, Gerodontics 4(6):321, 1988.
10. Bowles L, Portnoi V, and Kenny R: Wear and tear: common biologic changes of aging, Geriatrics 36:77, 1981.
11. Boyne P and James R: Grafting of the maxillary sinus floor with autogenous marrow and bone, J Oral Surg 38:613, 1980.
12. Brånemark P-I: Osseointegration and its experimental background, J Prosthet Dent 50:399, 1983.
13. Brånemark P-I, Adell R, Albrektson T, et al: Osseointe-grated titanium fixtures in the treatment of edentulousness, Biomaterials 4:25, 1983.
14. Brånemark P-I, Lindström J, Hallén O, et al: Osseointe-grated implants in the treatment of the edentulous jaw: experience from a ten year period, Scand J Plast Reconstr Surg (suppl 16):1, 1977.
15. Breakstone G: Maxillary sinus: common difficulties and complications, NY Dent J 23:473, 1957.
16. Bullamore J: Effect of age of calcium absorption, Lancet 2:535, 1970.
17. Clark H: Deepening of the labial sulcus by mucosa flap advancement: report of case, J Oral Surg 11:165, 1953.
18. Clark JW: (See ref. 65a.)
19. Crolius W: Use of gold plate for the closure of oro-antral fistulas, Oral Surg 9:836, 1956.
20. Davis W, Delo R, and Weiner J: Transoral bone graft for atrophy of the mandible, J Oral Surg 28:760, 1970.
21. Dengam E: Mandibular fracture in the geriatric patient: problems in treatment planning: report of a case, J Oral Surg 28:438, 1970.
22. Eriksson AR and Adell R: Temperatures during drilling for the placement of implants using the osseointegration technique, J Oral Maxillofac Surg 44:4, 1986.
23. Eriksson AR and Albrektsson T: Temperature threshold levels for heat-induced bone tissue injury: a vital-micro-scopic study in the rabbit, J Prosthet Dent 50:101, 1983.
24. Fazile M et al: Follow-up investigation of reconstruction of the alveolar process of the atrophic mandible, Int J Oral Surg 7:400, 1978.
25. Fonseca R and Davis W: Reconstructive preprosthetic oral and maxillofacial surgery, Philadelphia, 1986, WB Saunders Co.
26. Franks A and Hedegard B: Geriatric dentistry, Oxford, 1973, Blackwell Scientific Publications, Ltd.
27. Fredrics H, Scopp I, Gerstman E, and Morgan F: Closure of oro-antral fistula with gold plate: report of case, J Oral Surg 23:650, 1965.
28. Gerber J: Drug usage in the elderly. In Schrier R, editor: Clinical internal medicine in the aged, Philadelphia, 1982, WB Saunders Co.
29. Gift H: Issues of aging and oral health promotion, Gerodontics 4(5):194, 1988.
30. Goldberd M: Mucosal grafts for denture preparation, J Conn Dent Assoc 41:24, 1967.
31. Goldberg M and Gershkoff A: Implant lower denture, Dent Dig 5:11, 1974.
32. Hall H and O'Steen A: Free grafts of palatal mucosa in mandibular vestibuloplasty, J Oral Surg 28:565, 1970.
33. Harle F: Visor osteotomy to increase the absolute height of the atrophied mandible: a preliminary report, J Maxillofac Surg 3:257, 1975.
34. Hickey T: Health and aging, Monterey, Calif, 1980, Wadsworth, Inc, p. 102.
35. Holroyd S and Clark B: Local anesthetics. In Wynn R, editor: Holroyd's clinical pharmacology in dental practice, ed 3, St. Louis, 1983, The CV Mosby Co.
36. Kazanjian V: Surgical operations as related to satisfactory dentures, Dent Cosmos, 66:387, 1924.
37. Keithley J and Gamble J: The lip switch: a modification of Kazanjian's labial vestibuloplasty, J Oral Surg 36:701, 1978.
38. Kent JN and Block MS: Simultaneous maxillary sinus floor bone grafting and placement of hydroxylapatite-coated implants, J Oral Maxillofac Surg 47:283, 1989.

39. Kent J, Quinn JH, Zide MF, et al: Correction of alveolar ridge deficiencies with nonresorbable hydroxylapatite, J Am Dent Assoc 105:993, 1982.
40. Kent J, Quinn JH, Zide MF, et al: Alveolar ridge augmentation using nonresorbable hydroxylapatite with or without autogenous cancellous bone, J Oral Maxillofac Surg 41:629, 1983.
41. Khedroo, L: External pin fixation for treatment of mandibular fractures: a reappraisal, J Oral Surg 28:101, 1970.
42. Kirsh A and Mentag P: The IMZ endosseous two-phase implant system: a complete oral rehabilitation treatment concept, J Oral Implant 12:576, 1986.
43. Kruger G: Textbook of oral and maxillofacial surgery, ed 6, St. Louis, 1984, The CV Mosby Co.
44. Laskin D: Oral and maxillofacial surgery, vol 1, Chapters 18, 20, St. Louis, 1985, The CV Mosby Co.
45. Laskin D: Oral and maxillofacial surgery, vol 2, Chapter 18: Surgery in the geriatric patient, St. Louis, 1985, The CV Mosby Co.
46. Laskin D and Robinson I: Surgical closure of the oro-antral fistula, J Oral Surg 14:201, 1956.
47. Levy S, Baker K, Selma T, and Kahout F: Medications with dental significance: usage in an elderly population, IADR Abstr 1339, J Dent Res 66(special issue):274, 1987.
48. Levy S, Baker K, Semla T, and Kohout F: Use of medications with dental significance by a non-institutionalized elderly population, Gerodontics 4(3):119, 1988.
49. Linkow L and Cherchive R: Theories and techniques of oral implantology, St. Louis, 1970, The CV Mosby Co.
50. MacIntosh R and Obwegeser H: Preprosthetic surgery: a scheme for its effective employment, J Oral Surg 25:397, 1967.
51. Malamed S: Handbook of local anesthesia, ed 2, St. Louis, 1986, The CV Mosby Co.
52. Malamed SF: Sedation: a guide to patient management, ed 2, St. Louis, 1989, The CV Mosby Co.
53. Maloney P and Doku HC: Maxillary sinusitis of odontogenic origin, J Can Dent Assoc 34(11):592, 1968.
54. Maloney P, Doku HC, and Shepherd N: Mucosal grafting in oral reconstructive surgery, J Oral Surg 32:705, 1974.
55. Maloney P, Shepherd N, Doku HC, and Murnane T: Free buccal mucosal grafts for vestibuloplasty, J Oral Surg 30:716, 1972.
56. Martin E: Hazards of medication, Philadelphia, 1971, JB Lippincott Co.
57. Meenaghan M and Natiella J: Evaluation of the crypt surface adjacent to metal endosseous implants: an electron microscopic study, J Prosthet Dent 31:574, 1974.
58. Mercier P and Lanfontant R: Residual alveolar ridge atrophy: classification and influence of facial morphology, J Prosthet Dent 41:90, 1979.
59. Mercier P and Vinet A: Local and systemic factors in residual alveolar ridge atrophy, Int J Oral Surg 10:65, 1981.
60. Mercier P and Vinet A: Factors involved in residual alveolar ridge atrophy of the mandible, J Am Dent Assoc 49:339, 1983.
61. Metz H: Mandibular staple implant for an atrophic mandibular ridge: solving retention difficulties of a denture, J Prosthet Dent 32(5):572, 1974.
62. Michocki R and Lamy P: A "risk" approach to adverse drug reactions, J Am Geriatr Soc 26:79, 1988.
63. Miller A, Brunelle J, Carlos J, Brown L, and Löe H: Oral health of United States adults: the national survey of oral health in U.S. employed adults and seniors: 1985-1986, U.S. Department of Health and Human Services, NIH Publ no 87-2868, Washington, DC, 1987.
64. Nelson JF, Barnes G, Tollefsbol RG, and Parker W: Prevalence and significance of prescription medication usage among gerodontic patients, Gerodontology 6(1):17, 1987.
65. Obwegeser H: Die submukose Vestibulumplastik, Dtsch Zahnaerztl Z 14:629, 1959.
65a. Peterson LJ: Augmentation of the bony residual ridge. Chapter 30 in vol 3 of Hardin JF, ed: Clark's clinical dentistry, rev ed, Philadelphia, 1989, JB Lippincott Co.
66. Peterson L, Ellis E III, Hupp J, and Tucker M: Contemporary oral and maxillofacial surgery, St. Louis, 1988, The CV Mosby Co.
67. Peterson L and Slade E: Mandibular ridge augmentation by a modified visor osteotomy: preliminary report, J Oral Surg 35:999, 1977.
68. Propper R: Simplified ridge extension using free mucosal grafts, J Oral Surg 22:469, 1964.
69. Rowe NL: Nonunion of the mandible and maxilla, J Oral Surg 27:520, 1969.
70. Rowe NL and Williams J: Maxillofacial injuries, Edinburgh and London, 1985, Churchill Livingstone.
71. Sanders B and Cox R: Inferior border rib grafting for augmentation of the atrophic edentulous mandible, J Oral Surg 34:897, 1976.
72. Schrier R: Clinical internal medicine in the aged, Philadelphia, 1982, WB Saunders Co.
73. Shafer W, Hine M, and Levy B: A textbook of oral pathology, ed 4, Philadelphia, 1983, WB Saunders Co.
74. Shulman L and Rogoff G: Dental implantology. In Peterson L, Ellis E III, Hupp J, and Tucker M: Contemporary oral and maxillofacial surgery, St. Louis, 1988, The CV Mosby Co.
75. Silverglade L and Stablein M: Diagnostic survey of 9,000 biopsies from three age groups: under 60 years, 60-69 and over 70, Gerodontics 4(6):285, 1988.
76. Skoglund LL, Pederson SS, and Holst E: Surgical management of 85 perforations to the maxillary sinus, Int J Oral Surg 12(1):1, 1983.
77. Small I: The mandibular staple bone plate: its use and advantages in reconstructive surgery, Dent Clin North Am 30:175, 1986.
78. Small I, Metz H, et al: The mandibular staple implant for the atrophic mandible, J Biomed Mater Res Symp 5(2):365, 1974.
79. Smiler D, Radack K, Bilovsky P, et al: Dermal graft—a versatile technique for oral surgery, Oral Surg 43:342, 1977.
80. Steinhauser E: Vestibuloplasty: skin grafts, J Oral Surg 29:777, 1971.
81. Talgren A: The continuing reduction of the residual alveolar ridge in complete denture wearers: a mixed longitudinal study for 25 years, J Prosthet Dent 32:13, 1972.
82. Tatum H: Maxillary and sinus implant reconstruction, Dent Clin North Am 30:207, 1986.
83. Terry B, Albright J, and Baker R: Alveolar ridge augmentation in the edentulous maxilla with use of autogenous ribs, J Oral Surg 32:429, 1974.

84. Thoma K and Holland D: Atrophy of the mandible, Oral Surg 4:1477, 1951.
85. Uhler I: Oral surgery and the geriatric patient, J Oral Surg 20:129, 1962.
86. U.S. Senate Special Committee of Aging: Aging Americans: trends and projections, PL3377, 584, 1983.
87. Visconti J, and Smith M: Reaction to prescribed drugs, J Am Pharm Assoc 9:210, 1969.
88. Wang J, Waite D, and Steinhauser E: Ridge augmentation: an evaluation and follow-up report, J Oral Surg 34:600, 1976.
89. Weintraub J and Burt B: Oral health status in the United States: tooth loss and edentulism, J Dent Educ 49:368, 1985.
90. Wynn R and Clark B: Drug interactions. In Holroyd S and Wynn R: Clinical pharmacology in dental practice, ed 3, St. Louis, 1983, The CV Mosby Co.
91. Yamazaki Y et al: The submucosal island flap in the closure of oroantral fistula, Br J Oral Maxillofac Surg 23:259, 1985.
92. Yih W, Merrill R, and Howerton D: Secondary closure of oroantral and oronasal fistulas: a modification of existing techniques, J Oral Maxillofac Surg 46:357, 1988.
93. Ziemba R: Combined buccal and reverse palatal flap for closure of oralantral fistula, Oral Surg 30:729, 1972.

# 14

## Maxillofacial Prosthetics

*Thomas J. Vergo, Jr.*

Maxillofacial prosthetics is the art and science that involves the anatomic, functional, and cosmetic reconstruction of tissues in the head and neck region using nonliving substitutes. Implicit in this definition is the concept that the dentists participates in the prosthetic reconstruction and rehabilitation of patients with either acquired or congenital defects, above and beyond the replacement of missing teeth. Herein the word "defect" is employed to denote the anatomic or cosmetic tissue loss as well as the functional loss.

The maxillofacial prosthodontist must deal with the special problems of deglutition (swallowing), mastication (chewing), phonation (speech), and esthetics attributable to the patient's defect. Patients seen in a typical maxillofacial prosthetic service may be grouped into one of four major categories based on the cause of their defect: tumor patients, congenital defect patients, developmental defect patients, and trauma patients.

Since there is a significant correlation between the aging process and the incidence of head and neck oncology, this chapter emphasizes cancer of the head and neck in the geriatric patient. According to the American Cancer Society[12-14] approximately 30% of all Americans will be diagnosed as having cancer in their lifetime. From among these patients, approximately one in four will eventually succumb to the disease without having undergone a 5-year survival period. Each year more than 27,000 patients are diagnosed and treated for head and neck cancer, with approximately 9000 succumbing to the disease. Cancer is ranked second to heart disease as a leading cause of death in males and females between 55 and 74 years of age. Over 75 years of age, cancer ranks second and third for males and females, respectfully, after cardiovascular and heart disease.[53]

Approximately 90% of all oral cancers are diagnosed as squamous cell carcinomas with adenocarcinomas and sarcomas accounting for the remaining 10%. Pharyngeal cancer is second to salivary gland and floor-of-the-mouth lesions, with 29% and 36% respectfully. Malignant lesions of the tongue account for 18%, whereas the lips represent 17% of the total.[53]

Data from the American Cancer Society[12-14] indicate that malignant skin tumors are the most common of all cancers and have a higher cure rate (excluding malignant melanomas) when an early diagnosis is made. More than 4 million cases of skin cancer will be reported in the United States each year. It is estimated[13] that 40% to 50% of persons who reach 65 years of age will have had at least one skin cancer during their lifetime. After the first occurrence, there is a 50% to 60% chance of recurrence. Even with an early diagnosis and the successful use of surgery, radiation, or chemosurgery, approximately 1% to 2% (almost 6000) of patients with skin cancer will die annually. The majority (4300) of these persons will have had malignant melanomas.

Except for malignant melanomas, 90% to 95% of skin cancers occur on the exposed surfaces of the body. Once diagnosed, approximately 90% are curable, if one assumes that adequate treatment is instituted at an early stage. Etiologic factors, such as exposure to sunlight and other radiation sources, chronic exposure to chemicals, molten metal burns, or ulcerated old burn scars, as well as irritants from industrial chemicals, tend to be the primary causative agents. Over 90% of diagnosed skin cancers are either basal cell carcinomas or squamous cell carcinomas. Both have a high cure rate if diagnosed early and properly treated. In addition to cancers originating from the skin, many tumors of the oral cavity, the maxillary sinus, or the nasal cavity will spread to the face and result in defects that arise from the surgical removal of these tumors.

There is a significant number of patients who have been diagnosed and treated for benign tumors of the head and neck region. Benign tumors are usually characterized by either limited or noninvasive growth into the normal surrounding tissues. They are generallly surrounded by a fibrous capsule, which limits their growth. Most often benign tumors resemble their parent tissue, grow slowly by expansion, and remain localized. Malignant tumors, however, are atypical in character, exhibiting rapid infiltrating growth patterns and generally spreading to distant areas of the body via metastases. The individual cells of the malignant tumor have an atypical appearance and usually obliterate the normal cellular architecture. Most malignant tumors tend to recur, either locally on a multifocal basis or as distant metastases. These features tend to make the treatment of malignant tumor more complex than that for benign tumors.[21,45]

## HEAD AND NECK CANCER: TREATMENT MODALITIES

Because benign tumors are less aggressive, they are usually treated by surgical intervention. Because of the complex behavior of malignant tumors, surgical removal, radiation therapy, chemotherapy, or a combination of the three modalities is used to eradicate these lesions.

### Surgery

Historically, surgery was the treatment of choice when one treated a head and neck malignant tumor. If the malignant tumor was deemed resectable, the tumor mass with a wide safety margin of normal tissues was removed. There are obvious limits to the amount of tissue that can surgically be removed based on the complex anatomic structures of the head and neck region. Large surgical defects could significantly affect or totally eliminate normal oral functions such as speech, swallowing, and chew-

ing; in addition, sensory losses of smell, taste, hearing, and vision can be affected.

### Radiation therapy

Although surgery is considered to be the most specific method of removing a malignant tumor, radiation therapy has become more widely utilized because of its increasing predictability. Radiation therapy can be used either as a primary treatment to shrink a large, inoperative tumor or as a secondary mode of treatment in conjunction with surgery. Cancer cells are more sensitive to ionizing radiation than the cells of the surrounding normal tissues are. In general, the more abnormal the cancer cell, that is, the more atypical the tumor, the more sensitive it is to radiation therapy.

Although the use of radiation therapy may appear to be more conservative than surgical removal, it has specific side effects that can cause severe complication. In extreme cases, complications from radiation may even result in the death of the patient. Ionizing radiation kills cancer cells, but also affects other normal cells that divide rapidly.

Patients receiving radiation to the head and neck region will develop permanent xerostomia (dry mouth) if the field of radiation includes the major salivary glands. There are other external (skin) and internal (mucous membrane) changes that can complicate the patient's oral hygiene. Radiation can cause great discomfort during treatment and for 6 to 12 weeks subsequent to treatment (Fig. 14-1). This condition, known as "mucositis," in its more severe presentation, may limit treatment with the ultimate prognosis being compromised.

Because the muscles of mastication are very sensitive to simple contact prematurities that the dentist may create in restoring the patient's teeth, exposing these muscles to ionizing radiation may cause trismus (muscle spasms). Thus the triad of dry mouth, acute mucositis, and trismus can lead to rampant caries as well as severe periodontal disease[56,60] (Fig. 14-2).

Another side effect of radiation therapy is scarring of the major blood vessels supplying the maxilla and mandible. This, in turn, may cause osteoradionecrosis, or necrotic nonhealing lesions of the bone. The onset of osteoradionecrosis may be spontaneous, or it may be enhanced by the extrac-

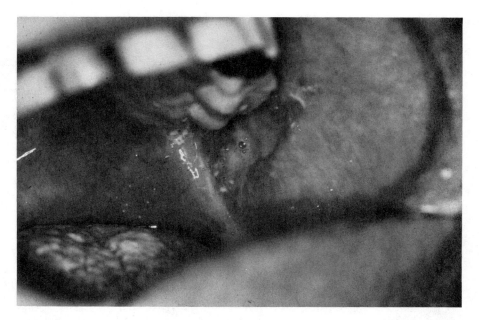

**Fig. 14-1** Typical mucositis with very painful deeply eroded ulcers in the buccal mucosa of the cheek.

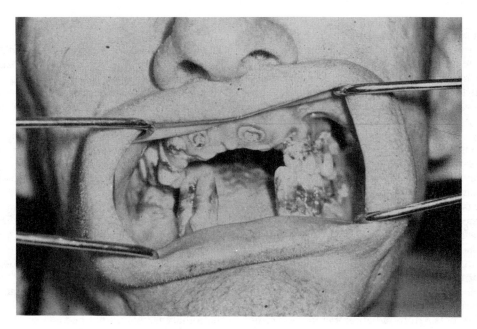

**Fig. 14-2** Rampant caries, advanced periodontal disease, retained roots secondary to radiation caries.

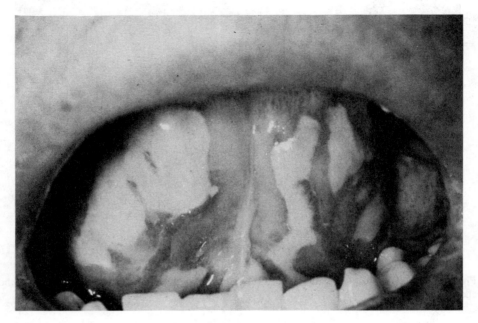

**Fig. 14-3** Undersurface of tongue and floor of the mouth significantly affected by stomatitis secondary to the testicular chemotherapy treatment protocol.

tion of teeth in the irradiated area. Even a simple denture sore may eventually erode into the bone and create an infection with neurosis. Osteoradionecrosis has been so feared in the past that it was common to have all remaining teeth extracted in patients who were scheduled to receive radiation therapy, regardless of the prognosis for a cure or their age. It was considered easier to manage the edentulous patient than to deal with the problems of aggressive decay and potential osteoradionecrosis. Today, with the establishment of treatment protocols containing good oral hygiene, daily fluoride treatments with custom-prepared trays, continuous dental checks, and the use of artificial saliva, it is possible for the patient to retain his or her teeth during and subsequent to radiation therapy.[17,23,44]

Although use of a remineralizing solution consisting of a supersaturated solution of calcium and phosphate has strengthened the dental-radiation armamentarium, it is the responsibility of the dentist to treat patients before radiation therapy and eliminate all dental disease that might complicate the patient's ultimate medical treatment.[17,23,30,31,44]

## Chemotherapy

The *third* modality of treatment reserved for cancer patients is chemotherapy. Chemotherapeutic drugs have a toxic effect on rapidly dividing cells. Although toxic effects of the drugs have a greater effect on cancer cells because the reproduction potential is different from that of normal cells, the systemic treatment of cancer by this mode can be devastating and is usually reserved for metatastic disease or systemic malignancies.[30,56]

Depression of the antibody and blood-clotting systems of the body are significant side effects of chemotherapy. Bleeding and infection in patients undergoing chemotherapy can be life threatening. As with radiation therapy, an acute reaction to chemotherapeutic drugs may result in stomatitis (Fig. 14-3). The breakdown of the oral mucosa, coupled with a decrease in the blood-clotting factors, can lead to spontaneous and sometimes fatal hemorrhages. The systemic spread of simple infection that otherwise would not become serious can also occur. These complications may limit the chemotherapeutic regimen as well as the prognosis for

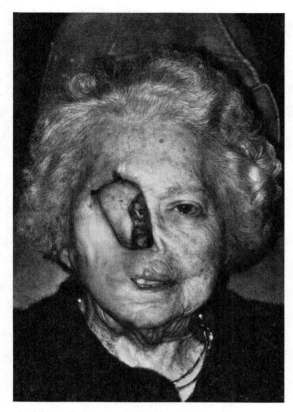

**Fig. 14-4** Large orbitofacial defect resulting in facial deformity and loss of vision in the affected eye.

cure. In their most extreme form, these side effects can lead to death.[30]

## PSYCHOSOCIAL CONSIDERATIONS

The majority of the patients seen in a maxillofacial prosthetic clinic have either anatomic or functional defects with which the prosthodontist must deal (Fig. 14-4). Anatomic defects of the head and neck region not only present esthetic and social problems, but also may induce significant physiologic and functional problems relative to the patient's oral function.

Disfigurement of the head and neck area may cause a dramatic psychologic disturbance in the patient, which affects both the quality and dignity of life. These complications can limit the potential of the patient as a viable participant in our society. The face, in our society, remains uncovered at all times, and it is of great importance to be considered "normal" in a society where great emphasis is placed on interpersonal relationships and a youthful, beautiful look.[8,19,24,32,35-38]

In our society the individual primarily presents him- or herself through the face, which can mirror the emotions[35] or, alternatively, represent a mask behind which the individual's emotions are concealed.[38] If the individual is unable to express his or her emotions because of orofacial dysfunctions, this aspect of his or her ability to communicate can become restricted.[19]

A link is purported to exist between beauty, attractiveness, and success,[8] and extensive research on the psychologic impact of facial disfigurement has been conducted.[35-37] Unlike congenital craniofacial anomalies, disfigurement of the face or oral dysfunction occurring later in life does not appear to have the same degree of impact on the victim's self-image.[24,32] Although a significant degree of body image may be damaged, the occurrence of orofacial defects after the period during which the individual's personality is shaped appears to limit the reaction to a brief but painful period until that person is rehabilitated, and the deep disturbances observed in children with congenital anomalies usually do not occur. The reactions of society to the new deformity are of great importance to patients with newly acquired defects.[36] The avoidance reaction exhibited by others such as averted eyes and hurried and embarrassed conversations contributes to a strong feeling of isolation in the orofacially deformed persons, who may compensate through withdrawal by exaggerated friendliness or complacent behavior.[37]

## MANDIBULECTOMY DEFECTS

Malignant tumors of the mandible account for 0.5% of all deaths attributable to cancer.[12-14,21,45,53] The mandible consists of several distinct histologic tissues, each of which may give rise to malignant tumors: osteosarcoma, Ewing's sarcoma, ameloblastoma, and, rarely, osteochondroma.[20] In addition to these primary tumors, the mandible is a common site for metastatic carcinoma of the breast, the mandible frequently becomes involved, through direct extension, with various types of carcinomas from the floor of the mouth, tongue, buccal mucosa, or gingiva. These factors appear to support the clinical impression that malignancies of the mandible are far more prevalent than the figures indicate.[12]

Vergo and Schaaf[57] have shown that partial surgical resection of the mandible has become common practice in the treatment of "oromandibular" sarcoma and carcinoma. In an attempt to eliminate microscopic tumors and achieve an improved cure rate, the current treatment of choice is a combination of surgery and radiation therapy. This often leaves the patient in a debilitated state. The surgical rehabilitation of the partial mandibulectomy patient often consists in a "wait-and-see" attitude by the surgeon. If the patient does not have a recurrence within a given time period, reconstruction with bone or synthetic implants may be considered so as to restore the continuity of the mandible. In reality, either as a result of tumor recurrence or a reluctance by the surgeon to reconstruct the previously irradiated mandible, partial mandibulectomy patients usually are forced to remain in mandibular discontinuity.

According to Guichet,[28] there are four main determinants of mandibular motion. The temporomandibular joints (TMJ) and their associated muscles and ligaments constitute the first two determinants. They are considered to be fixed in the intact mandible. The interocclusal contacts of the teeth and the neuromuscular system are considered the other two variable determinants of mandibular motion. Since the intact, nonembryonic mandible is one bone, the joint of each side must act in a coordinated effort to accomplish every mandibular movement. This system is further complicated by the fact that the TMJ is characterized as being ginglymoid diarthrodial, which accounts for the freely movable, sliding-hinge nature of the joint. Even though the combination of two joints restricts the motion of the mandible, remarkable freedom of movement in all planes of space are achieved.[26]

Although the definition of an occlusal centric relation is specific with respect to the posterior limit of the joint, controversy still exists as to its true nature.[6,27,47] Regardless of which theory of posterior limit is accepted, the concept that an occlusal centric relation exists as a stable, reproducible starting position from which prostheses can be constructed is clinically important.[1,4,6,27,39,42,46,47,52,62,63]

The windmill motion of a ball-and-socket joint of the shoulder is one example of a joint that is capable of circumduction. The mandible and its joints, as a unit, approximate a freely movable joint, but it is more complicated than the shoulder.[52] The degree of circumduction is limited by the ligaments, muscles, and neuromuscular input of both joints working together. In the partial mandibulectomized patient, the "hemijoint" has a greater degree of circumduction in the horizontal plane than the intact mandible.[57]

After surgery, the remaining mandibular segment deviates medially and returns laterally when the jaw is opened and closed. Alternating contraction of either pair of pterygoid muscles will cause a side-to-side, or triturating, motion of the mandible during mastication.[46] The rest position of the mandible, acquired as a result of the remaining muscle pull, scarring of tissue, and flap procedures, is medial to the opposing maxillary arch.[10] After a partial mandibulectomy, it is difficult for the remaining muscles to maintain a proper jaw relationship because of the breakdown of the neural conduction and the resulting associated muscle fatigue.[50] Swoope[54] states that in the deviated position a maxillomandibular relationship cannot be recorded with any degree of accuracy and a satisfactory occlusion is difficult to obtain. He implies that it is impossible to obtain a centric relation record. Sharry[50] has indicated that nonanatomic teeth should be used for relative freedom of the jaw to accommodate the unstable, nonrepeatable motion. Atkinson and Shepherd[5] studied the masticatory movements of partial mandibulectomy patients in an anterior coronal plane of reference and noted that there was a constant lack of return to the "centric occlusal position." Most of the chewing cyles showed a diagonal pattern with some degree of lateral movement.[22]

Curtis et al.[22] studied vertical sagittal tracings from patients with partial mandibulectomies. The TMJ on the unaffected side was, at best, considered a limited universal joint having the characteristic of circumduction. Even though the lateral movements are distorted and a diagonal closure exists, there appears to be a repeatable posterior range consistent with a universal joint.[57] In summary,[57] patients having undergone a partial mandibulectomy are unable to consistently close their mouth in one position. Since the mandible is not continuous, a centric starting position is not present and there is no accurate, repeatable position from which to construct the prosthesis. Since the mandible is incomplete, prosthetic rehabilitation is difficult because of the limited availability of tissues to provide support, stability, and retention. The more teeth remaining in the mouth that can support the prosthesis, the greater is the degree of success in rehabilitating the patient.[4,46]

When teeth are present in either the maxillary or the mandibular arch, there generally is an inability to close into maximum intercuspation because of the residual muscle pull. Placement of immediate interarch fixation at the time of surgery has proved only partially successful, and many patients have various degrees of deviation.

Based on the amount of scarring present, the maxillofacial prosthodontist may be able to develop a "guide-flange prosthesis" to assist in the repositioning of the mandible to permit maximal closure efficiency with maximal intercuspation. The guide flange prosthesis usually consists of a framework on the maxillary arch with a buccal bar (Fig. 14-5) and a mandibular cast framework containing a vertical component that is guided by the buccal bar (Fig. 14-6). The prostheses together force the mandible back into its proper position and act as a training device, worn for a specific period of time, for achieving a consistent closure (Fig. 14-7). The patient usually functions with this prosthesis from 6 months to 1 year, followed by a slow "weaning period," during which the residual musculature is strengthened (Fig. 14-8). Once a stable occlusion is achieved, the remaining teeth in the defect area are replaced utilizing a special framework design for a removable partial denture.

Another form of a mandibular resection guide flange prosthesis is used for patients with only man-

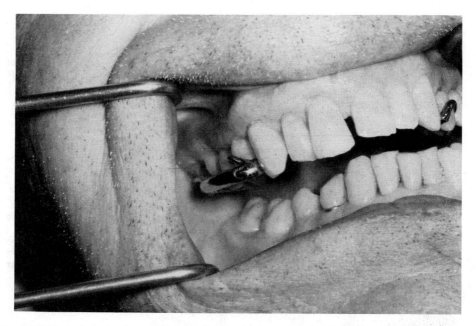

**Fig. 14-5** Typical deviated mandible associated with a partial mandibulectomy surgical procedure. The buccal bar of the maxillary component of the guide flange prosthesis is positioned on the contralateral maxillary arch to the surgical mandibular defect.

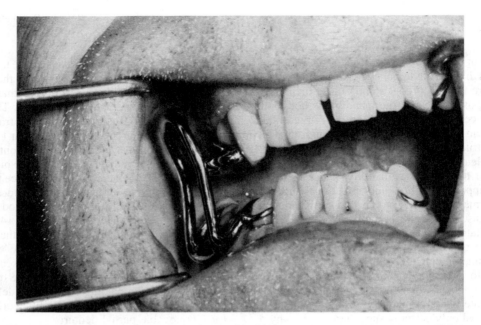

**Fig. 14-6** The mandibular component of the guide flange prosthesis repositions the mandible into a more favorable maxillomandibular position. The length of the vertical guide bar is determined by the height of the buccal vestibule.

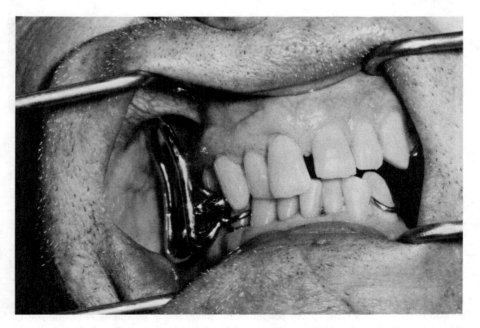

**Fig. 14-7** The maxillary and mandibular components of the guide flange prosthesis act together to assure the patient near-normal maximum intercuspal position upon contact of the teeth.

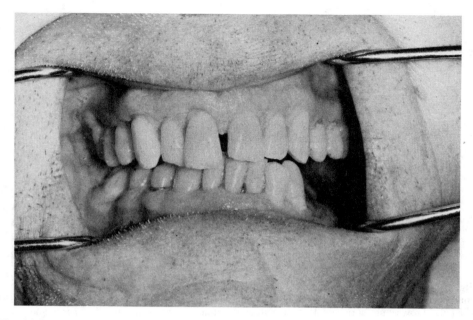

**Fig. 14-8** Unassisted closure into maximum intercuspal position. The muscles on the contralateral side to the mandibular defect have strengthened with the use of the guide flange prosthesis allowing the patient to function without the prosthesis for up to 18 hours per day.

dibular teeth. The maxillary denture must be fabricated to accommodate mandibular deviation and inconsistent occlusal patterns. The maxillary denture can be fabricated with monoplane occlusion that is extended onto the palatal aspects of the denture to accommodate for different closure positions (Fig. 14-9). This accommodation can be achieved by use of a double row of posterior teeth or an acrylic ramp. As a result, when closing, the patient will occlude unilaterally on one portion of the denture (Fig. 14-10) and then move into a final resting position with more stable bilateral contact (Fig. 14-11).

Schaaf[48] has enumerated several factors that must be considered when one is fabricating an intraoral prosthesis for the totally edentulous partial mandibulectomized patient. Previous denture experience and the patient's overall vigor and awareness of his or her limitations are important guiding factors. The amount of denture-bearing area, the presurgical interridge relationship, the amount of postsurgical deviation, and the patient's kinesthetic

sense and muscle control are relevant factors. In addition, the treatment modalities used and the status of the patient's disease are of great importance. Because of these limiting factors, a great number of part-mandibular prosthesis fail (Figs. 14-12 and 14-13).

## DEFECTS OF THE TONGUE

A high proportion of the patients with oral cancer have a history of chronic alcohol or tobacco use (smoking, chewing, or snuff), or other chronic conditions that irritate the oral cavity. Malignancies of the tongue, floor of the mouth, alveolar mucosa, and buccal mucosa account for the majority of malignant tumors in the head and neck region.[12-14]

The tongue ranks second only to the lips as the most frequent site of oral cancer. The posterior two thirds and lateral borders of the tongue exhibit the highest prevalence. Early detection of these lesions and refined surgical techniques have increased the survival rate.[12-14] Cancer of the tongue and the floor

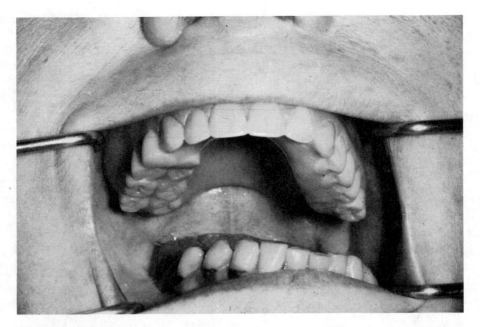

**Fig. 14-9** Maxillary complete denture with palatal and occlusal extensions to accommodate atypical, nonrepeatable closure of a partial mandibulectomy patient. These palatal extensions may consist of a palatal row of prefabricated denture teeth or a continuation of the denture-base acrylic polymer.

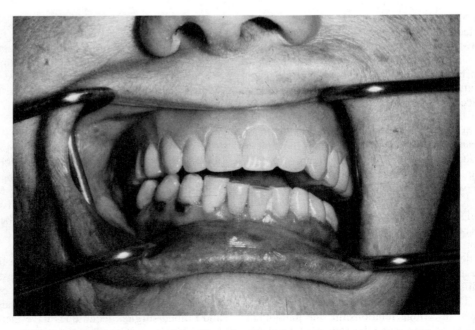

**Fig. 14-10** Initial closure with unilateral occlusal contact on the nonresected side.

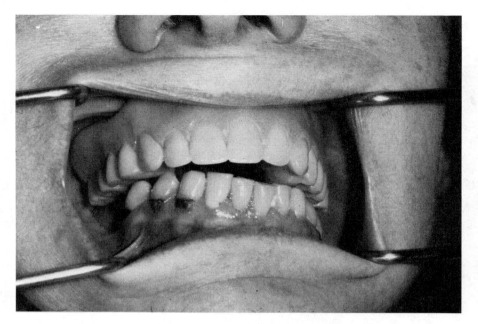

**Fig. 14-11** Final stable occlusal closure achieved by means of the guide ramps of the maxillary complete denture.

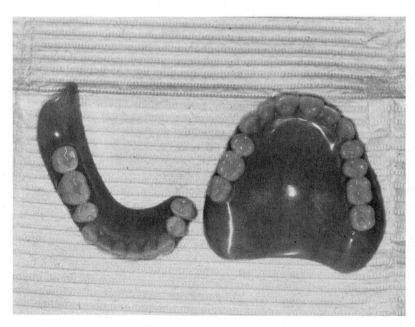

**Fig. 14-12** Maxillary and mandibular removable prosthesis for a patient with a partial mandibulectomy. Palatal guide ramps were not necessary, since the patient could make repeatable closures despite the mandibular defect.

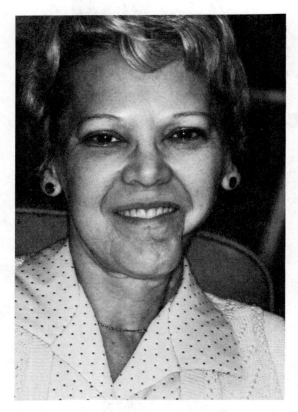

**Fig. 14-13** Final esthetic result after prosthetic rehabilitation.

of the mouth can be devastating because of its highly malignant nature and frequent incidence of metastasis. Taking into consideration tumor location, size and degree of malignancy, and the treatment modalities used, one should attempt to conserve the oral structures maximally. The remaining teeth and the amount of alveolar bone present can make the difference between success and failure in prosthetic rehabilitation.

Lauciello et al.[33] have outlined the three basic oral functions in which the tongue plays an integral part: mastication, deglutition, and speech.

### Mastication

The tongue has several important functions during mastication. It aids in the "chewing" process by working in a coordinated manner with the muscles of the cheeks to position and maintain the food bolus on the occlusal surfaces of the teeth. Sensory nerve endings in the tongue signal food texture and consistency and determine when the bolus is ready for swallowing. The tongue subsequently aids in the débridement of the buccal vestibule and floor of the mouth.

### Deglutition

The swallowing movement is a composite of three stages: oral, pharyngeal, and esophageal. During the oral stage the tongue manipulates the masticated food into a bolus and manipulates it into a position between the dorsum of the tongue and the hard palate. The tongue is then elevated by the contraction of the mylohyoid muscle and the soft palate is depressed, forcing the food bolus into the pharynx. During the pharyngeal stage, the tongue releases the bolus, while the palatopharyngeal closure prevents food from entering the nasopharynx. As a bolus of food is transported from the pharynx into the lumen of the esophagus, the pulmonary opening is protected by the epiglottis.

### Speech

Speech is a learned neuromuscular function. Speech rehabilitation for the patient with a glossectomy requires a basic knowledge of the parameters involved in phonation. Human speech is produced by an airstream that first passes through a vibrating mechanism, then into a resonating system, and finally through the partially or totally occluded oral cavity. Speech is produced by various combinations of these structures.

Speech sounds may be labeled as vowels or consonants. Vowel sounds are produced by modification of the size and shape of the resonating cavities of the vocal tract. By a combination of these vowels, diphthongs such as /ai/ or /ei/ or /ou/ are produced. All vowels and diphthongs are produced as continuous sounds with no check or stop in the airstream. They are always associated with laryngeal vibration. A consonant is a speech sound chiefly characterized by a complete or partial check of the airflow in the oral cavity by various combinations of the articulators. Laryngeal vibration may or may not be associated with the different sounds. Consonants may be classified as plosive,

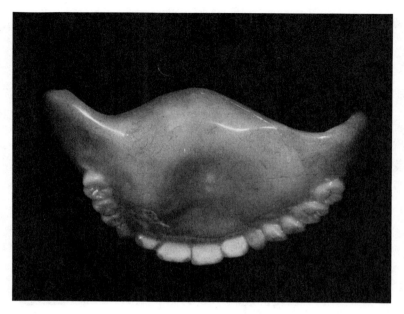

**Fig. 14-14** Typical palatal-augmentation component of a maxillary complete denture. Selective thickening of the palate of the denture allows for improved function of the tongue during speech, swallowing, and mastication.

fricative, affricative, or nasal sounds. A plosive sound is characterized by complete occlusion of the oral channel followed by a sudden release of air, resulting in the intended sound. If the airstream is only partially interrupted, with the air being forced through a narrow orifice, a fricative sound is produced. The affricative sound is actually a combination of the plosive and fricative formats. The airflow is completely checked and then released through a narrow orifice as in the sounds /ch/ and /j/. When the oral channel is completely blocked and the airflow is directed through the nasal pharynx to exit through the nasal passage, the results are referred to as "nasal sounds."

Within each of the sound classifications there generally is more than one sound, and the same oral format may have both a voiced and a voiceless counterpart. For example, the /z/ sound is voiced (laryngeal vibration), and the /s/ sound is voiceless. During the production of all sounds, except for bilabial and labiodental sounds, the tongue is the major articulator. It is the ability of the lingual musculature to modify the shape of the oral cavity and thus change the resonance characteristics that produces the various vowels and diphthongs. The ability of the tongue to completely or partially occlude the vocal tract results in the different consonant sounds.

In the patient with a glossectomy the altered size of the oral cavity often produces a change in the resonance associated with certain sounds. Normal articulation patterns between the tongue, the hard and soft palates, and the teeth may be interrupted. Depending on the remaining function of the residual portion of the tongue, speech rehabilitation may involve the simple reestablishment of near-normal articulation, with utilization of a modified dental prosthesis (Fig. 14-14), or may involve the relearning of compensatory substituted movements with the aid of a modified dental prosthesis[15,34,40] (Fig. 14-15).

When considering the prosthetic rehabilitation of patients with a glossectomy, one must carefully evaluate residual oral function. Each patient presents with an individual problem, and rehabilitative efforts must be geared to that particular person.

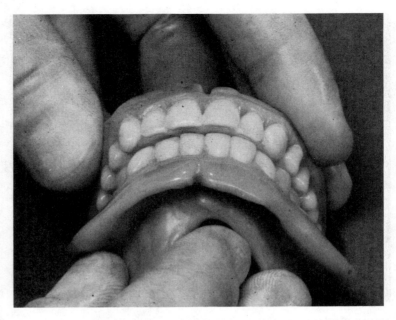

**Fig. 14-15** If the residual tongue is nonmovable or if little or no tongue remains after glossectomy, substitute formats of speech and swallowing must be made by special modifications of the intraoral prosthesis. In addition to the palatal-augmentation component shown in Fig. 14-14, an artificial articulation of the lower anterior teeth to the acrylic palatal to the upper anterior teeth will allow the patient to make the /s/, /sh/, /z/, /zh/ speech sounds.

Considerable variation can exist among a group of patients who may appear to have the same residual defect. Factors such as the mobility of the remaining oral and paraoral tissues, degree of neuromuscular coordination, mental competence, and motivation are vital parameters that influence the degree to which the patient's oral functions may be rehabilitated.[33]

## PATIENTS WITH A MAXILLARY DEFECT

The hard and soft palates rank fourth with respect to tumor occurrence.[12-14, 21,45,53] This area contains several tissue types, which may become tumorous. The hard palate contains the gingival epithelium and attached mucosa, minor salivary glands, calcified structures, and the epithelium lining of the nasal cavity and the maxillary sinus. The soft palate is composed of oral and nasopharyngeal mucosa (epithelium) and muscle. Thus tumors may arise from the mucosal, glandular, muscular, or calcified tissues.

The hard and soft palates provide a physical barrier that separates the oral cavity from the nasal cavity, maxillary sinus, and oral and nasal pharynx. The hard palate is a fixed structure that permanently separates these cavities, whereas the soft palate separates various of these areas depending on its position during speech and swallowing.[59] Because there are only three sounds in the English language that do not require intraoral pressure buildup (/m/, /n/, and /ng/), the hard and soft palates play an extremely important role in maintaining proper speech capability.

Functional or anatomic disruption of this area may cause major speech problems. Speech formats have often a nasal quality, which can seriously alter intelligibility. A void in the hard or soft palate will further distort speech. In addition, intraoral defects

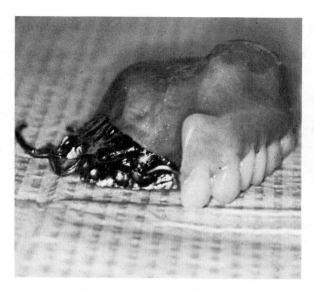

**Fig. 14-16** Typical all-acrylic maxillary obturator prosthesis.

of the hard and soft palates involving the nasal cavity, the maxillary sinus, or the orbital bone may cause significant facial deformation. Many times the intraoral defect may extend onto the face, requiring an independent facial prosthesis.

The maxillofacial prosthodontist, from necessity, must deal with tissues that normally would not be used to provide support, retention, and stability to a prosthesis. The residual intraoral structures (teeth, alveolar ridge, and remaining hard palate), and the bony and soft-tissue structures within the defect itself must be used. An obturator or speech bulb may help reestablish the integrity of the oral cavity (Figs. 14-16 and 14-17).

There is a long history of prosthetic obturation dating back several centuries.[2,3,7,11,18,25,43] Recently methylmethacrylate has been the material of choice for fabrication of obturator prostheses.[2,3,11,25] Desjardins[25] and Aramany[3] in discussing the objectives of obturator design have comprehensively applied the principles of support, retention, and

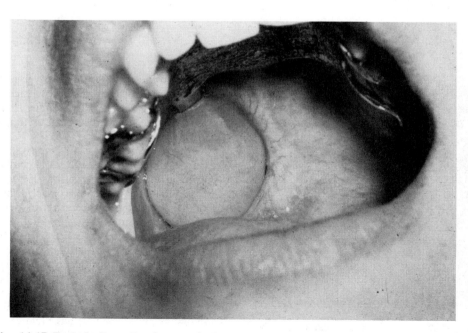

**Fig. 14-17** Typical all-acrylic pharyngeal obturator (speech bulb) prosthesis closing a surgical defect of the soft palate.

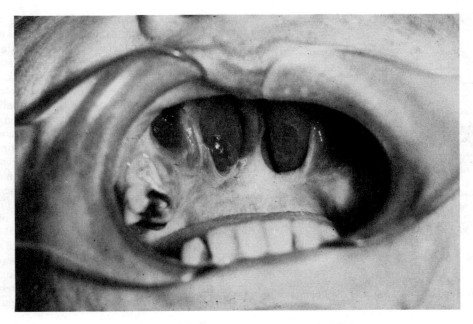

**Fig. 14-18** Large bilateral maxillary surgical defect.

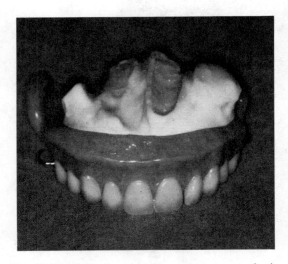

**Fig. 14-19** Medical-grade silicone obturator prosthesis. Maximum support, retention, and stability can be achieved by use of the "within-the-defect" residual structures.

stability to the residual maxillary tissues. Obturators consisting of rigid materials, such as methylmethacrylate, may impose certain limitations on these principles and in turn may compromise the patient's function.[2,11,16,29,41,48,51,55,59,61]

If there is an inability to employ the available tissue to support the prosthesis, it may necessitate dependence on fixed splinting of the remaining teeth, plus a complicated clasp design, or the swing-lock retention to ensure an optimum biomechanical design of the obturator.[43] However, the structures within the defect often can be used independently of the oral structures. This is accomplished by use of medical-grade silicone (Dow Corning Corp., Midland, MI) that is attached to the obturator connecting it to all the structures in the defect (Figs. 14-18 and 14-19). Several authors[9,16,18,41,43,49,51,55,58,61] have had excellent clinical success using detachable medical-grade silicone obturators.

Vergo and Chapman[59] have showed that two

types of maxillary obturator can be prepared: (1) where support is obtained from the residual oral structures and (2) where support is gained from the calcified and soft-tissues within the defect area. The quality of support provided by each modality differs, but by using all potentially available support areas, one can provide the obturator with a significantly increased support. Up to 38% more support for the maxillary obturator can be realized by the latter type.

The obturator prosthesis must be designed so that it is comfortable as well as esthetic. It must restore the physiologic functions of speech, swallowing, and mastication yet help maintain the remaining oral structures in "optimum" health.

Carl[16] has emphasized the importance of fabricating immediate or postsurgical obturators. Once the tumor is diagnosed, it is important that the maxillofacial prosthodontist make preliminary diagnostic models capturing a maximum of the soft and hard palates as well as the supporting structures so that mounted presurgical diagnostic casts can be prepared. For most patients, surgery is followed by the placement of an iodoform gauze pack that obturated the defect for 4 to 7 days. By utilizing the preliminary diagnostic model and visualizing the defect postsurgically, one can prepare a mockup of the surgical site on the cast and fabricate a temporary obturator. This can be delivered at the time of pack removal and refitted using temporary relining materials (Fig. 14-20). If radiation therapy is to be instituted, the obturator allows the patient oral function during his or her course of treatment. Once healing has occurred and the tissues have stabilized, the definitive maxillary obturator prosthesis can be fabricated.

## PATIENTS WITH A FACIAL DEFECT

The prosthetic reconstruction of facial defects involves correction of both anatomic and functional deficits. Obviously, defects of the face that communicate with intraoral defects involve the functional component associated with speech, chewing, swallowing, and esthetics. Tumors that involve the orbital region, the nasal region, or the auricular region can affect the functions of sight, smell, or hearing.

Depending on the practitioner's training, patient's need, and available materials, the following

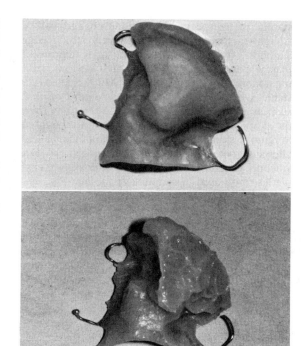

**Fig. 14-20** Postsurgical transitional obturator prosthesis. Using presurgical casts, visualizing the surgical defect, performing cast surgery, and using temporary reline material to make accurate the fit of the prosthesis directly in the mouth at time of surgical pack removal.

may be utilized: acrylic resins, acrylic copolymers, polyvinylchloride, polyurethane elastomers, polyethylene, and silicone elastomers.[9] The most popular materials used to fabricate facial prostheses are the polyurethane elastomers, polyethylene, and the silicone elastomers.[9]

Bemmer[9] and Vergo[58] have described the advantages of MDX4-4210 (MDX), a silicone elastomer. Although each of the available materials has advantages and disadvantages, MDX silicone elastomer possesses most of the properties desired by both the maxillofacial prosthodontist and the patient. This material allows for an esthetic result utilizing several coloring techniques. MDX is easy to fabricate by utilization of stone molds in either regular or giant Hanau flasks. It is flexible but stabile, with respect to dimensional changes. MDX is lighweight; it possesses relatively strong edge strength, which permits thinning or feathering of margins; and its thermal conductivity is low, making it more comfortable to wear.[9] MDX is relatively stable when exposed to environmental "insults" such as ultraviolet light, oxygen, secretions from the skin and skin adhesives, and the solvents used to remove skin adhesives. It is nontoxic, has a low allergenic potential, and is not carcinogenic. MDX silicone generally resists stains and allows cosmetics to be used to camouflage the margins.

MDX silicone elastomer will maintain its physical and chemical properties and esthetic value from 6 months to 2 years.[9] Most facial prostheses are retained with specialized skin adhesives or biphasic adhesive tapes. The final color characterization of the prosthesis is undertaken by the following[58]:

1. Intrinsic coloring involves mixing of earth colors or nylon flocks in the base material before it is cured to obtain final characterization.
2. Silicone adhesives can be used with color mixtures to paint on surface color on an extrinsic level.
3. Last, tattooing with oil paints and a standard tattoo machine can be used to achieve extrinsic coloring. It is generally accepted that the most esthetic facial prostheses are produced from a combination of various techniques utilizing intrinsic as well as extrinsic coloring to achieve the most lifelike prosthesis.

### Nasal prostheses

Since the nose has a high exposure to sunlight and the other carcinogenic elements enumerated, it frequently develps squamous cell or basal cell carcinoma. Depending on the size and extent of the tumor, the treatment of choice for irradication is either surgery or radiation, or both. The surgeon is usually reluctant to reconstruct this area with skin grafts or free-standing partial-thickness skin grafts when these tumors are of a recurrent nature. The fabrication of a silicone nasal prosthesis will allow the patient to return to society (Figs. 14-21 and 14-22). The prosthesis can be characterized both intrinsically and extrinsically, and an accept-

able esthetic result achieved, even to the extent of replicating blood vessels that continue from the natural tissues onto the prosthesis. Total nose replacements can be complicated by adjunctive treatment with radiation therapy or a surgical communication into the oral cavity, which affects the functional competence of the patient. After an intraoral obturator, which maximizes the lip and lateral check contours, is placed, the total nose prosthesis can be fabricated.

### Orbital prostheses

Orbital prostheses are difficult to prepare because they must correspond to the average opening of the nature eye. The prosthetic eye remains in a static position, while the functional eye moves accompanied by variations in eyelid movements. The natural eye exhibits movement, especially when the person exhibits various emotions. Thus orbital prostheses frequently have limited esthetics; the patient tends to stare straight forward using direct vision with movement of the total head to avoid obvious asymmetry (Fig. 14-23).

### Auricular prostheses

Partial ear defects are usually more difficult to reconstruct than if the total ear is missing because the margins of the prosthesis are more difficult to conceal. Various shades of oil-based paints can be used to tattoo the final color characterization into the prosthetic ear. The desired color is first painted on the surface of the prosthesis, and then the tattoo machine is passed over it to allow the needles to pierce the surface and deposit paint into the silicone. The quick elastic memory of the MDX silicone "wipes off" the needles as they withdraw from the surface, and small points of color remain. The final prosthesis (Figs. 14-24 and 14-25) can be very esthetically acceptable. The color is permanent, unlike most extrinsic techniques of coloring, which are removed as a result of the repeated cleaning procedures used for skin-adhesive removal.

### Combination facial prostheses

Combination facial prostheses (Figs. 14-26 and 14-27) can be very difficult to fabricate because they are an attempt to cover larger facial defects. The larger the prosthesis, the less animated is the face

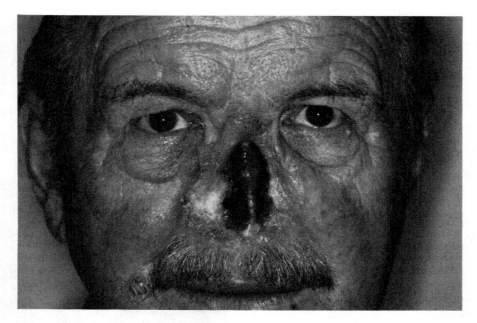

**Fig. 14-21** Large nasal defect after total rhinectomy with adjunctive radiation therapy.

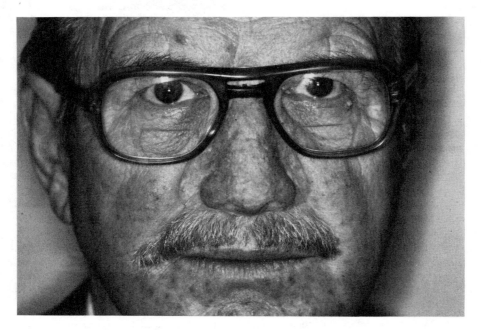

**Fig. 14-22** Total nasal prosthesis made of medical-grade silicone.

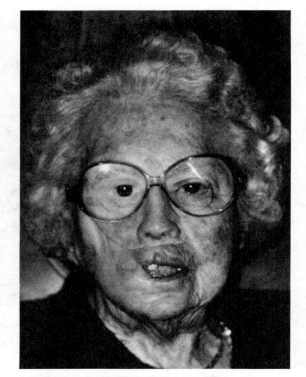

**Fig. 14-23** Orbitofacial prosthesis concealing large defect as seen in Fig. 14-4.

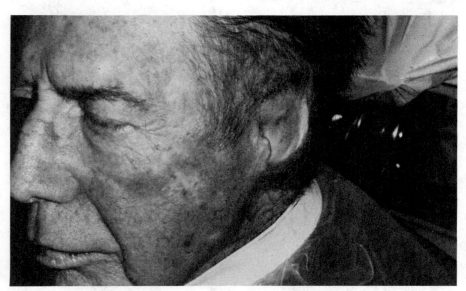

**Fig. 14-24** Surgical defect after total ear removal so that a squamous cell carcinoma could be eradicated.

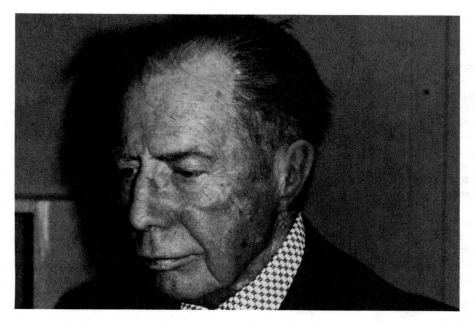

**Fig. 14-25** Total ear replacement using a removable medical-grade silicone prosthesis.

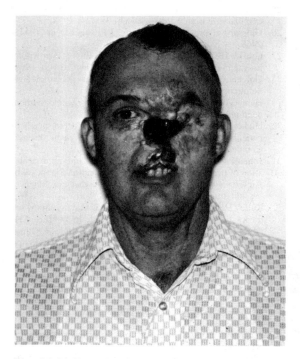

**Fig. 14-26** Extensive facial defect of the orbit, nose, cheek, and upper lip.

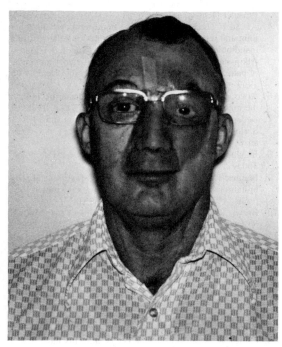

**Fig. 14-27** Large facial prostheses are more difficult to "mask" even if a satisfactory esthetic result is achieved.

and the more obvious is the prosthetic replacement. The asymmetric character of the face attributable to the surgical procedure is much more difficult to mask. With a smaller facial prosthesis (nasal, orbital, or auricular), the use of eyeglasses to hide the margins helps to make the prosthesis blend into the living tissues.

One goal of the maxillofacial prosthodontist, in addition to the restoration of an esthetic appearance, is to provide psychologic assistance to the patient and to afford greater dignity and an improved quality of life. With the use of currently available materials that exhibit greater chemical and physical stability, the patient with a facial prosthesis is able to return to society and function productively.

## REFERENCES

1. Aprile H and Saizar P: Gothic arch tracing and temporomandibular anatomy, J Am Dent Assoc 35:266, 1947.
2. Aramany MA: A history of prosthetic management of cleft palate: Paré to Swensen, Cleft Palate J 8:415, 1971.
3. Aramany MA: Basic principles of obturator design for partially edentulous patients. Part II: Design principles, J Prosthet Dent 40:656, 1978.
4. Arstad T: The capsular ligaments of the temporomandibular joint and retrusion facets of the dentition in relationship to mandibular movement, Oslo, 1954, Akademisk Forlag.
5. Atkinson HJ and Shepherd RW: The masticatory movement of patients after major oral surgery, J Prosthet Dent 21:86, 1969.
6. Atwood D: A critique of research of the posterior limits of the mandibular position, J Prosthet Dent 20:21, 1968.
7. Beder OE: Fundamental for maxillofacial prosthetics, Springfield, Ill, 1974, Charles C Thomas, Publisher, Chapter 8.
8. Bershied E and Walster E: Beauty and the best, Psychology Today 5:10, 42, 74, 94, 1982.
9. Beumer J, Curtis TA, and Firtell DN: Maxillofacial rehabilitation: prosthodontic and surgical considerations, St. Louis, 1979, The CV Mosby Co, pp 331-371.
10. Brown KE: Complete denture treatment in patients with resected mandibles, J Prosthet Dent 21:443, 1969.
11. Bulbulian AH: Maxillofacial prosthetics: evaluation and practical application in patient rehabilitation, J Prosthet Dent 15:554, 1965.
12. Cancer facts and figures: New York, 1984, American Cancer Society.
13. A cancer source book for nurses, New York, 1981, American Cancer Society, Professional Education Publications.
14. Cancer statistics, New York, 1983, American Cancer Society, Professional Education Publications.
15. Cantor R, Curtis TA, Ship T, et al: Maxillary speech prostheses for mandibular surgical defects, J Prosthet Dent 22:253, 1969.
16. Carl W: Preoperative and immediate postoperative obturators, J Prosthet Dent 36:298, 1976.
17. Carl W, Schaaf NG, and Chen TY: Oral care for patients irradiated for cancer of the head and neck, Cancer 30:448, 1972.
18. Chalian VA, Drane JB, and Standish SM: Maxillofacial prosthetics multidisciplinary practice, Baltimore, 1971, The Williams & Wilkins Co.
19. Clifford E: Psychosocial aspects of orificial anomalies: specialties in search of data in orificial anomalies, clinical and research implications, Proc Conference—ASHA Rep 8, Washington, DC, 1973, American Speech-Language-Hearing Association.
20. Clinical oncology for medical students and physicians: a multidisciplinary approach, ed 4, The University of Rochester, School of Medicine and Dentistry, Rochester, NY, New York, 1974, American Cancer Society.
21. Colby RA et al: Color atlas of oral pathology, ed 2, Philadelphia, 1961, JB Lippincott Co, pp 135-168.
22. Curtis TA, Taylor RC, and Rositano SA: Physical problems in obtaining records of the maxillofacial patient, J Prosthet Dent 34:539, 1975.
23. Daily TE: Dental care in the irradiated patient. In Fletcher GH, editor: Textbook of radiotherapy, ed 2, Philadelphia, 1973, Lea & Febiger, pp 157-165.
24. Dembo T et al: Adjustment to misfortune: a problem of sociopsychological rehabilitation, Artif limbs 3:4, 1956.
25. Desjardins RP: Obturator prosthesis design for acquired maxillary defects, J Prosthet Dent 39:424, 1978.
26. Glossary of prosthodontic terms, J Prosthet Dent 20:443, 1968.
27. Grasso JE and Sharry J: The duplicability of arrowpoint tracing in dentulous subjects, J Prosthet Dent 20:106, 1968.
28. Guichet N: Gnathology, everyday dentistry, Gnathological Seminar, Santa Ana, Calif, 1966.
29. Hahn GW: A comfortable silicone obturator with or without dentures, J Prosthet Dent 28:313, 1972.
30. Hickey AJ and Vergo TJ: Survey of oral/dental needs of patients receiving chemotherapy for malignant disease, Compend Contin Educ Dent 2:92, 1981.
31. Johansen E, Taves PR, and Olsen TO: Continuing evaluation of the use of fluorides, AAAS Selection Symposium, American Association for the Advancement of Science, Washington, D.C. 1979.
32. Kelley HH et al: Some implications of social psychological theory for research on the handicapped. In Lofquist LH, editor: Psychological research and rehabilitation, Washington, DC, 1960, American Psychological Association, pp 172-204.
33. Lauciello FR, Vergo T, Schaaf NG, and Zimmerman R: Prosthodontics and speech rehabilitation after partial and complete glossectomy, J Prosthet Dent 43:204, 1980.
34. Leham WL, Hulicka IM, and Mehringer EJ: Prosthetic treatment following complete glossectomy, J Prosthet Dent 16:344, 1964.
35. McGregor FC:L Source psychosocial problems associated with facial deformities, Am Soc Rev 16:629, 1951.
36. McGregor FC: Social and psychological implications of dentofacial disfigurement, Angle Orthodont 40:231, 1970.

37. McGregor F, Abel T, et al: Facial deformities and plaster surgery: a psychosocial study, Springfield, Ill, 1953, Charles C Thomas, Publisher.

38. Meiloo, JAM: The fate of one's face, Psychiatr Q 30:31, 1956.

39. Meyer H: Das Kiefergelenk, Arch Anat, Physiol Wissenschaft Med, Sept 1865, p. 719.

40. Moore DJ: Glossectomy rehabilitation by mandibular tongue prosthesis, J Prosthet Dent 28:429, 1972.

41. Parr GR: A combination obturator, J Prosthet Dent 41:329, 1979.

42. Posselt U: Studies on the mobility of the human mandible, Acta Odontol Scand 10:19, 1952.

43. Rahn AO and Boucher LJ: Maxillofacial prosthetics: principles and concepts, Philadelphia, 1970, WB Saunders Co, Chap 7.

44. Rahn AO and Drane JB: Dental aspects of the problems, care, and treatment of the irradiated oral cancer patient, J Am Dent Assoc 74(5):957, 1967.

45. Robbins SL: Pathology, ed 3, Philadelphia, 1967, WB Saunders Co, pp 88-132.

46. Rosenthal LE: The edentulous patient with jaw defects, Dent Clin North Am 8:773, 1964.

47. Saizar P: Centric relation and condylar movement: anatomic mechanism, J Prosthet Dent 26:581, 1971.

48. Schaaf NG: Oral reconstruction of the edentulous partial mandibulectomy patient, J Prosthet Dent 36:292, 1976.

49. Schaaf NG: Obturators on complete dentures, Dent Clin North Am 21:395, 1977.

50. Sharry JJ: Complete denture prosthodontics, ed 2, New York, 1968, McGraw-Hill Book Co.

51. Shipman B and McCasland J: Occlusally oriented impressions for large maxillary stomas, J Prosthet Dent 38:632, 1977.

52. Sicher H: Oral anatomy, ed 4, St. Louis, 1965, The CV Mosby Co.

53. Silberberg E: Cancer statistics 1984, CA 34:7, 1984.

54. Swoope CC: Prosthetic management of the resected edentulous mandible, J Prosthet Dent 21:197, 1969.

55. Vergo TJ: Detachable silicone obturators for closure of maxillary defects. In Lefkowitz W, editor: Proc Second International Prosthodontic Congress, St. Louis, 1979, The CV Mosby Co, pp 253-255.

56. Vergo TJ Jr and Andrews R: Maxillofacial prosthetics: rehabilitation of head and neck cancer patient (I), Quintessence Dent Technol 8:289, 1984.

57. Vergo TJ Jr and Andrews R: Maxillofacial prosthodontics: rehabilitation of the head and neck cancer patients (II). Quintessence Dent Technol 8:349, 1984.

58. Vergo TJ Jr and Andrews R: Maxillofacial prosthetics: rehabilitation of the head and neck cancer patient (III), Quintessence Dent Technol 8:427, 1984.

59. Vergo TJ Jr and Chapman JR: Maximizing support for maxillary defects, J Prosthet Dent 45:179, 1981.

60. Vergo TJ Jr and Kadish S: Dentures as artificial saliva reservoirs in the irradiated edentulous patient with xerostomia: a pilot study, Oral Surg 51(3):229, 1981.

61. Wood RH and Carl W: Hollow silicone obturators for patients after total maxillectomy, J Prosthet Dent 38:643, 1977.

62. Zenker W: Das retro-articular plastische Polster des Kiefergelenkes und seine mechanische Bedeutung, Z Anat 119:357, 1956.

63. Zola A: Morphologic limiting factors in the temporomandibular joint, J Prosthet Dent 13:732, 1963.

# 15

# Nutrition and Oral Health of the Elderly

*Carole A. Palmer*

As average life expectancy increases, greater attention is being focused on ways of improving the health and quality of life of the aging population. The elderly are an especially vulnerable group because of the spectrum of physiologic and psychosocial challenges that commonly confront them. The increasing cost of providing medical and social services for the elderly is an important incentive for directing efforts to assist them to assume an independent life style.[124]

Adequate nutrition is a vital factor in promoting the health and well-being of the aged. Inadequate nutrition may contribute to an accelerated physical and mental degeneration. Poor oral health can be a detrimental factor to nutritional status and health. Disorders of the oral cavity have been reported to be major contributors to poor eating habits in the elderly.[64] Loose, painful teeth or ill-fitting dentures may result in a reduced desire or ability to eat. A compromised nutritional status, in turn, can further undermine the integrity of the oral tissues. Since nutritional status and the health of the oral cavity are closely interrelated, diet and nutrition should be considered as an integral part of the oral health assessment and management of the elderly.

## NUTRITION AND THE AGING PROCESS

In the field of gerontology theories of aging related to nutrition can be frequently found. One popular theory, that toxins secreted by intestinal bacteria caused aging, was satirized by Aldous Huxley in a novel in which a raw carp was eaten to populate the intestine with bacteria. More recent theories that relate aging to the gradual oxidation of lipid membranes have led to the increased consumption of foods with antioxidant properties such as vitamins A, C, and E and selenium.[118,134]

Not only is there no evidence that supplementation with excessive quantities of vitamins and minerals or the use of special diets prolongs the human life span, but also high doses of these materials can be toxic.[118]

More importantly, a proper diet will prevent malnutrition, may help increase resistance to infection, and may assist in delaying the onset of cardiovascular disease and osteoporosis.[36,112] A compromised nutritional status in the elderly can contribute to a decreased ability to respond to physiologic challenges by impairing the immune response and thus the ability to heal and resist infection.[79] The relationship between life expectancy and nutritional status has been difficult to delineate, except in animal models.[75,125] In humans, a body weight 10% below average has been associated with low mortality, but the optimal body weight for a maximum life span has not been determined.[73] Observations on groups, such as Mormons, who have specific dietary practices and a longer life expectancy than the average, may imply that nutrition can play an important role in longevity.[32]

## NUTRITIONAL STATUS AND REQUIREMENTS OF THE ELDERLY

Evidence exists that the elderly are at special risk for developing malnutrition and that vulnerability to nutrient deficiencies increases with age.[22] Conditioning factors, common to the elderly, that can contribute to a compromised nutritional status are presented in Table 15-1.[77]

The variety of chronic diseases associated with

**Table 15-1** Factors contributing to nutritional problems in the elderly

**Oral**

Changes in ability to chew food
Changes in taste and smell
Drug-induced xerostomia

**Physical**

Changes in ability to absorb and utilize nutrients
Changes in ability to metabolize nutrients
Changes in energy requirements and activity
Effects of medications on appetite and nutrient absorption and utilization

**Functional**

Changes in eyesight and hearing
Physical disability such as arthritis and stroke
Inability to shop and carry groceries

**Psychosocial**

Loneliness and isolation
Loss of appetite and interest in eating
Lack of financial resources
Depression

---

aging and the dearth of nutritional data specific to this segment of our population have contributed to an increasing interest in the nutritional status, nutrient requirements, and other relevant problems of the elderly.

## ASSESSMENT OF NUTRITIONAL STATUS IN THE ELDERLY

The effect of nutritional status on the well-being of the elderly has been difficult to determine, since differences in study populations, diet-assessment methodology, and the standards used to assess dietary adequacy have made the comparison between studies difficult. Various biochemical indices have been used to identify malnutrition, particularly in institutionalized patients. However, since the normal nutrient levels for the elderly are unknown and serum levels may be unrelated to total body status, this type of analysis is open to misinterpretation.[59] Where malnutrition does occur, it must be determined whether it is the result of an insufficient dietary intake or of secondary factors such as disease or malabsorption. Nutrient depletion induced

by an inadequate diet usually occurs slowly over a period of years. Therefore overt clinical signs of malnutrition generally appear only in cases of severe deficiency[88] or when exacerbated by stress. One severe problem is that nutritional aberrations often are not recognized early enough in the depletion process to provide a meaningful corrective intervention.

Most of the current information on the nutritional needs of the elderly is based upon extrapolation from data on other age groups, rather than information specific to this group.[33,82] Diet adequacy is usually assessed when one compares nutrient ingestion to the recommended intake for a specific age group according to standards, such as the Recommended Dietary Allowances. The criteria used for assessing adequacy may vary, since some researchers may use 100% of the RDA as their standard for nutrient adequacy whereas others consider that diets achieving 50% or more of the RDA are adequate.[59] Although a dietary intake below the recommended level does not always indicate that a deficiency will develop, the risk of deficiency increases as if intake persists at low levels. Thus diet assessment and comparison to published standards may indicate the potential for risk, but it is not always proof of a deficiency.

## NUTRITIONAL STATUS AND ASSOCIATED RECOMMENDATIONS

Current findings from dietary and nutritional status studies show that many persons over 65 years of age consume inadequate diets,[37,65,76,98] and such diets place them at risk for nutritional deficiency. Malnutrition in hospitalized elderly patients has been a major cause of morbidity in the past.[112] In the ambulatory elderly there is evidence of suboptimal nutrient levels and the significance of this is under active study.[112]

In the National Health and Nutrition Examination Survey I (NHANES I, a comprehensive, periodic, random survey of American dietary habits and patterns), 50% or more elderly black and white men and women below the poverty level consumed less than two thirds of the RDA for calories, calcium and vitamin A, whereas 30% to 50% ingested less than two thirds of the RDA for vitamin C, iron, thiamine ($B_1$), and niacin ($B_2$).[83] Several other studies, based upon random population samples, have found that less than optimal intakes of calcium, vitamin $B_6$, zinc, copper, and magnesium occurred in more than 50% of the population studied.[9,58,78] Others have reported the inadequate intake of vitamins D, C, $B_1$ (thiamine), $B_2$ (riboflavin), and $B_3$ (niacin) and folic acid.[69,71,106] In a large-scale Tennessee study, low intakes of several nutrients were reported in about 10% of the populace with a high income.[128]

### Calories and protein

Caloric requirements usually decrease in the elderly because of a decline in their basal metabolic rate (BMR), brought on by reduced lean muscle mass and lower exercise levels.[33,69,80,82] Although the BMR generally decreases approximately 30% between 30 and 60 years of age,[112] appetite and food intake may also decrease, occasionally leading to an insufficient caloric intake.[41,69,72,80] With a reduced nutrient intake, diet quality becomes very important, and as a result of the decrease in calories the consumption of calcium, iron, and zinc frequently are insufficient, especially among elderly females.[82] In addition, calorie and protein requirements can be increased by the stress associated with fever, trauma, surgery, or disease.

The lower energy requirements of the elderly may also lead to obesity in some persons.[24] Increased physical activity should be encouraged because it allows a higher caloric intake, making it easier to meet nutrient needs and to control weight and body composition.[82]

Protein requirements do not seem to be a problem in the elderly population, except in hospitalized patients.[24] Despite a reduced lean body mass in the elderly, protein recommendations for persons over 60 years of age are the same as those for other adults; 12% to 14% of their caloric intake should be from proteins.[81]

### Vitamins

Although numerous studies have indicated an inadequate consumption of vitamin A by the elderly, few persons exhibit signs of a biochemical deficiency, such as depleted liver stores or decreased circulating retinol levels. It may be that vitamin A absorption is increased in the elderly or that the requirement is lower than that for young adults.[126] There is also little evidence of vitamin E deficien-

cies occurring in this population. Vitamin A and E toxicity from oversupplementation may be more of a problem than a deficiency would be.[13]

Vitamin D deficiency may represent a problem in the elderly, since older persons may have a limited exposure to sunlight (which activates vitamin D in the skin), a decreased ability of the skin to produce the vitamin D precursor, and a reduced dietary intake of vitamin D.[24,57,70] Between 62% and 74% of healthy elderly may be achieving less than two thirds of the RDA for vitamin D.[86] Since vitamin D is required for the absorption of calcium, deficiency can precipitate a calcium deficit and initiate osteoporosis. Increased vitamin D intake will induce an increase in calcium absorption and reduced bone loss in elderly women.[34,89] Vitamin D supplements generally are not advised because of their potential for toxicity, but increased exposure to sunlight and an increased intake by food or daily supplementation (400 IU) may be indicated.[13] Ascorbic acid intake tends to decline in the elderly with an inverse correlation noted between age and the plasma and leukocyte vitamin C level, but no change in the RDA has been suggested. The elderly are encouraged to consume more vitamin C–rich fruits and vegetables.

Inadequate thiamin and riboflavin intake occur in 0 to 53% of the populations studied, an indication of a broad variability among individuals.[21,45,63]

Vitamin $B_{12}$ deficiency and the occurrence of associated pernicious anemia varies widely in the elderly population and is most often associated with malabsorption because of a decrease in intrinsic factor.[30] Vitamin $B_6$ also may be inadequate in 50% to 90% of the elderly, and there may be an altered metabolism of this vitamin. However, no changes in the RDA are recommended at this time.[39,46]

As with vitamin A, there is evidence that the requirement for folic acid decreases with age.[24,126]

Although up to 80% of the elderly consume less than two thirds of the RDA for folic acid, the maintenance of adequate folate by this group implies that the RDA for folate may have been set too high for this group. Although it has been suggested that the RDA for folate should be lowered, others argue that increased intake may be indicated in the face of the achlorhydria and the associated malabsorption that occurs in many older persons.[55]

## Minerals

Calcium intake may also be deficient in the elderly. One study of free-living healthy persons over 60 years of age found that 43% of women and 30% of men received less than 75% of their RDA for calcium, and 12% of women and 9% of men received less than 50% of the RDA for calcium from their daily diet.[39] Increasing the calcium intake by the ingestion of milk or milk products is often hampered by the lactose intolerance often found in this group. A National Institutes of Health (NIH) consensus conference recommended a daily calcium consumption of 1500 mg/day in postmenopausal estrogen-deprived women.[84]

Iron deficiency seems to be related more to blood loss than diet in the elderly.[40] Zinc is an element that may be of particular importance in the elderly. Although the information relating to clinical zinc deficiency is limited, zinc status has been associated with impaired wound healing, anorexia, and taste changes.[97]

In summary, the nutritional status and requirements of the elderly segment of the population are an area of great interest and concern.

Although poor nutrition may result from inappropriate eating habits, the spectrum of physiologic and psychosocial factors that conspire to increase the elder's risk of malnutrition should not be overlooked. These factors are discussed below.

## FACTORS CONTRIBUTING TO COMPROMISED NUTRITIONAL STATUS IN THE ELDERLY
### Physiologic changes

The progressive decline in function noted in many organs and tissues of the elderly may lead to subsequent changes in their ability to digest, absorb, utilize, and excrete nutrients. The rate at which these age-associated physical changes occur varies among persons and organ systems.[106] The slow depletion of nutrient reserves caused by malabsorption thus can contribute to malnutrition even when nutrient intake is adequate.

The effect of aging on the person's ability to digest food is controversial. Both increases and decreases in digestive capability have been reported.[35,74] The secretion of digestive enzymes often decreases in the aged.[20] Ptyalin secretion may decrease by 20%, trypsin by 30%, and pepsin by 20%,[1] resulting in reduced absorption of calcium and proteins.[70,98] Atrophy of the intestinal mucosa, leading to achlorhydria, has been found in up to 25% of persons over 60 years of age and can lead to bacterial overgrowth and malabsorptions of folic acid and nonheme iron, as well as calcium.[67] The enzyme deficiencies may result in a decline in the intrinsic factor associated with pernicious anemia, a decrease in lactase function to lactose intolerance, a decrease in fat absorption capability to the complaint of abdominal discomfort, and a decreased absorption of fat-soluble vitamins. Alterations in digestive capacity associated with the aging process may be also the result of drug therapy, gastrointestinal surgery, or alimentary tract disease.

Changes in gastrointestinal tract motility can lead to constipation and laxative abuse.[98] Overuse of laxation products in turn can lead to excessive nutrient loss through malabsorption. A decrease in the number of kidney nephrons and the general loss of body water with aging increase the risk of fluid imbalances and dehydration.[103] It has been estimated that 86% of all elderly suffer from at least one chronic disease such as coronary heart disease, diabetes, cancer, and osteoporosis.[130]

Adequate nutrition can play a role in the progression or prevention of these disorders. On the other hand, chronic diseases can affect nutritional status through their effect on such factors as appetite, nutrient utilization, and physical mobility.[91]

### Functional and sensory changes

Any physical disability such as arthritis or hearing or vision impairment can indirectly affect nutritional status. The physically handicapped person may have difficulty obtaining food, opening cans and packages, and preparing meals. These handicaps may impair their ability and reduce their desire to eat, and the embarrassment caused by their inability to handle eating implements properly, see food clearly, or hear others may lead to social isolation, which can further contribute to malnutrition.[112]

Decreases in taste and smell sensitivity are also associated with the aging process.[26,117] Contrary to earlier beliefs that all the gustatory senses decline with age, recent research has indicated that although salt and bitter taste acuity decline with age, sweet or sour perceptivity do not.[135]

Olfactory acuity has been reported to decline with age. Many older persons have a lessened smell acuity than younger persons have and greater difficulty in differentiation between food odors.[116] Food palatability influences appetite, and an altered gustatory or olfactory capability can contribute to a poor diet. Diminished taste and smell acuity may result from disease, drugs, poor nutrition, or dental problems as well as the aging process.[31,87] Suggestions for improving appetite in persons with sensory deficits include increased use of flavorful spices and herbs, providing a variety of flavors and textures, and encouragement with adequate chewing to release a maximum of gustatory and olfactory stimuli.[115]

### Psychosocial factors

The importance of factors other than physiologic may be overlooked in the study of elder health. However, these factors may play an even greater role in determining health and well-being than the commonly considered physical, medical, and dental issues.[62] The elder is at risk for a variety of psychosocial problems that can undermine health and well-being.[25,54,98,106] Poverty can be a major contributor to malnutrition. The elderly have an economic status lower than that of other American adults as a result of retirement, inflation, death of a wage earner, and health care costs. When resources are low, rent and utilities may take precedence over food purchases. The NHANES I study showed widespread deficiencies in nutrient intake associated with poverty.[48,83]

The embarrassment of vision or hearing problems can lead the elderly to isolate themselves from eating with others.[91] Impairments in manual dexterity resulting from stroke, arthritis, or other disability may affect the elderly person's ability to get to grocery stores and carry groceries.

A common physiologic factor affecting the nutritional status of the elderly is depression. Depression, anxiety, and loneliness can result in decreased appetite and lack of desire to prepare food.[38,68] Depression has been estimated to occur in 12% to 14% of the elderly and has been associated with anorexia, weight loss, and increased mortality and morbidity. Depression often occurs in persons with chronic diseases and in persons who have lost a spouse, friend, or other close family member.[12]

Changes in living arrangements can also contribute to eating behavior problems.[28] When confronted with unfamiliar foods in nursing homes, the elder may refuse to eat. The elderly who are socially isolated tend to have poorer diets. Living alone seems to have the greatest impact on elderly men,[29,58] whereas diets of women living alone tend to equal or exceed those of women living with their spouses. These findings extended to biochemical studies of nutriture as well, with men living alone having poorer vitamin $B_1$ and vitamin C status than those living with others.[15] Companionship at mealtimes affected nutrition in 20% to 40% of those surveyed in a Tennessee study, as did income and education levels.[128] Missing meals is not a common problem with the elderly. Most who live alone or get home-delivered meals eat three times a day.[14,58] However, preoccupation with other difficulties such as health issues can lead older persons to relegate eating to a low priority, thereby contributing to the risk of malnutrition.

### Alcohol abuse

It has been estimated that at least 50% of Americans over 60 years of age consume alcoholic beverages on a regular basis, and 5% to 10% heavily. Alcohol abuse may be a response to stress, unwanted changes in their life situation, or social isolation.[11] Alcohol, which provides calories but is of little or no nutritional value, can undermine the nutritional status by decreasing appetite and by being used in place of foods that provide essential nutrients. Multiple clinical nutrient deficiencies that involve thiamin, riboflavin, niacin, pyridoxine, folic acid, vitamin A, zinc, and magnesium are common in alcoholics.

### Drug and nutrient interactions

Multiple medication use is a very frequent occurrence in the elderly. People over 70 years of age have been reported to receive more than 18 drug prescriptions yearly. The overuse of medications may alter food intake or nutrient digestion, absorption, and utilization.[24,43,65,98,105,118] Some drugs can stimulate appetite,[106] whereas others may contribute to anorexia.[118] Antacids can hinder the absorption of folic acid and iron, coumarin can inhibit vitamin K synthesis, cholestyramine can bind folic acid, fat, and fat-soluble vitamins, and mineral oil, commonly used for laxation, can bind and prevent absorption of fat-soluble vitamins and essential fatty acids. In turn, the absorption of certain medicaments can be impaired by various nutrients. Calcium, iron, zinc, and magnesium can inhibit antibiotic absorption.[136] Drug and nutrient interactions are common because of the inefficient metabolization of drugs by the elderly, which allows them to remain in the body for longer periods.[65,68,91]

### Use and abuse of nutritional supplements

The elderly are highly susceptible to advertisements that promise to help combat degenerative or chronic diseases or increase longevity.[50,102] For these reasons, the use of vitamin and mineral supplements is common among older persons. It has been estimated that between 30% to 70% of healthy elderly persons regularly take self-prescribed vitamins that are unrelated to any specific need.[39,45,53,100] There are several dangers associated with arbitrary self-supplementation. High doses of nutrients (10 times RDA or higher) are potentially toxic, especially in older persons who have a diminished renal tubular secretion capacity.[6,113] Also large doses of one nutrient may cause a deficiency of others because of nutrient interactions.[111] The cost of such products is often high and their use may divert limited funds from the purchase of foods.[102] In addition, supplements may give a false sense of security, and so the user pays less attention to nutritious eating.

Evaluation of the supplements used by the elderly indicated that the most popular were vitamins C and E, neither of which are usually deficient in the diets of the elderly.[39] The nutrients at risk, calcium, zinc, vitamin $B_6$, are rarely used as supplements.[49] Thus current supplementation practices do not appear to alleviate the most common dietary deficiencies of the elderly.[78]

Supplements may play an important role in health promotion for persons who get insufficient sunlight (such as vitamin D), are taking drugs that can cause nutrient depletion (such as potassium), are malnourished, or unable to eat properly.[59,61] However, most healthy elderly should be encouraged to purchase nutritious foods, rather than waste money on inappropriate or unneeded supplements.

## RELATIONSHIPS BETWEEN NUTRITIONAL AND DENTAL STATUS AND ORAL HEALTH

Dental status is considered to be an important contributing factor to health and adequate nutrition in the elderly. Masticatory problems may result in a reluctance to eat meals with other persons and cause a self-imposed isolation.[2] Persons who have lost a denture or teeth and who have not obtained a replacement denture may refuse to speak, smile, or eat with others for fear of revealing "gap teeth." A poorly fitting denture may result in a reluctance to talk or engage in social contact for fear of "whistling." Without social interaction, a downward spiral of health may ensue.

Recent research has indicated that dentures can have an effect on nutritional status as well.[19,87] Missing dentition has been associated with decreased chewing efficiency.[23,133] Although chewing efficiency and nutritional status improve when inadequate dentition or edentulousness is corrected with partial or complete dentures,[44] with these replacements, mastication is less efficient than with intact natural dentition.[23] The United States Department of Agriculture's Human Nutrition Research Center on Aging (HNRC) at Tufts University conducted the Nutritional Status Survey (NSS) of 691 free-living healthy elderly persons ages 60 to 98. Analysis of 3-day food diaries revealed low intakes of vitamins D, $B_6$, and $B_{12}$, folic acid, zinc, and calcium. Three life-style characteristics were associated with low dietary quality—low educational attainment, low median family income, and wearing of full or partial dentures.

Tufts University School of Dental Medicine conducted a study on a subsample (181) of the NSS population; it was found that persons who had at least one full denture exhibited a significantly lower dietary intake (approximately 20%).[94] Denture status may contribute to dietary risk when persons who have dentures find that they have difficulty masticating certain foods and must make dietary changes to soft, easily masticated foods, which are often high in fermentable carbohydrates. These diets are often low in nutritional value.

Study participants were asked if they had problems chewing the following foods:

| Food Item | Percent of difficulty |
| --- | --- |
| Raw carrot | 28 |
| Corn on cob | 25 |
| Steak or chops | 19 |
| Apples | 15 |

Of those who wore dentures, 28% reported chewing problems.[93]

Although dental problems usually are not considered life threatening, Anderson[8] found that a dental factor was implicated in the vast majority of cases of death because of food asphyxiation. Schweiger[120] observed that primary gastritis was eight times more prevalent in edentulous people than in those having an efficient masticatory apparatus. The elderly who experience digestive difficulties may turn to a soft diet, often high in easily digested sweets, and may adopt a pattern of frequent small meals. This is a pattern that will promote decay of the root surfaces and can aggravate periodontal disease.

## NUTRITION AND PERIODONTAL DISEASE

The precise role of nutritional factors in the cause, progression, and prevention of periodontal disease has been difficult to delineate up to now. Although malnutrition does not cause chronic inflammatory periodontal disease, nutritional factors can affect both the host susceptibility to this disease and its progression. A malnourished person has increased susceptibility to infection because of a compromised host defense. The epithelial barrier is particularly sensitive to nutrient restrictions because of its rapid cellular turnover rate. Nutritional stress during this "continuous critical period" can impair the renewal of the sulcular epithelium.[4]

Ascorbic acid has been studied extensively as a result of its essential role in collagen synthesis. Since the collagen in the gingival tissue has a high turnover rate, optimal ascorbic acid intake may be higher than that suggested by the Recommended Dietary Allowances. In monkeys, it has been found that marginal as well as clinical ascorbic acid deficiencies can affect host defense to periodontal irritation.[7] In animals with a suboptimal ascorbic acid intake but without clinical signs of ascorbate deficiency or spontaneous gingivitis, experimentally induced periodontitis resulted in impairment in polymorphonuclear leukocyte chemotoxins and phagocytosis. These animals had significantly greater pocket depth and gingival index scores than the control group. This finding has led some persons to hypothesize that "end-organ" deficiencies may occur at the level of the sulcular epithelial barrier even though no systemic deficiency exists. These "end-organ" deficiencies may adversely affect host defense mechanisms.[4]

The stress of infection and the associated increase in cell turnover increase folic acid requirements. Folate deficiency may result in an impairment of the sulcular epithelial barrier.[4] A decrease in host immunocompetence and mucosal permeability also have been associated with human folate deficiency.[5,131]

Tissue levels of zinc, which are often deficient in elderly persons, may modify periodontal disease defenses. Deficiencies can inhibit leukocyte activity, inhibit collagen formation, and increase sulcular epithelial permeability.[95-96]

Osteoporosis is one of the most prevalent age-related health problems in the elderly.[90] The alveolar bone may be the first area affected by osteoporosis.[3,137] The result may be a premature loss of bone, causing tooth loss or problems with denture fit.

The importance of saliva for immunologic, remineralizing, and oral-cleansing purposes cannot be overemphasized. Xerostomia (dry mouth from lack of saliva) is a condition commonly found in older persons.[66,123] Xerostomia is not a direct consequence of the aging process but may result from one or more organic functional causes or drugs. At least 400 drugs produce xerostomia as a side effect.[10,123] These drugs include antihypertensives, anticonvulsants, antiparkinsonian drugs, antidepressants, and tranquilizers. Xerostomia, in turn, is one of the important risk factors for caries formation in adults. (See Chapter 17.)

## LOCAL FOOD FACTORS THAT AFFECT CARIES

Among Americans sugar consumption has been observed to rise in the elderly (males and females in the 65 to 74 year age group consumed 53% and

47% more sugar-containing foods than young adults in the 19 to 24 year age group).

Over the past century, many epidemiologic and clinical studies have established the causal relationship between the consumption of fermentable carbohydrates and caries incidence. These studies have identified several factors that are associated with caries:

1. Amount of fermentable carbohydrate consumed
2. Sugar concentration of food item
3. Physical form of carbohydrate
4. Oral retentiveness (length of time teeth are exposed to decreased plaque pH)
5. Frequency of eating meals and snacks
6. Length of interval between eating events and proximity of eating to bedtime
7. Sequence of food consumption (for example, if cheese is eaten after sugar exposure, the pH drop is reduced)

Factors that make studies in this area difficult include the many variables that affect cariogenicity and the high interindividual and intraindividual variability in food intake, the fluoridation of water supplies, and the high level of "hidden sugars" in the diet; these make differences between dietary patterns difficult to discern. Any one of these factors contributes to the complexity of such investigations, necessitating large sample size, multivariate analysis, and careful training of the participant to prepare food records.

In a longitudinal study of a teenage cohort, Burt et al.[18] reported that the average daily consumption of sugar was strongly related to proximal and smooth-surface caries and the weekly consumption was related to total caries incidence. Teenagers who developed two or more carious lesions reported more snacking on at least one high-sugar food and consumed more carbohydrate-rich snacks and more calories after 9:00 P.M. When high- and low-sugar groups were compared for caries incidences, there were statistically significant differences between the groups for proximal surface caries. The average number of eating occasions was not significant. Rugg-Gunn et al.[110] also found that the total amount of sugar consumed was more strongly associated with caries incidence than with frequency of consumption.

Studies employing the NHANES I[129] data have shown that in persons 1 to 74 years of age the three independent variables that more highly correlated with caries experience are total sweets consumed, sweets consumed between meals, and the frequency of sweet consumption between meals.[16] The strongest correlation was between DMFS (decayed, missing, and filled surfaces) and the consumption frequency of between-meal snacks such as sugar products and cereals or grains.

Mixing starch with sugars may increase the cariogenicity of the sugar. In the Vipeholm study, bread given at meals was more cariogenic than twice the amount of sugar provided in liquid form.[47] Several animal studies have shown that a starch base can actually enhance cariogenicity by increasing retentiveness in the oral cavity. Starch-sugar combinations, such as cakes, cookies, waffles with syrup, have been found to be associated with increased caries prevalence.[85]

Efforts to determine the cariogenic potential of specific foods have encountered methodologic difficulties because of a variety of factors. The cariogenic potential of a particular food is determined by the retention time of the food in the mouth, its physical form, its pH, the buffering capacity of saliva, the capacity of the oral bacteria, and the presence of other foods, which may interact.[99]

At this time foods may be categorized as potentially cariogenic (sugar-containing foods and starch-sugar combinations) or noncariogenic (proteins, fats, and fiber). However, cariogenic foods cannot be ranked as to more or less cariogenic because of the complex factors mentioned.[27] In vitro studies are complicated by the fact that the sucrose content of a food may not be related to its acidogenic potential, nor is acid production by the oral flora always related to enamel dissolution.[127]

The cariogenic potential of fermentable carbohydrate-containing foods can be altered when their consumption patterns are changed.[108] Nonadherent, sugar-containing foods eaten at meals (rather than between meals), consumed at infrequent intervals, or eaten with other foods that reduce the oral contact time or raise the plaque pH have a lower cariogenic potential.[109] Presweetened cereals consumed with milk are less cariogenic than when they are consumed dry as a snack. Apples and bananas contain fermentable carbohydrates, but the banana has a slower rate of oral clearance. Thus the term "effective cariogenicity," that is, the total exposure time of the teeth to a fermentable carbohydrate challenge is a more appropriate manner of assessing the cariogenic potential of a diet than the wholesale condemnation of specific foods.[17]

For these reasons, the patient should be informed that all simple carbohydrates, not just sucrose, can and do contribute to dental caries and that factors other than the amount or type of sugar consumed are also important in caries development. Other habits such as sucking slowly dissolving vitamin C tablets or constant sipping of acid-containing beverages such as carbonated beverages can also lead to enamel decalcification.[42]

Food components other than carbohydrates may help to mitigate the cariogenic potential of these items. Most fermentable carbohydrates are found in association with other constituents—starch, fiber, protein, fats and oils, water, and minerals. The presence of these other factors in foods can alter the cariogenicity of the carbohydrate.[60]

Dairy products (especially cheeses) can exert a cariostatic effect. This has been demonstrated in studies using in vitro dentin demineralization,[60] in vitro and in vivo enamel demineralization,[121,122] plaque pH, and intraoral cariogenicity tests,[114] experimental animals,[104] and epidemiologic studies of children.[110] Many mechanisms of action for the caries-protective effect of dairy products have been proposed. Dairy products can lower the critical pH of plaque by the diffusion of calcium and phosphate into plaque. They may also stimulate salivary secretion rate, affect salivary composition, increase salivary urea, buffer plaque pH, and increase the rate of oral clearance.[121] Caseinates and other organic phosphates found in dairy products can reduce demineralization by adsorption onto the tooth surface (acting as an artificial pellicle), by inhibiting the adhesion of normal microbial flora, and by reducing mineral susceptibility to acid dissolution.[51,52] Lipids in dairy products may provide a protective coating over tooth surfaces, and bactericidal activity has been associated with the lactoperoxidase in milk.[119]

Rosen et al.[107] have shown in animal studies that the consumption of cheddar cheese can significantly lower caries activity in rats fed sucrose-containing diets. The consumption of cheese along with other food items offering a cariogenic challenge can totally obliterate any cariogenic effect of that item.[114] Silva et al.[121,122] have found that cheese extracts reduce acid demineralization in vitro. Papas et al.[92,94] found similar results for root caries in two adult populations. Additionally, Rugg-Gunn et al.[110] found that caries-free children consumed twice the amount of cheese than children with the highest caries rate did ($p > 0.02$).

## DIET AND ROOT CARIES

It has been suggested that the dietary factors involved in the causes of root caries may be similar to those responsible for coronal caries. Dietary studies on patients with periodontal disease[56,101] have found a statistically significant correlation between the frequency of fermentable carbohydrate consumption and root-caries prevalence.[132] When sugars were separated into categories based on form and retention, those who developed root caries consumed almost twice the amount of sugary liquids and 25% more solid sugars than those who did not have root caries in two different studies— 45 to 64 age group and 65-and-over age group.[94]

## STRATEGY FOR DIETARY SCREENING AND MANAGEMENT BY THE DENTAL TEAM

The dental problems of the elderly can affect food intake and subsequent nutritional status. In turn, nutritional problems can help to undermine oral health. The dental team is in an ideal position to screen older patients for nutritional risk and provide guidance or referral to nutrition professionals when indicated. Often simple suggestions or appropriate referrals can contribute immeasurably to improving health and the quality of life for this ever-increasing segment of the population.

To provide meaningful nutrition care to the elderly, it is essential to have a systematic approach to assessing dietary and possible nutritional factors and making appropriate recommendations.

Since overt clinical signs and symptoms are apparent in only the most advanced stages of nutritional problems, it would be inappropriate to base the assessment on merely a visual inspection. Likewise, the simple question "How are you eating" may evoke a subjective response such as "Fine," which is also not a qualitative, objective response.

The following is a simple, comprehensive, diet-screening technique that can be adapted to any dental setting. Questions to consider include the following: Is there any reason to suspect nutritional problems? If so, what is the nutritional area of concern? What is the extent of the problem? What physiologic mechanisms are involved (such as alterations in intake, digestion and absorption, metabolism, and excretion requirement)? What factors underlie the physiologic mechanisms (such as dental problems, psychosocial factors)? Is this a problem for which counseling can be provided in the office (poor food choices) or does the patient need to be referred to a physician and dietitian (diabetes, cardiovascular disease)?

### Step 1. Observations for clinical signs of nutritional problems

It is essential that the elder be questioned clearly and carefully about his or her health and living status. The medical and dental and social histories will provide important clues to any physiologic oral, psychosocial, and environmental problems that may interfere with eating habits and nutritional status. Nutritional problems in the elderly, as in any person, can be either primary (because of chronically deficient intake of food) or secondary or conditioned (because of malabsorptions, decreased ability to utilize nutrients, increased nu-

trient excretion or destruction, or increased nutrient requirements).

The social history can reveal important social, emotional, economic, and environmental factors that can impinge on the elder's eating habits. The simplest most effective way to elicit this information is to ask the elder to describe the routine of a "usual day." The daily routine will provide clues and information about:

- Eating habits (meals and snacks—how many, when, where eaten, with whom, who prepares)
- Social activities and exercise
- Stresses and problems (financial, loneliness, lack of ability to get out to the store, lack of desire to cook, and so on)

### Step 2. Determine dental, medical, personal, and social history

Clinically manifested nutritional disease represents only the tip of the iceberg of inadequate nutrition, since only the most severe deficiency states have clinically observable signs (Fig. 15-1). "Latent" nutritional deficiencies not visibly manifested can seriously affect and impair physiologic functioning. Many of the biochemical impairments to healing, resistance to infection, and so on result from decreased serum levels of nutrients before clinical signs are observable. Thus nutritional deficiencies should not be ruled out in the elderly patient with

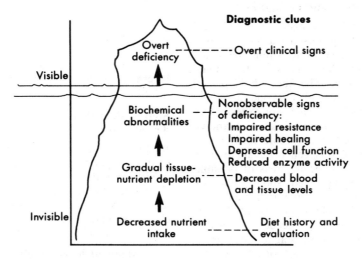

**Fig. 15-1** Progress of nutritional deficiencies.

poor eating habits who does not have clinical signs of malnutrition; the possibility of "latent" nutritional deficiency disease should be explored.

*Signs and symptoms of overt malnutrition.* It is important to realize that no one clinical sign or symptom is sufficient to diagnose malnutrition. In many cases, the same symptoms or signs can be caused by a variety of factors. Such signs or symptoms should be seen as *clues* to possible problems. In general, any sign of true nutritional deficiency will be bilateral (appear equally on both sides of the body).

Table 15-2 describes some common signs of nutritional deficiency as well as other possible causes of such signs.

*Symptoms of latent malnutrition.* The earliest symptoms of malnutrition are vague and nonspecific and may be mistaken for the aging process. Reported symptoms that serve to reinforce the importance of individual assessment include anorexia (lack of appetite), anxiety, abdominal discomfort, backache, decreased work output, depression, confusion, fatigue, dyspepsia (acid indigestion), insomnia (inability to sleep), irritability, lassitude (weakness), muscle pain, palpitations, paresthesia (numbness), and poor concentration. Vitamin deficiencies can contribute to mental confusion, neurologic symptoms, anemia, increased susceptibility to infection, and a host of other problems.

### Step 3. Dietary history and evaluation

In addition to the subjective histories and clinical examination, the elderly person's actual diet pattern should be ascertained to determine the actual diet intake and quality. Once it has been determined as accurately as possible what the elderly person actually eats for one or several days, one can screen the diet for adequacy (deficiencies or excesses) by comparing the reported food intake to a known standard such as a food guide (Table 15-3).

Upon completion of this general evaluation of the elderly person's diet recall, areas of possible nutritional risk can be pinpointed. Too few portions of the four basic food groups may indicate lack of important nutrients. Too many servings of the four food groups may be providing needed calories *or* may be contributing to excess weight. There is no recommended number of servings of fats, sweets, or alcohol. These foods should be consumed only in moderation; they provide little nutritional value,

they may contribute excess calories, and they may be taking the place of more nutritious foods.

### Step 4. Dietary diagnosis

Once the medicodental and personal-social histories and dietary habits have been evaluated and clinical observations have been made, a management strategy can be determined.

| | Yes | No |
|---|---|---|
| Are there any medical problems that may affect diet or nutritional status? | | |
| Are there any clinical signs that may indicate nutritional problems? | | |
| Are there any emotional, psychologic, economic, or environmental problems that are affecting eating? | | |
| Does the diet appear inadequate in any way? | | |

If the answer to all of the above is *no,* nutrition can be ruled out as a problem. If the answer to one or more of the above is *yes*, the elderly person should be provided with counseling to rectify the problem or referred to a physician or nutritionist (if the problem is complex or if there is an underlying medical complication) according to the following flow diagram:

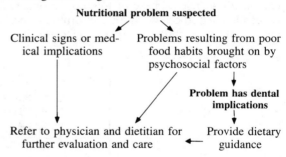

### Step 5. Provide dietary guidance in the dental office

Balance and variety are important for optimum nutrition and palatability for the elderly. A variety of foods from the four food groups (Table 15-4) should be combined at each meal, and the textures and colors should be varied. Wisdom in food choices should be stressed and adherence to dietary guidelines should be promoted as follows:

1. Maintain ideal weight. Excess weight is a stress on the body and may contribute to a variety of medical problems.

**Table 15-2** Components of the clinical exam suggestive of nutritional problems

| Component | Alteration | Possible inadequacy* |
|---|---|---|
| Weight | Excessive or inadequate fat storage | Excessive or inadequate calorie intake |
| Head | Bossing | Vitamin D |
| Hair | Brittle, pluckable, sparse, depigmentation | Protein |
| Eyes | Xerophthalmia, photophobia, night blindness, Blind spots, keratomalacia | Vitamin A |
| | Circumcorneal injection, canthal fissures | Riboflavin |
| Nose | Nasolabial seborrhea | Riboflavin |
| Skin | Edema | Protein |
| | Dyssebacea | Riboflavin |
| | Xerosis, follicular hyperkeratosis | Vitamin A |
| | Perifolliculitis, petechiae, purpura | Ascorbate |
| | Pellagrous dermatitis | Niacin |
| Neck | Casal's necklace | Niacin |
| | Goiter | Iodine |
| Fingernails | Fragility, bands, lines | Protein |
| Lips | Angular cheilosis, angular scars | Riboflavin, B complex |
| | Pallor | Iron |
| Tongue | Pallor, magenta color, red color, papillary hypertrophy, papillary atrophy | Iron, B complex, particularly thiamin and riboflavin |
| Oral mucosa | Pallor | Iron, folate, $B_{12}$ |
| | Hyperkeratosis | Vitamin A |
| Gingiva | Red and spongy | Ascorbate |
| | Gingivitis | Multiple nutrient deficiencies |
| | Pallor | Iron, folate, $B_{12}$ |
| Teeth | Caries | Fluoride, excessive sugar intake |
| | Linear hypoplasia, melanodontia, malposition | Developmental nutrient deficiencies |
| Oral bioassay | Excessive periodontal destruction relative to amount of local irritation | Multiple nutrient deficiencies |

From Palmer C, Cassidy M, and Larsen C: Nutrition, diet, and dental health: concepts and methods (self-study course), Chicago, 1981, American Dental Hygienists Association.
*It should be noted that the deficiencies listed are only suggested by the tissue alterations described. Confirmatory data must be obtained to determine the exact cause of the tissue changes, which may be attributable strictly to local factors as well as nutritional or other systemic problems.

**Table 15-3** Guidelines for a healthy diet

| Food | Portion size considered as one serving | Adult | Comments |
|---|---|---|---|
| Milk | 1 cup milk or<br>1 cup yogurt<br>1½+ oz. cheddar cheese*<br>1½ slices American cheese<br>2 cups cottage cheese | 2+ | Lowfat or skim (lowfat milk products have approximately the same nutrient content as whole milk but fewer calories. |
| Meat | 2 oz. cooked lean meat, fish, poultry or 2 eggs<br>4 tbsp. peanut butter<br>1 cup dried beans or peas<br>2 oz. cheddar cheese*<br>½ cup cottage cheese* | 2 | Protein from plant sources is a lower quality protein than animal protein but can provide good sources of protein when combined with other protein foods. |
| Fruit/vegetable | ½ cup cooked fruit or vegetable<br>(1 cup if raw or portion size as usually served)<br>½ cup juice | 4 | A citrus fruit is recommended daily; dark, green, leafy, or orange vegetables or fruit are recommended 3-4 times weekly for vitamins. |
| Grain,<br>whole grain,<br>fortified,<br>or enriched | 1 slice of bread<br>1 cup dry, ready to eat cereal,<br>½ cup cooked cereal,<br>rice, pasta, or grits | 4 | Whole grain products may have greater trace mineral content and fiber than enriched products. |

*Count cheese as a serving of milk or meat, not as both simultaneously.

**The elderly should go easy on extra sweets, fats, and alcohol:**

| Sweets | Fats | Alcohol |
|---|---|---|
| cake | butter | wine, sherry, brandy |
| candy | margarine | beer |
| cookies | oil | "hard" liquor |
| pastry | salad dressing | mixed drinks |
| honey, molasses | mayonnaise | |
| corn syrup | | |
| jam, jelly | | |
| sugar | | |
| carbonated beverages | | |

- Small amounts of these foods make eating enjoyable.
- However, since they are high in calories and low in nutrient value, they provide primarily calories and should not be used in place of more nutritious foods.
- Liquid is important if constipation is to be avoided; 6 to 8 glasses (8 oz.) daily are recommended and may include the liquid in hot bouillon, soups, coffee, teas, fruit, and vegetable juices as well as water.

From Palmer C, Cassidy M, and Larsen C: Nutrition, diet and dental health: concepts and methods, Chicago, 1981, American Dental Hygienists Association.

**Table 15-4** Managing the diet of the elderly

| | Food Groups | | | |
|---|---|---|---|---|
| | **Milk**<br>2 servings minimum | **Meat**<br>2 servings minimum | **Fruit and vegetable**<br>4 servings minimum | **Bread and cereal**<br>4 servings minimum |
| **Problems and suggestions** | | | | |
| Mastication | Instant breakfast, high protein milk, eggnog,* cottage cheese | Chop/grind meat, blenderize, peanut butter, eggs, fish | Canned fruits and vegetables, cooked vegetables with soups | Softer breads (avoid hard crusts), crackers, pasta |
| Taste | Flavored milk, yogurt, buttermilk | Chewing slowly and thoroughly; add spices | Fruits with skin, raw vegetables | Whole-grain breads (rye, pumpernickel), pasta with spicy sauce |
| Arthritis | Cheese pieces, use of straw for drinking | Prepare stews and soups; freeze extras, tender meats | Finger foods, cut up into pieces — raw fruits and vegetables | Crackers, muffins, breads |
| Dehydration | Milk, cocoa, yogurt, eggnog,* buttermilk, creamed cottage cheese | Stews, soups | Vegetable soups, fruit sauce (applesauce) | Whole grains (high fiber binds water), crackers, cereal with milk |
| Food intolerance | Lactose — Use yogurt, cheese, milk, buttermilk as tolerated (usually small amounts) | Lean foods (not fried), chicken, fish | Cooked vegetables, fruit sauces | Cereal, plain breads (others as tolerated), pasta |

**Other suggestions**

- Osteoporosis — Recommend increased calcium intake, i.e., milk products, green, leafy vegetables.
- Eating alone — Plan interesting meals, plan other activities around mealtimes (listen to radio show, watch TV, read newspaper, sit on porch, eat in park).
- Taste — Instead of using salt, use other herbs and spices, e.g., oregano, garlic, onion, basil.
- Sweets — Encourage elderly persons to decrease intake. Sweets are concentrated sources of calories with low nutritive value.
- Alcohol — Encourage elderly persons to limit intake. Alcohol may interfere with the action of blood-pressure medications amd may be used in place of foods needed for an adequate diet. In some cases, use of an alcoholic beverage before a meal may stimulate the appetite. (Wine is usually the beverage of choice).

From Palmer C, Cassidy M, and Larsen C: Nutrition, diet, and dental health: concepts and methods, Chicago, 1981, American Dental Hygienists Association.
*Do not use raw egg.

2. Avoid too much fat, saturated fat, and cholesterol. Low-fat milk is a good choice. Emphasize poultry and fish, which are generally inexpensive and easy to chew.
3. Eat foods with adequate starch and fiber. One tablespoon of raw bran may be added to each serving of cereal. Other complex carbohydrates, fresh fruits, and vegetables should be eaten daily.
4. Avoid too much sugar. Simple desserts (custards, fruit) are best.
5. Avoid too much sodium. Herbs and spices enhance flavors. Highly salted foods should be limited.
6. If the elder drinks alcohol, it should be used in moderation.

The elderly should be encouraged to include foods that require chewing whenever possible. In addition, high-fiber foods can help reduce the risk of bowel disease and promote bowel function as well.

*Adapting the diet plan when changes in consistency or texture are needed as in liquid and soft diets.* If for any reason the elderly person cannot consume a normal diet and must have soft or liquid foods, it is important that sufficient nutrient intake be maintained. The following suggestion may be helpful under such circumstances:

For extra protein and calories recommend adding powdered skim milk to milk drinks and milk soups and suggest commercially prepared supplemental milk drinks like liquid breakfast drinks instead of plain milk (they are high in nutritional quality and provide approximately 250 calories per 8 ounces). In addition, recommend making eggnogs with powdered egg, milk, ice cream, and orange juice (approximately 350 calories) and suggest blenderizing meats, fruits, vegetables, and so on, making sure that the foods the elderly person chooses are moderate in temperature and not too spicy, so as to prevent irritation to tender oral tissues (Table 15-4).

### Step 6. Community services to assist nutrition care

If an elderly person requires professional nutrition care, the services of a qualified nutritionist should be sought. In most states, there is no legislation

that assures the qualifications of those who call themselves "nutritionists"; therefore a registered dietitian (RD) is the most reliably creditable resource. A registered dietitian is a licensed, professionally educated nutrition specialist who may be found in hospitals, ambulatory clinics, and private practice as well. Although other non-RDs, such as those with nutrition doctorates, may be well qualified, the plethora of unsound nutrition practitioners requires that the credentials of potential nutrition care providers be carefully scrutinized before they are engaged for patient referral.

For patients living alone, most communities provide communal meal programs in local senior centers or churches that provide hot meals at noontime several days a week. These meals are federally subsidized, free to the elderly (a small donation is requested), and meets one third of the RDA for the day. The meals program is specifically designed to help improve the nutritional status of the elderly by providing a nutritious meal in a social environment that will enhance appetite.

For patients who are homebound, home-delivered meals are also available through state departments of elderly affairs.

### SUMMARY

It is clear that diet and nutrition can affect health and well-being on a variety of levels. Oral health status can contribute to improved nutrition and general health status or can undermine both. The dental team is in an ideal position to contribute to the well-being of the elderly population even beyond dental concerns. Dental team members can and should be alert to nutritional risk factors in the elderly population and, by careful screening and referral for care, can intervene in the early stages of nutritional problems when such interventions can be most valuable and effective.

### REFERENCES

1. Aging and nutrition, Columbus, Ohio, 1982, Ross Laboratories.
2. Albanese AA: Nutrition of the elderly: introduction, Postgrad Med 63:117, 1978.
3. Albanese AA, Edelson AH, Lorenze EJ Jr, et al: Problems of bone health in elderly, NY State J Med 75:326, 1975.
4. Alfano MD: Controversies, perspectives, and clinical implications of nutrition in periodontal disease, Dent Clin North Am 20:519, 1976.

5. Alfano M and Masi C: Effect of acute folic acid deficiency on oral mucosal permeability, J Dent Res 57(special issue A):949, 1978.
6. Alhadeff L, Gualtieri CT, and Lipton M: Toxic effects of water-soluble vitamins, Nutr Rev 42:33, 1984.
7. Alvares O, Altman LC, Springmeyer S, et al: The effect of subclinical ascorbate deficiency on periodontal health in nonhuman primates, J Periodont Res 16:628, 1981.
8. Anderson DL: Death from improper mastication, Int Dent J 27:349, 1977.
9. Baghurst KI and Record SJ: The vitamin and mineral intake of a free-living young elderly Australian population in relation to total diet and supplementation practices, Hum Nutr Appl Nutr 41A:327, 1987.
10. Bahn SL: Drug related dental destruction, Oral Surg Oral Med Oral Pathol 33:49, 1972.
11. Barboriak JJ and Rooney CB: Alcohol and its effect on the nutrition of the elderly. In Watson WR, editor: Handbook of nutrition in the aged, Boca Raton, Fla, 1985, CRC Press, Inc.
12. Bidlack WR and Smith CH: Nutritional requirements of the aged, Crit Rev Food Sci Nutr 27(3):189, 1988.
13. Blumberg JB: Nutrient requirements for the healthy elderly, Contemp Nutr 11(6), 1986, and Bol Asoc Med PR 78(11):494, 1986.
14. Bonner MH, Fox KM, and Williams PK: An evaluation of the Christchurch meals-on-wheels service, Christchurch, New Zealand, 1985, Canterbury Hospital Board of Health Planning and Research Unit.
15. Burr ML, Mibank JE, and Gibbs D: The nutritional status of the elderly, Aging 11:89, 1982.
16. Burt BA and Eklund SA: Sugar consumption and dental caries: some epidemiological patterns in the United States. In Hefferren JJ, Ayer W, and Koeler H, editors: Food nutrition and dental health, vol 3, Minneapolis, 1981, American Dental Association Health Foundation.
17. Burt BA and Ismail AI: Diet, nutrition and food cariogenicity, J Dent Res 65(special issue):1475, 1986.
18. Burt BA, Eklund SA, Morgan KJ, et al: The effects of sugar intake and frequency of ingestion on dental caries increment in a 3-year longitudinal study, J Dent Res 67(11):1422, 1988.
19. Busse EW: How mind, body and environment influence nutrition in the elderly, Postgrad Med 63(3):118, 125, 1978.
20. Busse EW: Eating in later life: physiological and psychological factors, Contemp Nutr 4(1), Nov 1979, and Am Pharm 20(5):36, 1980.
21. Chang L et al: Vitamin C and the elderly. In Watson RR, editor: CRC handbook of nutrition in the aged, Boca Raton, Fla, 1985, CRC Press Inc.
22. Changing nutrient needs pose problems for people facing fifty, Environ Nutr 11(10):1, 1988.
23. Chauncey HH, Meunch M, Kapur KK, et al: The effect of the loss of teeth on diet and nutrition, Int Dent J 34:98, 1984.
24. Chernoff R and Lipschitz DA: In Shils ME and Young VR, editors: Modern nutrition in health and disease, ed 7, Philadelphia, 1988, Lea & Febiger.
25. Coe R and Miller D: Sociological factors that influence nutritional status in the elderly. In Armbrecht JH, Prendergast JM, and Coe RM, editors: Nutritional interventions in the aging process, New York, 1984, Springer-Verlag.
26. Cowart BJ: Development of taste perceptions in humans: sensitivity and preference throughout the life span, Psychol Bull 90:43, 1981.
27. Curzon MEJ: Integration of methods for determining the cariogenic potential of foods. Is this possible with present technologies? J Dent Res 65(special issue):1520, 1986.
28. Davis MA, Murphy SP, and Neuhaus JM: Living arrangements and eating behaviors of older adults in the United States, J Gerontol 43(3):S96-8, 1988.
29. Davis MA, Randall E, Forthofer RN, et al: Living arrangements and dietary patterns of older adults in the United States, J Gerontol 40:434, 1985.
30. Dawson DW et al: Malabsorption of protein bound vitamin $B_{12}$, Br Med J 288:675, 1984.
31. Dye C: Age related changes in taste and smell that affect nutritional adequacy. In Armbrecht JH, Prendergast JM, and Coe RM, editors: Nutritional interventions in the aging process, New York, 1984, Springer-Verlag.
32. Enstrom JE: Cancer and total mortality among active Mormons, Cancer 42:1943, 1978.
33. Food and Nutrition Board: Recommended Dietary Allowances, ed 9 revised, Washington, DC, 1980, National Academy of Sciences–National Research Council.
34. Francis RM and Peacock MM: Local action of oral 1,25-dihydroxycholecalciferol on calcium absorption in osteoporosis, Am J Clin Nutr 45:501, 1987.
35. Franks AST and Hedegard B: Geriatric dentistry, Oxford, England, 1973, Blackwell Scientific Publications.
36. Fries JF: Aging, natural death, and the compression of morbidity, N Engl J Med 303:130, 1980.
37. Gambert SR and Duthie EH Jr: Protein-calorie malnutrition in the elderly. In Watson RR, editor: CRC handbook of nutrition in the aged, Boca Raton, Fla, 1985, CRC Press, Inc.
38. Garetz K: Breaking the dangerous cycle of depression and faulty nutrition, Geriatrics 31:73, 1976.
39. Garry P et al: Nutritional status in a healthy elderly population: dietary and supplemental intakes, Am J Clin Nutr 36:319, 1982.
40. Garry P et al: Iron status and anemia in the elderly: new findings and a review of previous studies, J Am Geriatr Soc 31:389, 1983.
41. Garry P and Hunt W: Biochemical assessment of vitamin status in the elderly: effects of dietary supplemental intakes. In Hutchinson ML and Munro HN, editors: Nutrition and aging, Orlando, Fla, 1986, Academic Press Inc.
42. Giunta J: Dental erosion results from chewable vitamin C tablets, J Am Dent Assoc 107:253, 1983.
43. Good RA and Lorenz E: Nutrition, immunity, aging and cancer, Nutr Rev 46:62, 1988.
44. Gordon SR, Kelley SL, Sybyl JR, et al: Relationship in very elderly veterans of nutritional status, self-perceived chewing ability, dental status, and social isolation, J Am Geriatr Soc 33:334, 1985.
45. Gray GE, Paganini-Hill A, and Ross RK: Dietary intake and nutrient supplement use in a southern California retirement community, Am J Clin Nutr 38:122, 1983.

46. Guilland JC et al: Evaluation of pyridoxine intake and pyridoxine status among aged institutionalized people, Int J Vitam Nutr Res 54:185, 1984.

47. Gustafsson BE, Quensel CE, Lonke L, et al: The Vipeholm Dental Caries Study: effects of different levels of carbohydrate intake on caries activity in 436 individuals observed for 5 years, Acta Odontol Scand 11:232, 1954.

48. Guthrie HA, Black K, and Madden JP: Nutritional practices of elderly citizens in rural Pennsylvania, Gerontologist 12:330, 1972.

49. Hale WE, Stewart RB, Cerda JJ, et al: Use of nutritional supplements in ambulatory elderly population, Am Geriatr Soc 30:401, 1982.

50. Harrell I and Bowski MM: Relationship of age and sex to nutrient supplement usage in a group of adults in Colorado, J Nutr Elderly 1:51, 1981.

51. Harper DS, Osborn JC, Hefferren JJ, and Clayton R: Cariostatic potential of four cheeses evaluated in a programmed fed rat model, J Dent Res 62:283, 1983.

52. Harper DS, Osborn JC, Clayton R, and Hefferren JJ: Modification of food cariogenicity in rats by mineral-rich concentrates from milk, J Dent Res 66:42, 1987.

53. Hartz SC, Otradovec CL, McGandy RB, et al: Nutrient supplement use by healthy elderly, J Am Coll Nutr 7(2):119, 1988.

54. Hendricks J and Calasanti T: Social dimensions of nutrition. In Chen LH, editor: Nutritional aspects of aging, vol 1, Boca Raton, Fla, 1986, CRC Press Inc.

55. Herbert V: Recommended dietary intakes (RDI) of folate in humans, Am J Clin Nutr 45:661, 1987.

56. Hix JO III and O'Leary TJ: The relationship between cemental caries, oral hygiene status and fermentable carbohydrate intake, J Periodontol 47(7):398, 1976.

57. Holick M: Vitamin D synthesis by the aging skin. In Hutchinson ML and Munro HN, editors: Nutrition and aging, Orlando, Fla, 1986, Academic Press Inc.

58. Horwath CC: A random population study of dietary habits in elderly people, doctoral thesis, Adelaide, Australia, 1987, University of Adelaide.

59. Horwath CC: Dietary intake studies in elderly people. In Bourne GH, editor: Impact of nutrition on health and disease: world review of nutrition and dietetics, vol 1(59), Basel, 1989, S Karger, AG.

60. Jenkins GN and Harper DS: Protective effect of different cheeses in an in vitro demineralization system, J Dent Res 62:284, 1983 (abstract).

61. Katakity M, Webb JF, and Dickerson JW: Some effects of a food supplement in elderly hospital patients, a longitudinal study, Hum Nutr Appl Nutr 37A:85, 1983.

62. Kiyak HA: Psychosocial factors in dental needs of the elderly, Special Care in Dentistry 1(1):22, 1981.

63. Kohr MB, O'Neal R, Preston A, et al: Nutritional status in elderly residents in Missouri, Am J Clin Nutr 71:2186, 1978.

64. Krehl W: Changes and problems with aging, Geriatrics, p 65, May 1974.

65. Lamy PP: Drug nutrient interactions in the aged. In Watson RR, editor: CRC handbook of nutrition in the aged, Boca Raton, Fla, 1985, CRC Press, Inc.

66. Langer A: Oral signs of aging and their clinical significance, Geriatrics, p 63, Dec 1976.

67. Lemming JT, Webster SPG, and Dymock IW: Gastrointestinal systems. In Brocklehurst JC, editor: Textbook of geriatric medicine and gerontology, Edinburgh, 1973, Churchill Livingston.

68. Letsou AP and Price LS: Health, aging and nutrition: an overview, Clin Geriatr Med 3:253, 1987.

69. Lipson P and Bray G: Energy. In Chen L, editor: Nutritional aspects of aging, vol 1, Boca Raton, Fla, 1986, CRC Press Inc.

70. Lowenstein FW: Nutritional requirements of the elderly. In Young EA, editor: Nutrition, aging and health, New York, 1986, Alan R Liss, Inc.

71. Luros E: A rational approach to geriatric nutrition, Dietetic Currents 8(6):25, Columbus, Ohio, Nov-Dec 1981, Ross Laboratories.

72. McGandy RB: Nutrition and the aging cardiovascular system. In Hutchinson ML and Munro HN, editors: Nutrition and aging, Bristol-Meyers Nutrition Symposia, vol 5, Orlando, Fla, 1986, Academic Press Inc.

73. Manson JE, Stampher MJ, Hennekens CJ, and Willett WC: Body weight and longevity: a reassessment, JAMA 257:353, 1987.

74. Masoro EJ: Physiologic changes with aging. In Winick M, editor: Nutrition and aging, New York, 1976, Academic Press Inc.

75. Masoro EJ: Nutrition as a modulator of the aging process, Physiologist 27:98, 1984.

76. Mohs ME and Watson RR: Nutritional assessment for the elderly. In Watson RR, editor: CRC handbook of nutrition in the aged, Boca Raton, Fla, 1985, CRC Press, Inc.

77. Morely J: Nutritional status of the elderly, Am J Med 81:679, 1986.

78. Morgan KJ and Zabik ME: The influence of ready-to-eat cereal consumption at breakfast on nutrient intakes of individuals 62 years and older, J Am Coll Nutr 3:27, 1984.

79. Mullen JL, Gertner MH, Buzby GP et al: Implications of malnutrition in the surgical patient, Arch Surg 114:121, 1979.

80. Munro HN: Aging and nutrition: a multifaceted problem. In Hutchinson ML and Munro HN, editors: Nutrition and aging, Bristol-Meyers, Nutrition Symposia, vol 5, Orlando, Fla, 1986, Academic Press Inc.

81. Munro HN: Protein nutriture and requirements in elderly people, Bibl Nutr Dieta 33:61, Basel, 1983, S Karger, AG.

82. Munro HN, Suter PM, and Russell RM: Nutritional requirements of the elderly, Ann Rev Nutr 7:23, 1987.

83. National Center for Health Statistics: Dietary intake source data, United States 1971-1974, Hyattsville, Md, National Center for Health Statistics (DHEW publ no PHS 79-1221), 1979.

84. National Institutes of Health Consensus Conference: Osteoporosis, JAMA 252:799, 1984.

85. Navia JM: The value of animal models to predict the caries-promoting properties of human diet or dietary components, Cariology Today, p 154, 1983.

86. Newton HMV et al: The relationships between vitamin $D_2$ and $D_3$ in the diet and plasma 25OHD$_2$ and 25OHD$_3$ in elderly women in Great Britain, Am J Clin Nutr 41:760, 1985.

87. Niessen L and Jones SA: Oral health changes in the el-

derly: their relationship to nutrition, Postgrad Med 75(5):231, 1984.

88. Norden AM and Scherstén F: Chemical analyses of what old people eat and their states of health during 6 year follow-up: assessment of nutritional status, Scand J Gastroenterol 14(52):42, 1979.

89. Nordin BEC, Baker MR, Horseman A, and Peacock M: A prospective trial of the effect of vitamin D supplementation on metacarpal bone loss in elderly women, Am J Clin Nutr 42:470, 1985.

90. Osteoporosis: causes, treatment, prevention. National Institute of Arthritis and Musculoskeletal and Skin Diseases, National Institutes of Health, NIH publ no 86-2226, revised May 1986.

91. Owen A and Frankle RT: Nutrition in the community: the art of delivering services, St. Louis, 1986, Times-Mirror/Mosby College Publ, p 304.

92. Papas A, Herman J, Palmer C, et al: Oral health status of the elderly, with dietary and nutritional considerations, Gerodontology 3:147, 1984.

93. Papas A, Palmer C, McGandy R, Hartz S, and Russell R: Dietary and nutritional factors in relation to dental caries in elderly subjects, Gerodontics 3:30, 1987.

94. Papas AS, Palmer CA, Rounds ME, et al: Longitudinal relationship between nutrition and oral health, Ann NY Acad Sci 561:125, 1989.

95. Papisarda E and Long A: Effects of zinc and vitamin B$_6$ in caries in rats, Minerva Stomatol 30(4):317, 1981.

96. Pekarek R, Sandstead H, Jacob R, and Barcome D: Abnormal cellular immune responses during acquired zinc deficiency, Am J Clin Nutr 32:1466, 1979.

97. Pilch SM and Senti FR, editors: Assessment of the zinc nutritional status of the U.S. population based on data collected in the 2nd National Health and Nutrition Examination Survey 1976-1980, Bethesda, Md, 1984, Life Sciences Research Office, Federation of American Societies for Experimental Biology.

98. Position of the American Dietetic Association: Nutrition, aging, and the continuum of health care, J Am Diet Assoc 87(3):344, 1987.

99. Proceedings of the Scientific Consensus Conference on Methods for Assessment of the Cariogenic Potential of Foods, J Dent Res 65 (special issue), 1986.

100. Ranno BS, Wardlaw GM, and Gerger CJ: What characterizes elderly women who overuse vitamin and mineral supplements, J Am Diet Assoc 88:347, 1988.

101. Ravald R, Hamp S-E, and Birked D: Long-term evaluation of root surface caries in periodontally treated patients, J Clin Periodontol 13:758, 1986.

102. Read MH and Graney AS: Food supplement usage by the elderly, J Am Diet Assoc 80:250, 1982.

103. Reiff TR: Water and aging, Clin Geriatr Med 3:403, 1987.

104. Reynolds EC and del Rio A: Effect of casein and whey-protein solutions on caries experience and feeding patterns of the rat, Arch Oral Biol 29:927, 1984.

105. Rikans LE: Drugs. In Chen LH, editor: Nutritional aspects of aging, vol 2, Boca Raton, Fla, 1986, CRC Press, Inc.

106. Roe DA: Geriatric nutrition, ed 2, Englewood Cliffs, NJ, 1987, Prentice-Hall, Inc.

107. Rosen S, Min DB, Harper DS, et al: Effect of cheese with and without sucrose on dental caries and recovery

of *Streptococcus mutans* in rats, J Dent Res 63(6):894, 1984.

108. Rugg-Gunn AJ, Edgar W, et al: The effect of different meal patterns upon plaque pH in human subjects, Br Dent J 137:351, 1975.

109. Rugg-Gunn AJ, Edgar W, and Jenkins GN: The effect of altering the position of a sugary food in a meal upon plaque pH in human subjects, J Dent Res 60(5):867, 1981.

110. Rugg-Gunn AJ, Hackett AF, Appleton DR, et al: Correlations of dietary intake of calcium, phosphorus, and Ca/P ratio with caries data in children, Caries Res 18:149, 1984.

111. Sandstead HH: Trace element interactions, J Lab Clin Med 98:457, 1981.

112. Sandstead HH: Nutrition in the elderly, Gerodontics 3:3, 1987.

113. Schlenker ED: Nutrition in aging, St. Louis, 1984, The CV Mosby Co, p 150.

114. Schachtele CF and Jensen ME: The acidogenic potential of reference foods and snacks at interproximal sites in the human dentition, J Dent Res 62(8):889, 1983.

115. Schiffman SS: Changes in taste and smell in old persons: advances in research, vol 2, Durham, NC, 1978, Duke University Center for the Study of Aging and Human Development.

116. Schiffman SS and Pasternak M: Decreased discrimination of food odors in the elderly, J Gerontol 34:73, 1979.

117. Schiffman SS and Covey E: Changes in taste and smell with age: nutritional aspects. In Ordy JM, Harmon D, and Alfin-Slater RB, editors: Nutrition in gerontology, vol 43, New York, 1984, Raven Press.

118. Schneider EL and Reed JD Jr: Life extension, N Engl J Med 312:1159, 1985.

119. Shrestha BM, Mundorff SA, and Bibby BG: Preliminary studies on calcium lactate as an anticaries food additive, Caries Res 16:12, 1982.

120. Schweiger JW: Prosthetic considerations for the aging, J Prosthet Dent 9:55, 1959.

121. Silva MFdeA et al: Effects of cheese on experimental caries in human subjects, Caries Res 20(3):263, 1986.

122. Silva MFdeA et al: Effects of cheese extract and its fraction on enamel demineralization in vitro and in vivo in humans, J Dent Res 66(10):1527, 1987.

123. Spielman A, Ben-Aryeh H, et al: Xerostomia: diagnosis and treatment. In Litt J, editor: Oral medicine, St. Louis, 1981, The CV Mosby Co.

124. Steen B: Summary of the results of round table discussion (nutritional problems of the elderly), Bibl Nutr Dieta 33:192, Basel, 1983, S Karger, AG.

125. Stini WA: Early nutrition, growth, disease and human longevity, Nutr Cancer 1:31, 1979.

126. Suter PM and Russell RM: Vitamin requirements of the elderly, Am J Clin Nutr 45:501, 1987.

127. Ten Cate JM: Demineralization models: mechanistic aspect of the caries process with special emphasis on the possible role of foods, J Dent Res 65(special issue):1511, 1986.

128. Todhunter EN: Lifestyle and nutrient intake in the elderly. In Winick M, editor: Nutrition and aging, New York, 1976, John Wiley & Sons, Inc.

129. US Department of Health, Education and Welfare: Pre-

liminary findings of the first health and nutrition examination survey, United States, 1971-72. Dietary intake and biochemical findings, DHEW publ no (DHS) 79-1221, Washington, DC, 1974, US Government Printing Office.

130. US Senate Special Committee on Aging: 1988—Aging America: trends and projections, LR 3377(1880) D 12198, Washington, DC, 1988, US Department of Health and Human Services.

131. Vogel RI and Deasy M: The effect of folic acid on experimentally produced gingivitis, J Prevent Dent 5:30, 1978.

132. Vehkalahti MM and Paunio IK: Occurrence of root caries in relation to dental health behavior, J Dent Res 67(6):911, 1988.

133. Wayler AH and Chauncey HH: Impact of complete dentures and impaired natural dentition on masticatory performance and food choice in healthy aging men, J Prosthet Dent 49:427, 1983.

134. Weber H and Miguel J: In Chen LH, editor: Nutritional aspects of aging, vol 1, Boca Raton, Fla, 1986, CRC Press, Inc, p 42.

135. Weiffenbach JM, Baum BJ, and Binghauser R: Taste thresholds: quality specific variation with human aging, J Gerontol 37:372, 1982.

136. Welling PG, Koch PA, Lau CC, and Craig WA: Bioavailability of tetracycline and doxycycline in fasted and nonfasted subjects, Antimicrob Agents Chemother 11:462, 1977.

137. Winick M: Nutrition and aging, Contemp Nutr (newsletter) 2(6), June 1977, and J Am Pharm Assoc 17(9):585, 1977.

# PART THREE

# Practice Management

# 16

# Delivering Treatment to the Confined Elderly

## Mobile offices and portable equipment

*Charles M. Goldstein*
*Roseann Mulligan*

The majority of elderly patients are vigorous and capable both physically and mentally of receiving their dental care in the conventional fixed dental facility. There are, however, a substantial number of patients of all ages who, because of a variety of disabilities, are confined to caretaker facilities or their homes. Historically the only option for care for these patients was hospitalization. Today's care provider is more likely to be prepared to deliver dental treatment in a variety of settings outside the traditional office environment. Dental manufacturers have supported this diversification in dental care delivery options by providing a wide variety of equipment types and packages.

## NONTRADITIONAL DELIVERY CONSIDERATIONS

Before a dentist undertakes practicing in a nontraditional setting using a mobile dental unit or portable dental equipment it is important to have a thorough knowledge of the patient population to be served, the need and demand for dental services by that population, the amount of time to be devoted by the dentist for this practice, the mix of services that will be provided, the financial feasibility of the venture to ensure its success and continuity, and the most appropriate equipment to provide the chosen range of treatment efficiently and safely.

## The patient population

A description of the patient population that would be best served by a nontraditional dental care delivery system includes the 6.7 million people who are confined to their homes and the 1.3 million who reside in nursing facilities.[17,24] An additional 23% of elderly who are noninstitutionalized suffer from functional limitations that affect their abilities to walk and get outside as well as to perform personal hygiene tasks.[8]

Functional limitations are most prevalent to the over-85 age group, with 60% reporting limitations in daily activities.[20] It is the 85-and-over age group that will double in size in the next 30 years while the 65-and-over group will increase at a rate of 5% to 51 million by the year 2020.[35]

## Need and demand for services

The great unmet need for dental treatment of the confined elderly has frequently been cited in numerous reports.[5,10,11,22,24]

Many dentists do not feel comfortable interacting with the elderly.[31] A recent inquiry to several local component societies in Los Angeles to find a dentist for a homebound patient revealed that all but one component society had no referral list and although that society had a list of over 30 dentists who, by self-report, would make house calls, only one had any portable equipment to provide care.

Even when dental services are available through regularly scheduled visits and formalized contracts, as occur with some nursing home programs, many dental treatments are not offered as options. A recent Colorado study reviewing dental services to nursing home residents demonstrated that 38% of the consultant dentists provided no full dentures, 66% no partial dentures, 47% no oral surgery services, and 69% no periodontal services.[6]

The demand for dental care by the confined elderly, even though less than the need, is substantial.[13] Many of the frail or otherwise handicapped elderly have other problems that far outweigh their dental needs. Often elderly patients, because of diminished mental capacity such as that caused by dementias, are not aware of their own oral disease.

In-service training of nursing home personnel can increase the staff's awareness of the residents' urgent dental needs, as well as instruct the staff in techniques for maintaining good oral hygiene for the residents.[26] Screening patients for soft-tissue lesions and gross caries frequently increases the demand for care if the patient or the patient's family is made aware of the presence of oral disease. Family and staff usually are most anxious to engage a dentist's services to remove pain or infection in a resident's mouth and to promote a pleasant and socially pleasing breath. Many patients who are mentally alert want dental services if they are made available at the nursing facility.

The decision to treat or not to treat a patient may cause the dentist a difficult ethical dilemma.[31] The final decision for treatment should always place the patient's welfare first. If the desires of the family or others are not in the best interests of the patient, the dentist should not perform the service. Many nursing home residents may be able to tolerate only minimal care such as smoothing a rough tooth or adjusting a denture; others will need and want more comprehensive care. Treatment planning must involve consideration of both the cognitive and physiologic declines of the individual elderly patient.[22] The dentist who is serious about providing comprehensive care to these patients should be equipped to handle, at a minimum, examination of the soft and hard tissues of the mouth, extractions, metal and composite restorations, oral hygiene procedures including periodontal treatment, and prosthetic replacements, relines, and repairs.[34] Non-

surgical endodontic treatment should also be provided in some cases.

Because many of these patients are physically or mentally compromised, special attention should be given to consulting the mandatory medical chart maintained by the facility[26] within which will be described a history of the patient's medical condition, past or current, the medications ordered by the physician, and the patient's present physical capabilities and cognitive functioning level—information that is needed to be considered by the dentist before developing the appropriate treatment plan. Generally the new elderly (65 to 74 years of age) require more restorative and periodontal services than the old elderly (75 to 84 years of age) or the very old (85 and over), who are more likely to exhibit edentulism and require prosthetic services. However, there is more individual variation in the elderly than any other age group, and the oral status and health of each patient should be carefully evaluated before one makes treatment planning decisions and determines treatment priorities.[26]

Berkey[5] lists some of the advantages of providing care to this patient population on site, including minimizing the disruption of the operation of the nursing home and the patients' schedules, better management of the incontinent or catheterized patient, less fatigue for a frail patient undergoing care, and less apprehension for the emotionally fragile patient. To this list should be added the decreased chance of injury to the frail patient who is at risk when moved out of the protective nursing home environment.

## Amount of time designated

Dentists who wish to provide care for the confined elderly and handicapped in the community have several options. An individual dentist can acquire equipment and provide care personally either on a part-time or full-time basis. A young dentist just starting out in practice may find that portable dental care is appealing as an activity to expand a new practice and add additional income.[34] An established dentist with a conventional practice may also find portable dental care rewarding as a way of helping a very deserving and needy population and getting away from the confines of the fixed facility.[12,34] A retired dentist may look forward to continuing a professional career without the expense or time commitment required in a conventional practice.[18]

For some dentists, the opportunity to provide dental care full time to this population may be more satisfying than a conventional practice.[23] Moore[23] believes the physical advantages that encourage such a practice to be no large overhead for rent, staff, and so on and no large debt for a capital investment in equipment. He compares the setup costs for portable equipment of $10,000 to $15,000 as opposed to $150,000 to $250,000 for a fixed facility with operating overhead at 15% to 25% as opposed to 60% to 75%. When the dentist is on vacation, there is *no* overhead.

## Funding equipment purchases

In addition to self-funding there are other mechanisms to finance the purchase of portable dental equipment. A foundation can provide the equipment to be used by dentists in the community willing to provide mobile dental services. An example of one such service is operated by the National Foundation of Dentistry for the Handicapped (NFDH) in Denver, Colorado.[28] This foundation maintains a van fully equipped with dental and laboratory equipment for use by dentists in the community.[24] A driver who doubles as a dental assistant is provided. The cost to the dentist is 20% to 30% of the fee charged to the patient, or there is no charge if care is provided free to the patient.

Other similar programs are sponsored by the Illinois Foundation for the Handicapped (IFDH) and the Michigan Academy of Dentistry for the Handicapped (MADH).[7]

Not all dentists need to be involved in the actual delivery of treatment. Many older dentists may find it physically difficult to manage the transport and setup of the equipment at the facility. Such dentists may want to confine their efforts to screening nursing home patients and following up to be sure dental care is obtained for the patients. Established dentists who are very busy may not wish to take time away from their offices for fear of neglecting their patients of record. These people may be able to provide assistance by contacts in the community to help in raising funds for acquiring the portable dental equipment for their colleagues to use.

Other financing strategies may include a group

of solo-practice dentists or dentists in group practice who decide to share a mobile unit or portable equipment, or a dental society that acquires equipment for loan to its members wishing to provide such treatment.

## Professional association's position

Organized dentistry has long been aware of the growing problem of providing dental care for the institutionalized geriatric patient. In 1958 the American Dental Association established guidelines regarding the dental care requirements of nursing home residents.[29] In the guidelines were included the following dental recommendations:

1. A dental examination at the time of admission of the residents to the facility
2. The development of liaisons with the local dental societies to provide care in nursing homes
3. Transport of ambulatory residents to the dental office of their choice for treatment
4. The availability of portable dental equipment for dentists to treat patients in the nursing home
5. The development of a financing method for those not financially able to pay for dental care

Thirty years have elapsed since those initial guidelines were formulated, and no concerted effort has been mounted to address the above concerns. A few innovative and progressive dentists have shown that there is a solution to the problem.[12,18,23,34] In addition, dental schools are developing or have in place educational programs that prepare dental and hygiene students to competency in the treatment of the confined elderly.[9,15,30]

In 1979 and 1983 the American Dental Association prepared booklets that offer valuable resource information for individuals or groups interested in providing care to patients in long-term care facilities.[1,2]

## Financial feasibility for the practice

Before starting a portable or mobile dental practice a dentist should investigate the potential market for services in the community. For example, businesses and community services who have access to the homebound patient should be surveyed (see

---

### COMMUNITY BUSINESS SERVICES WITH ACCESS TO THE HOMEBOUND PATIENT

---

Utility companies, which may know who is homebound or permit stuffing of your information in the monthly billing as a public service

Medicab companies

Grocery stores that deliver food

Meals on Wheels

Automatic chair-lifter companies

Visiting Nurses Association

Libraries

Pharmacies

Laundromats

Medical supply houses, who provide wheel chairs, oxygen, and so on to the homebound

Newspapers/TV/radio. Let the health editor or an interested reporter know about your new practice.

Cooking services.

Hospital bed and bed modifier services.

Fast-foot delivery services (such as of pizza)

Emergency phone and alarm services, which enable the homebound to call for help on an emergency basis

---

Courtesy Dr. Peter Moore and M-DEC Inc. (Mobile Dental Equipment Corporation), Redmond, Washington.

box). A marketing strategy should be developed to ensure the appropriate-sized pool of patients according to a predetermined plan. Providing the screening visit at no cost[23] not only increases access to dental care by this population, but is also a practice builder. The locations of the populations to be served should be within reasonable distances to the dentist's home base and each other to minimize time spent in traveling. Written agreements to provide dental services to residents of live-in facilities should be made with the management of those facilities specifying the time to be spent at the facility, the role of the staff, and the space that will be available to the dentist.[19,34]

A bookkeeping system and a policy for billing and payment must be developed. An individual dentist may be able to manage the business record-keeping in a small card file such as those used for recipes, especially in a limited mobile practice.[34]

However, for large practices or in those areas of the country where extensive paperwork is required for the governmental funding of dental services,[12] a personal computer may be needed. An accountant should be consulted to determine the legitimate tax deductions and record-keeping requirements for expenses (such as locations and vehicles used in the practice, a portion of your residence, or a family car if your home is your base), travel expenses, dental equipment, computer equipment, telephone, and so on.

### Mix of services

A dentist needs to determine the type of dental care he or she feels comfortable delivering in a nontraditional setting. Screening examinations, periodic oral exams, emergency care, preventive care, restorative dentistry, prosthetics, periodontics, endodontics, and oral surgery are all needs of institutionalized or homebound senior citizens. The limitations that motivate a dentist to refer a patient in a traditional private practice to a specialist (such as the technical difficulty of the procedure, the availability of the proper instruments or equipment, or the medical status of the patient) should be considered just as carefully in this patient population, if not more so, than in a healthy, ambulatory one. Having a planned strategy for referrals will encourage the general practitioner to send the patient to the appropriate specialist when treatment is needed that the practitioner believes is beyond his capability.

Although comprehensive services are necessary for this patient population, the limitations just enumerated may dictate only limited treatment by a particular practitioner.[32] A practical plan to determine which procedures will be delivered by the practitioner at a facility and which will need to be referred out to other practitioners or specialists needs to be developed as part of the forecasting and planning strategy.

### Movable dental delivery systems

There is a wide variety of equipment available for both mobile and portable dental delivery systems, but there is much confusion as to which type of equipment is best suited for the dentist to achieve the expected goals most efficiently and economically with a given population. Many dentists have made poor decisions in their selection of equipment, resulting in great financial loss and often aborting a well-intentioned effort to treat a greatly underserved population.

To facilitate discussion, the term "mobile dental office" refers to a bus, motor home, camper, or trailer that has been furnished with dental equipment, x-ray equipment, and often laboratory facilities to create a dental office within the vehicle or trailer where patients will be treated, whereas "portable dental equipment" refers to free-standing equipment that can be readily set up and taken down and is moved into a building, with patients being treated in that structure. Such equipment must be operational without requiring any special electrical or plumbing alterations. At the University of Southern California School of Dentistry several extramural clinic sites, such as a four-chair clinic at a large senior citizens residential community, have been established using portable equipment without the need to alter the facility for plumbing or electrical needs (Fig. 16-1).

"Mobile dentistry" thus refers to the use of mobile dental offices (vehicles or trailers) for dental care delivery, and "portable dentistry" refers to the use of portable dental equipment used within a building that is in proximity to the confined elderly.

## MOBILE DENTAL OFFICES

At a minimum, the dental office within the mobile facility should contain a sterilizer, a sink with running water, an instrument cabinet with all the supplies and instruments necessary for the dentist to provide dental care, and a filing cabinet for records. The mobile dental unit also requires air conditioning, heating, and a source of water and electricity. For convenience the unit should have a self-contained water supply as well as the capability to connect to an external water source. It should also house a generator for a self-contained electrical source as well as the capability of connecting to the electrical supply of the building where the patients reside. To operate the dental units, an air compressor and a vacuum unit housed in a sound-insulated cabinet are also needed.

It is essential in a mobile unit to have adequate electrical power to run all the equipment. The air-conditioner and heating system, lights, and refrig-

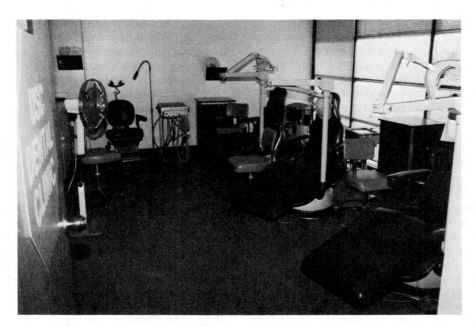

**Fig. 16-1** A four-chair dental clinic established in a senior citizens' residential community without any alterations being made to the plumbing or electrical systems of the building.

erator will require between 30 and 35 amps of power. Additional electrical power is needed to operate the vacuum system, compressor, dental lights, x-ray unit, automatic x-ray developer, sterilizer, and dental lathe. Therefore it is necessary to have a minimum of 50 amps to serve all the equipment and handle the power surges that occur when multiple pieces of equipment are turned on at the same time.[25] All equipment must be compatible with the 115-volt power source commonly used in the United States. For convenience a 50-amp/115-volt outlet should be installed at sites that are visited frequently, with the electrical outlets placed in a locked cabinet or room to prevent access and possible injury to the public.

In London, Ontario, a mobile clinic that visits several sites has electrical, water, and telephone services located underground and accessible through a manhole cover.[21] This method is convenient, and the services are protected against damage from weather changes.

When an elderly population is being served, it is necessary to outfit the mobile vehicle with a wheelchair lift to facilitate the entry of those seniors with ambulation problems. Once inside the mobile unit, it may be necessary to treat a patient in his or her wheelchair or to transfer the patient from the wheelchair to the dental chair. Providing adequate room for these maneuvers must be considered when the layout of the interior is being planned. Most state laws limit the width of a mobile vehicle to 8 feet for highway safety. Because of this, space must be made available between the inside doorway and the first dental chair to assist in maneuvering the wheelchair. This suggestion applies to all types of mobile dental units.

### Types of vehicles and trailers

*The motor home.* The motor home is similar to many of the recreational vehicles on the highways of this nation. It can be easily driven by most drivers because it is commonly equipped with power steering and power brakes. If the dentist plans to serve several different sites and has a heavy patient load, this type of unit is preferred. Because these units are very expensive, a known facility and patient base and commitment of the dentist's time must be a prerequisite for the success of this operation. If the dentist does not want to leave the unit at the work site for security reasons and there-

fore must return the vehicle to homebase at the end of the day, a motor home would be the mobile vehicle of choice.

*A bus or camper.* Bus or camper vehicles have basically the same uses and characteristics as a motor home with a few variations. A bus is usually more expensive to purchase and operate than a motor home and requires more driving skill to negotiate the road. The University of California School of Dentistry in San Francisco has had considerable experience with buses in providing care for children in northern California and in Israel as well as in other foreign countries.

A camper may be preferable if it is necessary to travel over unpaved roads or other rough terrain to reach patients. A camper mounted on a four-wheel truck equipped with heavy-duty springs, a winch, and a protective metal plate underneath to shield the engine from road hazards such as rocks would be suitable to work in any back country including underdeveloped regions of the world.

*The trailer.* A trailer provides the most space for the least financial expenditure, but it is not so easily moved as a motorized unit. It requires another vehicle such as a truck to transport it from one place to another. If a dentist plans to spend a week or more at each treatment site, a trailer and tow-truck combination would be a good choice for a vehicle, for once the trailer has been detached the truck may be used for personal transportation. Of course to leave a costly vehicle in an unknown environment such as a large retirement community for a week or more requires that inquiries be made as to security. If the truck needs servicing or repairs, another truck can always be rented to move the trailer. The trailer is therefore not dependent on the mechanical status or the life span of the tow vehicle. In fact, for certain hard-to-reach locations such as out-of-town clinics, hiring a truck service to provide a tow truck and driver to move the trailer may be wise. It is recommended that the trailer travel on well-paved roads only and, if it is large, it should be moved by a driver experienced in pulling such trailers. A small trailer might be more easily driven by the dentist.

The mobile dentistry program at the University of Southern California uses a fleet of vehicles including a bus, three motor homes, a camper, and a trailer, in providing care for needy children[16] (Fig. 16-2). There is such a great variety of ve-

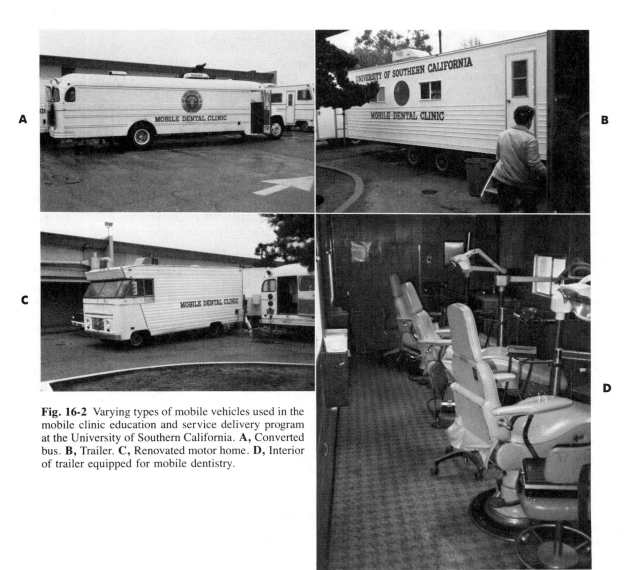

**Fig. 16-2** Varying types of mobile vehicles used in the mobile clinic education and service delivery program at the University of Southern California. **A,** Converted bus. **B,** Trailer. **C,** Renovated motor home. **D,** Interior of trailer equipped for mobile dentistry.

hicles because all the units were donated over time (except for the trailer, which was acquired in 1970 from a federal grant). All have been completely outfitted with dental equipment and work equally well in the USC mobile clinic program because the patients are physically robust and there are no problems regarding the patient's ability to climb into the vehicle.

### Moving the vehicle or trailer

In designing the operatory within the vehicle, it is necessary to place heavy metal hooks or loops in the walls in order to tie down dental units, lights, x-ray machines, and other equipment preparatory to moving. The dental chairs must be firmly secured to the floor. The counters should have protective barriers such as railings or lips to prevent equipment from falling when the vehicle is moving. All doors and cabinets must be firmly secured when in motion. Everything must be done to protect the valuable equipment and the driver before moving the unit. All the bolts securing the equipment should be periodically checked to be sure they have not loosened.

The sudden application of the brakes or the hitting of a bump in the road can destroy an x-ray unit or an operating light. Indeed, the dislodged equipment can act as a flying missile and cause severe bodily damage to the driver. One returning vehicle from a USC mobile clinic location was forced into a ditch to avoid a head-on collision with a vehicle driving toward it on the wrong side of the road. The jolt from hitting the ditch caused the units that were bolted to the floor to break loose. Fortunately, the student driver and his companion sustained only minor injuries, but it could have been a tragedy.

### Costs of the mobile office

A fully equipped mobile unit could cost anywhere between $25,000 and $500,000; an average price for one manufactured with two or three fully equipped operatories is between $150,000 and $250,000 (Medical Coaches, Inc., Mobile Dental Clinic, ProMobile). Utilizing a used motor home and equipment, a one-chair unit could be assembled for between $25,000 and $50,000, but it would require a dentist who is very handy in doing much of the conversion.

### Equipment selection

When selecting equipment for a mobile unit, an over-the-patient delivery system and an automatic dayloading type of x-ray developer are recommended because they take up the smallest amount of space.

For the practitioner who plans on combining mobile and portable dentistry delivery systems, a portable unit can be installed within a mobile dental unit by utilizing a "quick-connect" adaptor to the compressed air source. This would allow such a unit to be used within the mobile vehicle or easily disconnected for use at the patient's bedside within the facility with a compressed air cylinder or a portable compressor. (It is also possible to extend an air hose from the mobile unit for a distance of 50 to 100 feet.)

### Regulations

Many communities require a business license to practice dentistry. It is recommended that local ordinances be checked before one operates in a particular community.

To protect the public, many states have promulgated laws regulating the use of mobile dental units. Consult the dental board in the appropriate state or states for this information. Regardless of state regulations, a dentist using a mobile unit should observe the same precautions (such as radiation safety) to protect the patient's safety as in a fixed facility and should provide a plan for handling emergencies even when the mobile unit has physically left the geographic area.

### Mobile versus portable

There are many dentists and dental school programs using mobile units to treat the elderly; however there are many more involved in the delivery of care to the elderly who use portable equipment. Some dentists who have been successful in maintaining practices providing care for the confined elderly and other homebound patients have abandoned the use of mobile units in favor of portable equipment. This, however, does not negate the value of mobile units. For treating children and healthy adults of all ages, they are the ideal way to provide service to the patients at their schools or places where they congregate, eliminating access problems. The use of mobile units in the armed services, in small rural communities that cannot support a dentist full time, at residential communities with healthy adults, at senior centers, and in many other settings is most appropriate.

### PORTABLE DENTAL EQUIPMENT

Portable dental equipment should be *light weight* for ease in being transported by a slight person and easily installed for operation from conventional electrical outlets such as those in a home or live-in institution. Where ordinary electrical outlets are not available, a small generator or a gasoline-run compressor can be utilized for power.

For the remainder of this chapter those items of portable equipment that are normally heavy and bulky and are conventionally found fixed in a dental office are considered. They are the dental unit, dental chair, x-ray machine, compressor, dental light, and a portable developer or darkroom. Table

**Table 16-1** Types and sources of portable equipment

| Company | Chair | Compressors | Unit | Developer | Light | X-ray machine | Suction unit | Head-rest | Portable electric handpiece | Notes |
|---|---|---|---|---|---|---|---|---|---|---|
| A-dec, Inc | X | | | | | | | | | |
| Air Techniques, Inc. | | | X | X | | | X | | | Peri-pro |
| American Diversified | | | | X | | | | | | Self-developing film pack |
| Aseptico, Inc. | X | X | X | | | | | | | |
| DenDoc | | | X | | | | X | | | |
| Designs for Vision Inc. | | | | | X | | | | | |
| DNTL Corp. | X | X | X | | X | X | X | | | |
| Dremel | | | | | | | | | Lab motor and handpiece | Use for lab only |
| E.F. Brewer Co. | X | X | X | X | X | X | X | | | |
| Emesco | | | | | | | | | Lab motor and handpiece | Can be used in oral cavity |
| Foredom | | | | | | | | | Lab motor and handpiece | Can be used in oral cavity |
| Gomco | | | | | | | X | | | |
| Good-Lite | | | | | X | | | | | |
| Hampton Research | | | X | | | | | | | |
| Hi-Tech (Modern) Co. | | | | | | | | | X | |
| Honda | | | | | | | | | | Gasoline generator |
| Jayman Design, Inc. | X | | | | | | | | | |
| Lincoln Dental Supply Co. | | X | X | | | | X | | | |
| Metal Dynamics Corp. | | | | | | | | X | | |
| M-DEC Inc. | X | X | X | X | X | X | X | | | |
| MDT Biologic Co. | | | | | X | | | | | Rolux fiberoptic light |
| Microcopy | | | | X | | | | | | |
| Min-X-ray, Inc. | | | | | | X | | | | |
| NSK Nakamishi | | | | | | | | | X | Prophy handpiece 2000 RPM |

*Continued.*

Table 16-1 Types and sources of portable equipment—cont'd

| Company | Chair | Compressors | Unit | Developer | Light | X-ray machine | Suction unit | Head-rest | Portable electric handpiece | Notes |
|---|---|---|---|---|---|---|---|---|---|---|
| Osada Electric Co. | | | | | | | | | Cordless | |
| Parkell | | X | X | | | | X | | | Suction system is part of unit |
| Philips Dental Systems | | | | X | | X | | | | Milner chair Royal Conveni Type I |
| Portadontics, Inc. | X | | | | | | | | | |
| Posey Dental | | | | | | | | | Small rechargeable handpiece | |
| Prodonto Corp. | | | X | | | | | | | |
| Siemens Corp. | X | | | X | | X | | | | All in one carrying case |
| Steri-Dent Corp | | | | | | | | | | |
| Satelec | | | X | | | | X | | | Can be used with AC or DC |
| Spartan, USA | | X | X | | | | | | | |
| Therafin Corp. | | | | | | | X | X | | All in one cabinet |
| US Shizai | X | X | X | | | | X | | | |
| Warehouse #3 | X | | | | | | | | | |
| Yoshida/Kaycor | | | | | | X | | | Cordless | X-ray unit is mobile |

**Table 16-2** Mobile or portable equipment companies

A-dec, Inc., 2601 Crestview Drive, Newberg, OR 97132; (503) 538-7478.
Air Techniques, Inc., 70 Cantiaque Rock Road, Hicksville, NY 11801; (515) 433-7676.
American Diversified Dental Systems, Division of MDS, P.O. Box 6067C, Anaheim, CA 92806;
 (800) 637-2337.
Aseptico, Inc., P.O. Box 522, Kirkland, WA 98033; (800) 426-5913.
DenDoc Medical-Dental, 2-220 Third Avenue, Kamloops, BC V2C 3M3, Canada; (604) 372-2010.
Designs for Vision, Inc., 760 Koehler Ave., Ronkonkoma, NY 11779; (800) 345-4009.
DNTL Corp., 12742 E. Caley Ave., Unit E, Englewood, CO 80111;
 (800) 445-8765.
Dremel, Division of Emerson Electric Co., 4915 21st Street, Racine, WI 53406; (414) 554-1390.
E.F. Brewer Company, N 88 W 13901 Main St., Menomonee Falls, WI 53051; (414) 251-9530.
Emesco Products, Teledyne-Hanau, 80 Sonevil Drive, P.O. Box 203, Buffalo, NY 14225-0203;
 (800) 457-1700.
Foredom Electric Co., Route 6, Bethel, CT 06801; (203) 792-8622.
Gomco Division, Allied Healthcare Products, Inc., 828 East Ferry Street, Buffalo, NY 14211;
 (716) 894-6678.
Good-Lite, 1540 Hannah Avenue, Forest Park, IL 60130; (312) 366-3860.
Hampton Research, 4513 S. Pennsylvania, Oklahoma City, OK 73119; (405) 685-5501.
Hi-Tech (Modern) Company, 2315 E Street, Bakersfield, CA 93301; (805) 323-9000 or (800) 435-1900.
Honda, American Honda Motor Co., Inc., 1919 Torrance Blvd., Torrance, CA 90501; (213) 783-2000.
Jayman Design, Inc., 786 Northridge Road, Wichita, KS 67212; (316) 943-011.
D. Lincoln Dental Supply Co., P.O Box 12897, Philadelphia, PA 19108; (800) 523-1886.
Metal Dynamics Corporation, 9324 State Road, Philadelphia, PA 19114; (215) 632-8888.
M-DEC Inc. (Mobile Dental Equipment Corporation), 4224 172nd N.E., Redmond, WA 89052;
 (206) 882-0571.
MDT Biologic Co., 19645 Rancho Way, Rancho Dominguez, CA 90220; (213) 608-2290.
Microcopy, 1174 Tourmaline Drive, P.O. Box 977, Newbury Park, CA 91320; (800) 235-1863.
Min-X-ray, Inc., 3611 Commercial Ave., Northbrook, IL 60062; (312) 564-0323; (800) 221-2245.
NSK Nakanishi Dental Mfg. Co., Ltd., Tokyo, Japan. *Distributed by* Safco Dental Supply Co., 624 W.
 Adams Street, Chicago, IL 60606; (800) 621-2178 or (312) 332-0926.
Osada Electric Co., Inc., 3407 West 6th Street #702, Los Angeles, CA 90020; (213) 388-8128.
Parkell, 155 Schmitt Boulevard, Farmingdale, NY 11935; (516) 249-1134.
Philips Dental Systems, 102 Commerce Road, Stamford, CT 06902; (203) 357-8294.
Portadontics, Inc., P.O. Box 2152, Asheboro, NC 27203; (919) 625-8496.
Posey Dental, 306 Cactus Drive, Oxnard, CA 93030; (800) 421-3338; CA (800) 227-3448.
Prodonto Corporation, 7013 S.W. 46th Street, Miami, FL 33155; (305) 665-4587.
Siemens Corporation, 186 Wood Avenue South, Iselin, NJ 08830; (201) 494-1000.
Steri-Dent Corporation, 33 Reith Street, Copiague, NY 11726; (516) 842-4323.
Satelec, 159 Dwight Place, Fairfield, NJ 07006; (201) 882-1799.
Spartan, U.S.A., 1725 Larkin Williams Road, Fenton, MO 63026; (314) 343-8300.
Therafin Corporation, 3800 S. Union Avenue, Steger, IL 60475; (312) 755-1535.
US Shizai, 5261½ E. Beverly Boulevard, Los Angeles, CA 90022; (213) 722-2011.
Warehouse #3, Dept. B152, 3070 Ranchview Lane N, Minneapolis, MN 55447; (800) 872-4480.
Yoshida/Kaycor, 1732 Central Street, Evanston, IL 60201; (312) 869-4312 or (800) 323-4612.

**Mobile units**

Medical Coaches, Inc., Box 129, Oneonta, NY 13820-0129; (607) 432-1333.
Mobile Dental Clinic Division of Medical Support Systems, Inc., 9830 No. 32nd Street, A-205, Phoenix,
 AZ 85028; (602) 482-0257.
ProMobile, 16940 S.W. 94th Court, Miami, FL 33157; (305) 255-7575.

16-1 provides a graphic display of the types and sources for the major pieces of portable equipment. Table 16-2 provides the addresses of all manufacturers listed in the previous table and mentioned in the text. Table 16-3 lists examples of individual portable kits that could be put together depending on the procedures to be accomplished. Publications that cover in detail the various setups of instruments and supplies needed to conduct dentistry using portable equipment should be consulted for additional information.[3,33]

The portable equipment to be selected should be easily transported in a car trunk, station wagon, or possibly a van (Fig. 16-3).

### Dental units

The primary function of the dental unit is to provide power for a dental handpiece. All the other functions are convenient but not absolutely essential. For example, a bulb syringe can be used for a water source, a photographer's chip blower for the air supply, and a paper cup for oral evacuation. A source of power is needed to generate enough force to activate an effective dental handpiece. As recently as World War II a field unit consisted of a belt-driven handpiece that was powered by a corpsman working a treadle similar to that of an old sewing machine. Fortunately, there are available today a variety of dental units powered by electricity, compressed air, and batteries.

The simplest one-handpiece dental unit powered by compressed air has a rheostat, a pressure regulator, and an air hose with a connection for an air-turbine handpiece. The pressure regulator controls the pressure per square inch allowed to flow from a portable air compressor or compressed air tank to a rheostat, which when depressed allows the compressed air to flow and activate the air-turbine handpiece. This unit is very lightweight (less than 1 pound) and small ($4 \times 6 \times 3$ inches). It will operate any low-speed or high-speed handpiece (dry) and requires a source of compressed air

**Table 16-3** Portable kits

| | |
|---|---|
| **Examination kit** | Dental syringe, disposable needles (large and |
| Patient napkin and clip | small), anesthetic cartridges (3) |
| Mouth mirror or tongue blade | Hand instruments for cavity preparation (i.e., |
| High-intensity pocket light | hatchets, chisels, excavators) |
| Gauze squares | Cotton pliers |
| Explorer | Prepackaged in dose amounts: |
| Patient record |    Cotton rolls |
| Plus: Kit for medical emergencies |    Cotton pellets |
| |    Gauze squares |
| **Prophylaxis kit** | Alcohol |
| Scalers | Rubber mouth prop |
| Prophy paste | Mixing materials: |
| Rubber cups or brushes |    Glass slab |
| Dappen dish or finger holder |    Paper mixing pad |
| Dental floss |    Spatula |
| Portable engine with handpieces and prophy angle | Articulating paper |
| Fluoride for professional application | Dental floss |
| Plus: Examination kit | Cements and bases: |
|    Kit for medical emergencies |    Permanent cement powder and liquid |
| |    Calcium hydroxide |
| **Kit for restorative dentistry** |    Temporary cement (i.e., ZOE) |
| Electric or compressed air operated portable dental | Dappen dish |
|    unit | Plus: Kit for medical emergencies |
| Dental handpieces |    Examination kit |
| Dental burs and bur changers |    Carrying case (i.e., tackle box) |

**Table 16-3** Portable kits—cont'd

**Amalgam restoration kit**

Rubber-dam setup
Amalgamator and premixed capsules
Amalgam carrier
Amalgam plugger and burnishers
Carving instruments
Wedges (assorted)
Scissors, crown and bridge
Matrix retainers (2), straight and contra-angle
Matrix bands (assorted)

**Composite restoration**

Composite material
Celluloid strips
Wedges
Sandpaper disks and mandrel
Plastic placement instrument
Finishing burs
Finishing strips

**Oral surgery kit**

Sterile 2 × 2 inch gauzes
Dental syringe, disposable needles (large and small)
Anesthetic cartridges (3)
Forceps
Elevators
Periosteal elevators
Scalpel and blades (assorted)
Bone file(s)
Suture material and needles
Hemostats (curved and straight)
Surgical scissors
Cotton pliers
Alcohol
Gelfoam sponges
Plus: Examination kit
    Kit for medical emergencies

**Kit for prosthetic dentistry**

Hobby type of motor tool; burs and stones
Impression trays
Rubber bowl and spatula
Scissors
Alcohol torch and propane torch

Matches
Lab knives (for plaster and compound trimming)
Indelible pencil
Waxes
Petroleum jelly
Boley gauge
Wax spatula
Shade and mold guides
Adhesive powder
Articulating paper
Alginate, liquid and powder measures
Containers of dental stone and plaster
Tissue conditioner
Impression materials
Compound sticks
Orange solvent (for cleanup)
2 × 2 inch gauze pads
Tackle box
Plus: Examination kit
    Kit for medical emergencies

**Palliative emergency kit**

Mirror, explorer, tongue blades, 2 × 2 inch gauze squares
Temporary restorative material (Cavit, ZOE)
Spoon excavators
Cold-curing acrylic monomer and polymer (pink and clear)
Clasp adjustment pliers
Hobby type of motor tool: burs and stones
Plus: Kit for medical emergencies

**Special equipment (as needed)**

Radiographic unit
Developing system
Wheelchair headrest
Headlamp
Surface disinfectants
Handpiece lubricant and cleaner

**Kit for medical emergencies**

Specifics will depend on training of practitioner
Positive pressure oxygen delivery system
Emergency medications and delivery system

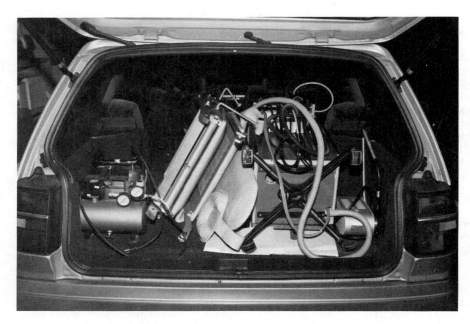

**Fig. 16-3** Portable equipment placed into the back of a midsized station wagon for transport to a care delivery site.

(Parkell). A small plastic spray bottle can be used as a source of water, a pressurized air can (used to clean photographic lenses for air), and a plastic container for expectoration. The pressurized air can must always be held upright so that the propellant is not expelled with the air.

*Multiple handpiece unit with air syringes.* At the University of Southern California Mobile Dental Clinic, students designed their own dental unit (The USC "Octopus") to power the handpieces (Fig. 16-4). Up to a total of eight handpieces and air syringes can be attached to the unit, which consists of a series of tubings with "quick connectors." The unit in turn is connected by an air hose to and powered by an air compressor with a pressure regulator.

*Lightweight units* (20 to 30 pounds without water supply) come equipped with air and water syringes (Fig. 16-5). These units need an external source of air in the form of a compressed nitrogen tank or a small air compressor and a separate mobile evacuation unit to form a complete dental unit. The water is supplied from a self-contained pressurized container. A half gallon of water is usually sufficient for a full day's supply of coolant for the handpiece spray and for the water syringe. This type of unit may be preferred by many dentists because of its light weight and portability. Some of these units have built-in brackets and regulators for use with small compressed nitrogen tanks. These units do not have suction (Hampton, U.S. Shizai, Lincoln, Aseptico, Prodonto).

*Medium-weight units* (35 to 45 pounds with carrying case) have evacuation systems in addition to the air-water syringe (Fig. 16-6). Such a unit stands on removable legs or wheels, which can be easily detached and stored in a carrying case that measures approximately 21 × 21 × 12 inches. This dental unit also contains a pressurized tank for water. (Distilled water is recommended to avoid mineral buildup in syringes or in the water-spray mechanism of handpieces.) A Venturi suction system has an evacuation tip with a valve that can be opened or closed to turn the system on or off. This unit requires only a compressed air source to operate. (A-dec, DenDoc.)

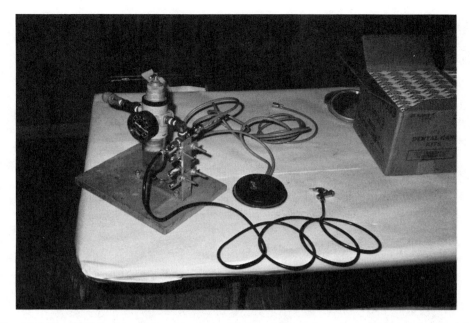

**Fig. 16-4** The USC "octopus" is a dental unit fabricated by students that will handle up to eight handpiece–air syringe combinations.

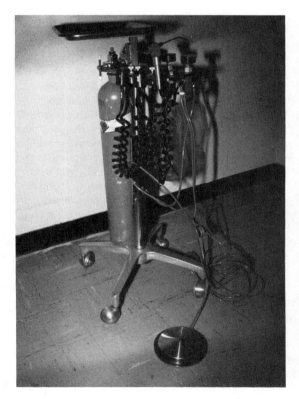

**Fig. 16-5** Lightweight dental units require an air source for power (notice compressed air tank). (Hampton Research & Engineering Inc., Oklahoma City, OK 73108.)

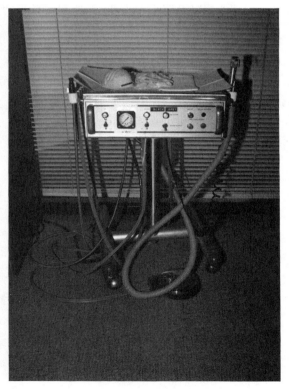

**Fig. 16-6** Medium weight unit with an evacuation system. (A-DEC Inc, Newberg OR 97132.)

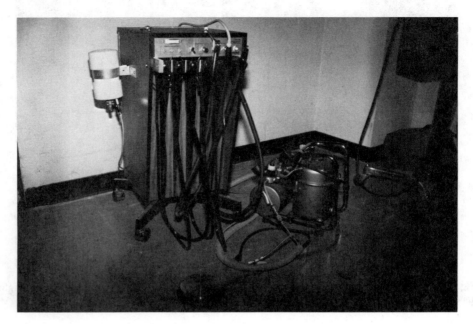

**Fig. 16-7** Cabinet unit on wheels with a portable compressor. (Parkell Products Inc, Farmingdale, NY 11735.)

*Cabinet unit on wheels* (60 pounds or more) has a built-in suction system, a pressurized water tank, three lines for handpieces, a three-way syringe, a high-volume evacuation tip, and a saliva ejector (Fig. 16-7). Such a system requires a portable compressor and a 115 amp electrical outlet to function. The unit measures in inches 30 high × 13½ wide × 18½ deep and weighs 60 pounds with a portable compressor weighing approximately 40 pounds more. Because it is on wheels, one person can move the unit around easily from room to room, with the cabinet doubling as a cart to move the portable compressor as well. It is, however, likely to take two people to move the unit in and out of a car trunk or station wagon. (Parkell.)

Another cabinet unit contains both a vacuum system and a compressor. The unit measures in inches 30 high × 26 wide × 18 deep and weighs 115 pounds. To function, it needs only an electrical outlet. This unit is definitely too heavy for one person to lift but would be very practical if stored in a van or mobile unit equipped with a lift or ramp. (Spartan USA.)

The *modular unit* delivery systems allow the dentist to disassemble the unit into separate sections that are small and lightweight enough to be hand carried and stored in a car trunk or in a light aircraft. They also can be assembled and transported intact because the lowest section has wheels.

One such unit is very esthetically attractive and can also be used in a conventional dental office. This unit is totally self-contained with a compressor, high-speed suction, a self-contained water supply, a view box, and a three-way syringe (Fig. 16-8). It has a bracket to hold a portable x-ray unit and is heavy enough when assembled to support the x-ray head when it is extended. The unit when assembled weighs 115 pounds. Each of the three modules weighs 30 to 40 pounds apiece. (DNTL.)

Another unit specifically designed for portable dentistry comes in three modules, which double as storage cases. The core module provides a full array of functional capabilities. It contains a compressor, vacuum pump, disk foot pedal, two handpiece tubings, adjustable water spray, operating light, three-way syringe, darkroom, high-volume

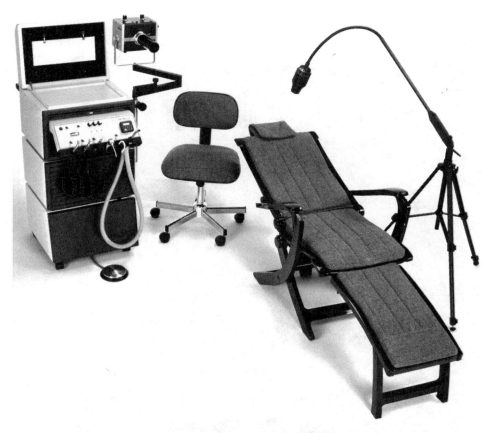

**Fig. 16-8** Assembled modular unit ready for service. (DNTL Corp., Englewood, CO 80111.)

suction, saliva ejector, work shelf, laboratory lathe, grinding wheel with arbor, buff wheel with arbor, pumice tray, x-ray viewer, amalgamator, water bottle, vacuum reservoir, auxiliary water outlet, cable drive for lab handpieces, and pressure gauge (Fig. 16-9). The first module weighs 44 pounds and is stored in a case that is in inches 16½ high × 14 wide × 14 deep. A second module is an instrument case and weighs 25 pounds. A third module contains an x-ray unit and weighs 55 pounds with the case. The case has wheels and acts as a weighted base for the x-ray unit, which is assembled from components all contained in the case. This system has the most functions available in the smallest package. Its developer, a dentist, has constantly worked to make the unit smaller and more versatile. (M-DEC.)

An over-the-patient delivery system with the unit and light attached to the chair bracket comes with a gasoline-powered compressor and generator that provides electricity and air for all systems and weighs 40 pounds. The entire unit also includes a suction module, water storage tank module, and air handpiece controller weighing an additional 12 pounds. (Brewer.)

An all-electric modular unit having an aspirator, water reservoir, and three-way air-water syringe, electrosurge, and electric scaler operates on 12-

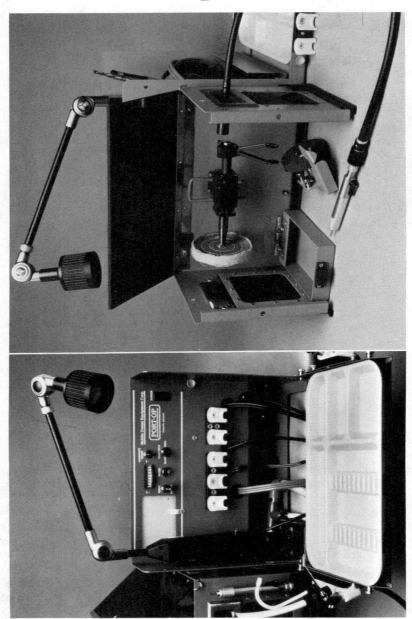

**Fig. 16-9 A,** Front of core module ready for patient care delivery. **B,** Rear of core module ready for laboratory activities. (Mobile Dental Equipment Corp, Bellevue, WA 98008.)

volt direct current or 110 alternating current. The electric micromotor handpiece in this unit operates at 26,000 or 40,000 rpm. The unit is housed in a waterproof, shock-resistant aluminum or polyester suitcase. The total weight of the listed equipment is 31 pounds. This unit can be used in most isolated areas with an ordinary car battery. (Satelec.)

Many fine portable units are available from various manufacturers. It is not the purpose of this chapter to endorse any particular unit. The above units are representative of the various types available. A partial list of additional manufacturers who offer portable units can be found in articles by Ettinger and Miller-Eldridge,[11] Goldstein,[15] and the ADA Council on Dental Health and Dental Health Planning.[3]

## Alternative handpiece ports

Handpiece ports are of course found on all the dental units just described. There are, however, power sources outside of the dental units for particular types of handpieces.

*Battery-powered rechargeable and electric devices.* Several battery-powered handpieces are available. They are the lightest in weight of any handpiece but have the least capacity for sustained operation. These units are very useful when one is seeing a single homebound or institutionalized patient for emergency care, and the need for the handpiece is expected to be brief.

There are two types of battery-powered handpieces. In one the power pack fits into a shirt pocket and supplies power to a slow-speed contra-angle or straight handpiece containing a micromotor with a lightweight cord (Posey). In the other, a nickel-cadmium battery in the handpiece (which recharges constantly when standing in the charger base) is the power source. This handpiece will operate continuously for 30 minutes when fully charged. The handpiece is 6 inches long and weighs 3.88 ounces. The base in inches is $3 \times 2 \times 4\frac{1}{2}$ and weighs 19.4 ounces. Variable speeds are attained by the use of interchangeable heads on the handpiece. It comes equipped with one straight-angle (right angle) head, two contra-angle heads, and one sealed prophy (prophylactic) angle head (which can be cold sterilized), with speeds ranging from 462 to 12,000 rpm. The torque is 150 g/cm. (Yoshida/Kaycor.)

Another cordless handpiece with a micromotor has a constant speed of 2000 rpm. It also has several interchangeable autoclavable heads—screwable and snap-on sealed prophy heads, a latched contra-angle head, and a quarter-turn endodontic head. The handpiece weighs 4.25 ounces and recharges constantly when placed in its charger base. (NSK Nakanishi.)

More powerful variable-speed, high-torque, slow-speed handpieces powered by alternating current are also available. These units are compact and have speeds in the 500 to 40,000 rpm range. The torque is over three times that of battery-powered units at 500 g/cm. The small size ($7\frac{1}{4} \times 6 \times 2\frac{3}{4}$ inches) of these handpieces make them very portable. These devices can be set at any constant speed within their range and used with an on-off foot switch (very small and lightweight) or with a variable-speed foot control (somewhat larger). The straight handpiece accepts burs, contra-angles, prophy angles, and so on without the need for tools. (Osada, Hi-Tech.)

Many dentists also have access to a laboratory engine and arm with a belt-driven handpiece that can be quite easily taken into a facility, placed on a countertop, and plugged in. Although the speed is not as high as the newer electric handpieces, when used with sharp burs it will suffice for many duties. (Emesco.)

*Hobby type of devices.* A hobby motor is a constant-speed handpiece (30,000 rpm), which is very handy for denture adjustments but not suitable for intraoral use. (Dremel.)

A more elaborate hobby type of unit has a small engine with a flexible cable to a straight handpiece. The engine can be hung on a hook providing the operator with a very lightweight handpiece. This unit is equipped with a rheostat and has a bur-speed range of 15,000 rpm. A variety of straight, contra-angle, and right-angle handpieces are available for this setup. (Foredom.)

## Radiographic units

The *mobile unit* is one particular unit mounted on a base with wheels allowing the unit to be easily moved from room to room to radiograph a patient in a bed or a wheelchair (Fig. 16-10). The base is designed to counterbalance the movement of the x-ray head when one is taking x-ray films. This

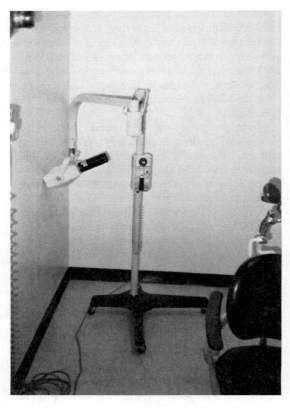

**Fig. 16-10** Mobile x-ray unit. (Yoshida/Kaycor International Ltd, Evanston, IL 60201.)

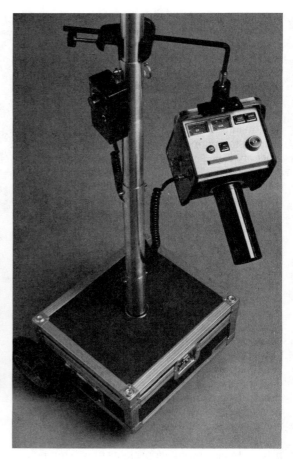

**Fig. 16-11** Radiographic unit with mounting and stabilizing features designed by Mobile Dental Equipment Corp, Bellevue, WA 98008.

type of unit can be used much like a conventional unit because it has an articulated arm with the x-ray head at the end. The base of this unit is quite heavy, and the unit with its stand might not fit into a car without being dismantled first, a feature that, although inconvenient, is possible. (Yoshida/ Kaycor.)

The *portable unit* is mounted on a tripod or lightweight stand. It is very lightweight (18 pounds) and easily transported by one person. The head and timer are carried in a case (2 pounds) for protection when not in use. One assembles the unit by attaching the head and timer to a tripod (3½ pounds) or other stabilizing device. It does not have an articulated arm; therefore the entire unit must be moved to obtain different angulations for each radiograph taken. By adapting an extension to the

cone, one can radiograph a bedridden patient. (M-DEC, Min-X-ray) (Fig. 16-11). A mobile floor stand weighing 21 pounds is also available (DNTL) as is a complete radiographic system (including stand, developer, and carrying case), weighing a total of 30 pounds (Brewer).

A third portable radiographic unit with a head that can be adjusted to several positions weighs 43 pounds and can be stored and carried in a water-resistant, high-density, foam-lined case that weighs 24 pounds. Because the combined weight of the machine and case is 67 pounds, the case comes equipped with handles and can be transported easily by two people. (Philips.)

There are other portable radiographic systems that are very sophisticated and, though they claim to be portable, are very bulky. One such system contains a chair, an x-ray unit, an automatic day-loading developer, all in a carrying trunk. It requires two people to carry it and is not suitable for portable dentistry for the homebound patient. It does have a place in dentistry in less-industrialized countries or for dentistry in the field. (Siemens.)

### Developing units and darkrooms

*Portable darkrooms.* The most commonly used unit of portable darkrooms has no need for electricity or plumbing. The unit has four beakers for the solutions to process the radiographs, a see-through lid that is made of light, safe plastic, and access holes that allow the operator to place both hands inside the unit without allowing light to leak into it. (Microcopy.)

*Automatic day-loading developers.* There are several automatic day-loading developers available. These require a 110-amp electrical outlet for power. The automatic day-loading developers are quite practical if they are set up for 1 day to take radiographs on several patients or left for several days in one location. It is not practical to move the developer to a different location for each patient; even when the machine is placed on a mobile chart and moved from room to room, sloshing of solutions and warm-up times may compromise the solutions or machine function. These machines require meticulous cleaning and solution changing and replenishment on a regular schedule to maintain their performance. They are, however, quite lightweight when empty, about 23 pounds. (Air Technique, Philips.)

The automatic developer is very popular in many fixed facilities because it requires little space and no darkroom. Most can be used freestanding and do not require special plumbing because they can be filled from containers.

A practical method of handling radiographs is to use a self-developing intraoral film pack for emergencies (American Diversified) and to use the portable unit only for planned radiographic sessions.

If one has chosen to use self-developing film, it is recommended that this film be used for emergencies only because the image will degrade with time. To supplement the self-developing film all other radiographs could then be developed away from the facility at the home base or office.

### Dental lights

The *headlight* is a light source worn like a hat and either battery powered or plugged in to an AC outlet to supply illumination (Design for Vision). Since one's head is a moving source, it requires some coordination to get used to this light source.

Lightweight *freestanding lights* that are easily portable and utilize a standard 110-amp outlet are available. These are of high intensity yet have a small beam to provide proper illumination without shining in the patient's eyes. (Goodlite.)

*Fiberoptic lights* can be mounted on a post that attaches to most portable dental chairs or are a unit that can be set on a table (MDT). Again, the high intensity and small beam make these lights quite useful.

A *halogen dental light* is a dental light that can be clamped onto a unit, chair, or table. It has a flexible arm and provides an adjustable, focused, high-intensity beam of light (M-DEC). Another halogen light on a tripod floor stand (total weight of 4 pounds) is also available (DNTL).

### Portable dental chairs

Portable dental chairs also come in a wide variety and are made from several materials. They should offer several positions to support the patient's head and back and have a thin enough headrest to allow room for the dentist's knees.[4]

The metal-frame portable chair has an adjustable back section so that the patient can be positioned from 90 to 180 degrees. Some of these chairs have a leg area that can also be raised or lowered. The chair can be folded to fit into the trunk of a car and can be set up very quickly. It usually weighs between 30 and 40 pounds and has a durable surface for easy care. (Aseptico, E.F. Brewer, A-dec.)

A wood-and-fabric chair can be dismantled and carried in a carrying case with a shoulder strap. As may be expected, a chair constructed out of these materials weighs more (48 pounds). However, it can be divided into parts for carrying. The backrest is adjustable though the height and slant of the seat are not. (Portadontics.)

A self-assembled chair can be pieced together by attachment of a portable headrest to a straight-backed chair or a wheelchair (Therafin, Metal Dynamics.)

A chair made out of an aluminum polycarbonate material weighs in at only 25 pounds (Jayman). One made of "indestructible" synthetic resin with four possible positions weighs 29 pounds (DNTL). A portable chair with a detached legrest that achieves only one position, the Trendelenburg, weighs 15 pounds (US Shizai.)

The cardboard chair is constructed out of 600-pound test corrugated cardboard. It weighs 8 pounds, will support a 200-pound person, and is easy to set up. With the addition of a thin pad for comfort, this chair might be used with elderly patients, particularly in screening settings. It is not adjustable, however, with the backrest fixed at about a 30-degree angle.[14]

There are also inexpensive lawn chaises or chairs, which, with some adjustments of the back portion, could be used for the delivery of dental care. One such chair out of tubular chromed steel weighs only 15 pounds and has an eight-position backrest and a footrest. It folds easily for carrying and storage and comes with a removable corduroy cover. (Warehouse.)

### Sources of power for equipment

Compressed air or nitrogen tanks for air-powered dental units is the simplest and quietest source of power. Because tanks contain only a fixed amount of air, they must be monitored so that they will not run out during a procedure. A supply agreement must be reached with a chemical company so that deliveries will be prompt and empty tanks will be replaced on a regular basis.

An air compressor with a holding tank can provide a continuous source of compressed air for an indefinite period of time as long as it has an electric power source. Some air compressors can be quite noisy and need to be located outside the room where the dental care is being delivered.

A dental compressor should provide clean air and should be reasonably quiet when running. The size of the compressor can vary according to the amount of compressed air needed to run the unit.

Generally the smallest portable compressors can power one portable dental unit. These compressors weigh 40 to 45 pounds, have an output of 2 to 3 cubic feet/minute at 100 psi, and are often equipped with an air-oil filter (Aseptico, E.F. Brewer, Parkell, D. Lincoln, US Shizai). If no electrical power is available, a small gasoline generator can be used for power (Honda).

### Evacuation systems

If the dental unit does not have a self-contained evacuation system, several portable evacuation systems are available. One is housed in a cabinet 12 × 15 × 26 inches in size, is on casters, and weighs approximately 40 pounds. Its motor has a 1-year warranty and can be replaced in minutes with a screwdriver. (Steri-Dent Corp., US Shizai, D. Lincoln, Aseptico.)

A hospital aspiration unit that is found in most nursing homes can be used for suction and is very lightweight and portable. It does not provide high-speed suction, however, but does a reasonable job of aspirating saliva. (Gomco.)

The simplest means of evacuation is the two-cup method. Using this method, the patient rinses with water from one disposable cup and expectorates into another.[27]

### CONCLUSIONS

In this chapter we consider the nontraditional delivery of care to geriatric patients by means of portable and mobile dental units. It is a discussion of the major factors that must be considered before a commitment is made to provide such care. These are the patient population to be served, the need and demand for dental services by that population, the amount of time the dentist can devote to the practice, the mix of services that will be provided, the fiscal feasibility of the venture, and the most appropriate equipment. The chapter is also a consideration of various types of mobile vehicles for mobile dental delivery and the major units of portable equipment. Before purchasing any equipment, one needs to investigate what is available and to field test the equipment whenever possible (Fig. 16-12). Dental manufacturers who produce portable equipment are listed for convenience. One should be aware that this is such a dynamic field, and manufacturers are constantly developing new

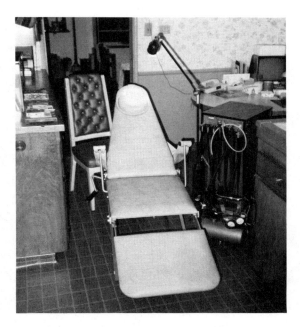

**Fig. 16-12** Portable dental equipment preparatory to being field tested in a kitchen during a home visit.

products. Therefore this list cannot be complete. Manufacturers are very happy to provide information about their products; however, consultation with dental colleagues who practice mobile and portable dentistry is also extremely helpful.

There is a great need to provide dental care for the homebound and institutionalized. With information and investigation new vistas can be opened in the dentist's professional life for the benefit of both the dentist and his or her patients.

## REFERENCES

1. American Dental Association: Oral health care in the long-term care facility, Chicago, 1983, the Association.
2. American Dental Association—Council on Dental Health and Health Planning: Oral health care for the geriatric patient in a long-term care facility, Chicago, 1979, the Association.
3. American Dental Association—Council on Dental Health and Health Planning: Manual on comprehensive dental care access programs, Chicago, 1981, the Association.
4. Baycar R, Aker F, and Serowski A: Portable dental chair, Special Care Dent 3:57, 1983.
5. Berkey DB: Improving dental access for the nursing home resident: portable dentistry interventions, Gerodontics 3:18, 1987.
6. Call R, Berkey D, and Gordon G: The activities of the advisory dentist in the long-term care facility, Gerodontics 2:35, 1986.
6a. Casamassimo PS, Coffee LM, and Leviton SJ: A comparison of two mobile treatment programs for the homebound and nursing home patient, Special Care Dent 8(2):77, 1988.
7. Combs HR: Dentists are reaching out to the homebound, Dent Econ 73:32, Nov 1983.
8. Dawson D, Hendershot G, and Fulton J: Aging in the eighties, functional limitations of individuals age 65 years and over, National Center for Health Statistics no 133, DHHS publ no (PHS) 87-1250, Hyattsville, Md, 1987.
9. Ellis RL and Ingham F: A mobile dental clinic program as part of the dental curriculum, J Can Dent Assoc 2:125, 1985.
10. Empey G, Kiyak HA, and Milgrom P: Oral health in nursing homes, Special Care Dent 3:65, 1983.
11. Ettinger RL and Miller-Eldridge J: An evaluation of dental programs and delivery systems for elderly isolated populations, Gerodontics 1:91, 1985.
12. Fleiner HL: The mobile dental practice: an insider's view, Can Dent Assoc J 14:43, 1986.
13. Giangrego E: Dentistry on the move, Special Care Dent 5:6, 1985.
14. Goldstein CM: Design of a practical dental chair made of corrugated cardboard, J Am Dent Assoc 97:996, 1978.
15. Goldstein CM: Portable dental equipment for treating the confined elderly, Can Dent Assoc J 12:38, Jan 1984.
16. Goldstein CM and Matosian G: USC's dental ambassadors, a voluntary student project, Can Dent Assoc J 4:35, Jan 1976.
17. Hing E: Use of nursing homes by the elderly: preliminary data from the 1985 national nursing home survey, National Center for Health Statistics no 135, DHHS publ no (PHS) 87-1250, Hyattsville, Md, 1987.
18. Jarmon P: Dentistry for the homebound: an inbound patient, NY State Dent J 4:276, 1980.
19. Kamen S: Organization of a dental service in long-term care facilities, Can Dent Assoc J 14:25, 1986.
20. Kovar MG: Aging in the eighties, preliminary data from the supplement on aging to the National Health Interview Survey, U.S., January-June, 1984, National Center for Health Statistics, no 115, DHHS publ no (PHS) 86-1250, Hyattsville, Md, 1986.
21. Leake JL: London's new clinic, Ontario Dentist, p 18, Sept 1974.
22. Mercer VH: Dentistry in the nursing home, Gerodontics 1:274, 1985.
23. Moore P: Mobile dentistry: the low cost, low overhead alternative, Can Dent Assoc J 14:31, 1986.
24. Most BW: Dentists who make house calls, Tic 39:1, March 1980.
25. Mulligan RA: Considerations in using mobile dental vans to deliver dental care to the elderly, Gerodontics 3:260, 1987.
26. Mulligan RA: Factors to be considered in the delivery of dental care to the geriatric residents of a skilled nursing home, Can Dent Assoc J 14:15, 1986.

27. Mulligan RA and Heaton S: Preventive oral health care for compromised individuals. In Harris NO and Christen AG, editors: Primary preventive dentistry, ed 2, Norwalk, Ct, 1987, Appleton & Lange.
28. See ref. 6a.
29. Ostergren WD and Wright RJ: The nursing home: a dental profile of the institutionalized geriatric patient and a concept for better geriatric oral health, Northwest Dent 53:142, May-June 1974.
30. Phair PW and Steele DK: The University of Iowa mobile dental unit project, Iowa Dent J 57:44, Aug 1971.
31. Pollick H: Ethics and geriatrics, Special Care Dent 1:149, 1981.
32. Randell S and Culp C: Financial profile of a home dental care program, Special Care Dent 5:68, 1985.
33. Shaver RO: Dentistry for the homebound, institutionalized and elderly, Lakewood, Col, 1982, Portable Dentistry Publications.
34. Shaver RO: Differences between the traditional and the mobile extended care facility practice, Can Dent Assoc J 14:34, 1986.
35. Spencer G: Projections of the population of the U.S., by age, sex, and race: 1983 to 2080, US Bureau of the Census no 952, series P-25, Washington, DC, 1984, US Government Printing Office.

# 17

# Preventive Dentistry for the Older Adult

*Maureen C. Rounds*
*Athena S. Papas*

The design and implementation of comprehensive preventive dentistry protocols for elders presents the dental professional with many challenges. Although a specific protocol must be tailored to the unique needs of the individual patient, there are certain factors common to the elderly segment of the population that may influence these protocols.

## NEED FOR PREVENTIVE SERVICES

Although the elderly in the United States are retaining their natural dentition longer than in the past,[43,47] dental morbidity (prevalence of dental disease) continues to be high.[14,15] A national epidemiologic survey of the United States employed adults and seniors in 1985 and 1986[47] indicated that 88% of males and females 65 years of age and older had gingival recession on at least one site with 2 mm or greater of attachment loss, but only 22% had pockets that were 5 mm or greater. Recent studies focused on elderly persons have revealed high prevalences of root caries: 61% of females and 67% of males 65 years of age or older[47]; 83% of terminally ill institutionalized elderly[1]; and 89% of patients with advanced periodontal disease.[53] Coronal caries (primary and recurrent) also are a major dental problem in the elderly. When the caries-prevalence rate is evaluated on a basis of 100 teeth present, the caries rate increases with age.[28]

One of the highest predictors for seeking dental care is past dental behavior.[4,7] The majority of those currently 65 years of age or older did not seek care to the same extent as middle-aged and younger populations. At the present time adults 45 to 64 years of age use dental services at a high rate; therefore it has been predicted that this cohort will continue to use dental services at a comparably high rate when they reach old age.[14]

Despite the fact that many of the oral diseases experienced by the elderly are either preventable or treatable, many of these persons do not avail themselves of the needed treatment. Thus the dental profession must endeavor to increase their use of preventive services. In doing so, the profession faces a dual challenge:

1. It must increase the preventive dentistry awareness of elders.
2. It must make both preventive and treatment services more accessible to those elders not currently using them.

Most persons currently older than 60 were not introduced to the concept of preventive dentistry at a young age and thus are not inclined to it. Many still hold the opinion that tooth loss is a normal part of the aging process and is not preventable. Others have adapted to a compromised oral health status and seek treatment only when an emergency arises. On the other hand, the elderly have been introduced to preventive dentistry modalities by their hygienist, dentist, friends or relatives, the media (informational articles or even advertisements for home care products), or dental education programs conducted at senior centers. This latter group appreciate the value of a preventive program and expect it from the dental practitioner.

## EVALUATION AND ASSESSMENT

A thorough oral assessment is the foundation of an effective comprehensive treatment plan including a preventive dentistry protocol. The evaluation of an elderly person, for the purpose of designing a comprehensive individualized preventive protocol, includes much of the following information routinely obtained during the initial history taking and treatment planning as well as certain additional information (see Chapter 7):

1. Present oral status and past dental treatment
2. Present medical status and medications
   (NOTE: Special attention should be given to systemic disorders and medication use that may directly or indirectly impinge on oral health status.)
3. Physical disabilities that might affect ability to carry out recommended home care procedures
4. Intellectual and educational level
5. Emotional status
6. Dietary adequacy and nutritional status
7. Life-style factors

### Present oral status and past dental treatment

This portion of the assessment is the same for an elderly person as for any adult and consists in both objective and subjective measures. Objective measures include radiographs and clinical examination and charting. Subjective measures might include a patient's reporting of dates and causes of tooth loss and history of fluoride use and a description of past and present oral home care practices.

### Medical status and medications

Systemic diseases can affect oral hygiene status and may require more frequent prophylaxes to prevent gingival inflammation and periodontal disease. Medications can cause xerostomia and thus increase the incidence and severity of oral disease.

### Physical disabilities

Assessment begins as soon as the dentist or hygienist greets the elderly person and observes obvious physical limitations such as complete or partial paralysis when a patient enters the operatory, severe arthritis in the hands and arms, tremors, and muscle weakness, noted on shaking hands. Upper extremity disabilities are of greatest concern, since these may affect a person's ability to perform oral hygiene procedures.

### Intellectual and education level

A good clinician assesses these factors of intellectual and educational level from the first contact with a patient. The appropriate level at which to address the patient becomes apparent during the history-taking interview. This is a very important aspect of the assessment because later efforts to inform and educate the patient will be successful to the degree that they are appropriate to the level of his or her comprehension.

### Emotional status

Assessment of a patient's emotional status may be more difficult than assessment of the level of physical ability or comprehension, but it is no less important. The clinician should observe affect. Is it appropriate? Is it consistent from appointment to appointment? Is the patient taking medications for psychiatric or emotional disorders? An elderly person who is suffering from anxiety or depression, for example, is likely to find it difficult to adhere to recommended home care procedures. If disorders are suspected, a consultation with the patient's primary physician may be in order.

### Dietary adequacy and nutritional status

(See Chapter 15.)

### Life-style factors

In learning something about an elderly person's life-style, the astute clinician is able to appreciate those values that are important to the patient. This, in turn, can enhance the dentist's or hygienist's efforts to motivate the patient to comply with recommendation for both oral home care procedures and specific treatment options. For example, an older patient who strives to maintain physical fitness through regular exercise is likely to relate more readily to the concept of maintaining oral health through diligent oral home care practices than one who accepts decline of health with aging as inevitable and makes no effort to prevent or slow the effects of this decline. The dental practitioner wants to discover some value held by the latter patient (such as freedom from pain or discomfort) and uses that as a basis for motivating him to comply with home care recommendations.

An appreciation of a patient's life-style can also help the dentist to design a treatment plan that is realistic and at the same time acceptable to an older patient. Consider the example of an edentulous patient who has insufficient alveolar bone to support a full lower denture. A patient who is socially active may be much more inclined to accept a treatment recommendation of ridge augmentation or implants in order that he or she may wear a lower denture than one who shuns social interaction and is content to function without a lower denture.

## PREVENTIVE DENTISTRY COMPONENTS
### Mechanical plaque removal

For the patient with natural teeth, effective plaque removal is the basic and essential oral home care procedure. Removal of plaque not only prevents caries and periodontal disease, but also enhances the overall sense of well-being by ensuring a mouth that feels and tastes good.

The preferred method of brushing for most elders is sulcular brushing with a soft toothbrush (Bass method).

Persons who have gingival recession should be instructed to observe certain precautions to avoid further recession or cemental abrasion. These may include use of an extra-soft toothbrush, use of very light pressure, or modification of the brushing method (such as a roll stroke, rather than the Bass method in areas of considerable recession). Those with recession on the canines should be advised to use extra caution when using a sulcular brushing method on the buccal surfaces of these teeth, which are in the corners of the arches. A preferred method of brushing the canines consists in placing the brush so that the bristles cover the lateral incisor and the mesial half of the canine, brushing those surfaces, and then lifting and placing the brush so that the bristles cover the distal half of the canine and the first premolar. Patients who are receiving chemotherapeutic agents, those who are immunosuppressed, and those in whom bacteremia would be dangerous (such as those with hip or valvular replacement) should be helped to minimize the possiblity of bacteremia. This can be done, for example, by teaching the patient to vibrate the toothbrush in position and to avoid any trauma to the gingiva when using floss, an interproximal brush, or a rubber tip. These patients should be cautioned against the use of any aids that might injure the gingiva (such as toothpicks).

The elderly person should be helped to develop the ability to brush both effectively and thoroughly (all accessible tooth surfaces and the hard palate and tongue, which are sites for bacterial and fungal growth). Those who have diminished manual dexterity may benefit from use of traditional mechanical toothbrushes, rotary electric toothbrushes, or manual brushes that have been adapted or customized for each person (these are discussed later).

Use of a dentifrice is recommended because it contains ingredients that help to loosen plaque and remove stains from the tooth surface, inhibit calculus formation (with tartar-control formulas), and serve as a vehicle for topical fluoride. (CAUTION: Use of dentifrice would be contraindicated for any patient likely to swallow or aspirate the dentifrice.)

### Interproximal plaque removal

Although dental floss remains the basic instrument for removal of plaque from proximal surfaces, other aids may be as effective or more effective for certain elderly persons.

*Dental floss* or *dental tape* is most effective when held and manipulated with the fingers. An elderly person who has impaired manual dexterity may find it easier to use a floss holder. However, there are certain drawbacks to the use of this device. If the floss is too taut, it will not "hug" the tooth surface, and thus only a portion of the proximal surface will be cleaned. Placing floss on the floss holder requires a certain level of manual dexterity. A patient who finds this a difficult task may be reluctant to constantly reposition the floss in order to provide a clean working area. In addition, some dentitions are too tight to allow use of a floss holder without difficulty.

An *interproximal brush* may be easier to use than floss and thus be more effective in removing interproximal plaque from large embrasures, exposed furcas, and a proximal surface adjacent to an edentulous area. Floss that has areas that are thicker and more abrasive than conventional floss may enhance plaque control from large interproximal spaces or under fixed bridges.

*Yarn, gauze,* or *pipe cleaners* may also be used for cleaning proximal surfaces where there is no adjacent tooth or lack of contact.

A *rubber tip* (preferably on a rubber-tip holder with an angled shaft, rather than on a toothbrush) may also be used to remove interproximal and marginal plaque.

*Balsa wood wedges* that are designed for interproximal cleaning may also be easier to use by an elderly person and hence more effective. If they are used properly (inserted between the teeth) and moved in a buccolingual direction with the broad surface against the tip of the papilla, there should be no trauma to the soft tissues. CAUTION: Many elderly persons have developed the habit of using wooden toothpicks after eating to clean between the teeth and around the gumline. This practice is not advisable because of the danger of injury to the soft tissues, and they should be cautioned about the potential for trauma. All these devices may be especially dangerous to elderly persons with precarious medical status because of the risk of bacteremia.

### Rinses

Many elderly persons habitually use a mouthwash or rinse as part of daily oral home care. Certain rinses may be beneficial to the individual's oral health, whereas others may be detrimental or may exacerbate existing pathologic conditions. It is important for the dental professional to determine what if any rinse an elderly person is using and whether it is enhancing oral health or having a questionable or deleterious effect.

In view of the large number of over-the-counter mouthrinses available today the dental practitioner should ask the elder what specific oral home care procedures he or she uses and make recommendations relative to the patient's oral condition and merits of a given product.

*"Cosmetic" rinses,* which are used primarily for a mouth-freshening effect, have major disadvantages:

1. They contain alcohol (from 6% to 29% of volume, depending on the brand), which can dry and irritate oral tissues and can exacerbate xerostomia induced by other factors. Second, alcoholism constitutes a major problem among the elderly population and so a general caution regarding use of any alcohol-containing rinse is appropriate.
2. The mouth-freshening effect by the rinse is transient and may serve to mask underlying causes of oral disease, such as halitosis, often an indicator of periodontal disease, and the person may delay seeking dental treatment for this condition.

A *"therapeutic" rinse* contains an agent that is beneficial to the tooth surface or oral environment. Therapeutic rinses may contain chlorhexidine, sodium benzoate, sanguinaria, a fluoride, or other remineralizing agents, which can enhance oral health and help to prevent oral disease and should be recommended to the elderly when appropriate.

*Chlorhexidine rinse.* A chlorhexidine-containing rinse (Peridex, available only by prescription) provides a form of chemical plaque control. Chlorhexidine is an effective broad-spectrum antimicrobial agent that not only kills oral bacteria initially, but also has substantivity, a prolonged bacteriostatic effect (ability to bind to surfaces in the oral cavity and continue its antibacterial effect).[5,9] CAUTION: Peridex contains alcohol, and this must be taken into consideration when one is prescribing it for the reasons cited here. The manufacturer recommends diluting the rinse by 50% with water for a patient whose oral tissues are alcohol sensitive.

Chlorhexidine rinse has numerous applications for treatment of the elderly. It is primarily indicated for gingivitis. However, it is effective against a variety of plaque bacteria,[8] thus enhancing the patient's mechanical plaque-control efforts. This is especially important for patients with physical or mental disabilities.

It has been used during dental treatment and is beneficial for the elderly who have undergone periodontal surgery.[44,57] It can be used during fixed prosthodontics treatment to maintain tissue integrity while the patient wears a temporary prosthesis.

Chlorhexidine can provide yet more benefits to the elderly. It has been shown to reduce oral mucositis and candidiasis in immunosuppressed patients who were undergoing bone marrow transplants and in oncology patients undergoing intensive chemotherapy.[6,21,22]

The dentist must monitor the elderly person's periodontal status both during and after treatment with chlorhexidine and may wish to prescribe additional courses of treatment if the patient's efforts to control plaque by other means are not sufficient.

*Fluoride.* There are three mechanisms by which fluoride acts to prevent the development of caries.

Although these can be separated for the purpose of discussion, keep in mind that usually two or more mechanisms of action are involved at a given time.[10,17,18,22,32,33,37,45,51,52,64]

The first way in which fluoride inhibits the development of caries is by being incorporated into the developing enamel in the form fluorapatite. A high concentration of fluorapatite in the outer surfaces of enamel increases the enamel's resistance to acid demineralization.[20] Fluoride promotes the formation of a more stable surface.

Second, fluoride acts to enhance or increase remineralization of enamel. As the pH of the oral cavity drops with acid formation subsequent to carbohydrate ingestion, demineralization occurs. When the pH rises again, there is a shift from demineralization to remineralization (caused by calcium and phosphate, which precipitate from saliva). Fluoride present topically in the oral cavity has the dual function of inhibiting mineral dissolution and enhancing remineralization. Levels of fluoride as low as 1 ppm enhance remineralization, and it has been found that higher concentrates of fluoride in plaque will result in increased remineralization. This is believed to be the principle means of caries protection by fluoride in adults. Additionally, research indicates that tooth structure that has been remineralized in the presence of fluoride and saliva is more resistant to subsequent acid attack.[52]

Third, fluoride has an antibacterial action. Fluoride may exert a bactericidal effect by inhibiting glycolysis (enzymatic breakdown of carbohydrates), thus rendering the bacteria unable to produce energy and causing them to die. Fluoride may also inhibit bacterial attachment and plaque formation by lowering the surface energy of the tooth. The antibacterial effect is dependent upon high concentration and frequent application of topical fluoride.[17,18,33,52]

Fluoride, topically supplied, can significantly enhance the oral health of the elderly.

*Role of systemic fluoride in the oral health of the elderly.* Systemic fluoride (once believed to be beneficial only for children) obtained from drinking water has been demonstrated to reduce the prevalence of coronal and root caries in adults.[24] A study of adults who had been lifelong residents of two communities in Ontario showed a significant difference in root caries prevalence as a result of flu-

oride intake. In this study the mean number of affected (decayed or filled) root surfaces was 0.64 for subjects residing in the community with a higher than optimal level of naturally occurring fluoride, whereas the mean number of decayed or filled root surfaces in residents of a community with a lower level of fluoride in the water was 1.36.[11,62]

In children, systemic fluoride is incorporated into the developing tooth. In adults, it is returned in the saliva to the oral cavity, where it can exert a cariostatic effect.

*Role of topical fluoride in the oral health of the elderly.* Topical fluoride in the form of gels, varnishes,[58] rinses, or dentifrices must play a significant role for the caries-prone older patient. At the very least, older patients with natural dentition should be advised to use a fluoride dentifrice daily. Those who show evidence of slight current or recent caries activity (both coronal and root caries) will benefit from daily use of a fluoride rinse or brush-on gel, both of which can provide the anticaries effects previously described. Some topical fluoride preparations are formulated for weekly rather than daily application; however it would seem that it might be easier and more beneficial for the older patient to adhere to a daily regimen. If one day is missed, the patient can rinse 6 out of 7 days. If a person misses a weekly rinse, protection for the week is lost.

In the case of an elderly person who is experiencing increased caries activity, a more aggressive fluoride regimen may be indicated. Daily application of a 1% gel in a custom tray for a limited period of time (usually 1 month at a time) can produce significant levels of remineralization.[18,63] The patient should be monitored by the dentist to determine whether an additional course of fluoride therapy is indicated. The use of fluoride in custom trays with remineralizing solution has proved successful in remineralizing severe or rampant caries.[34]

All patients should be advised to avoid ingesting topical fluoride as much as possible because of the possibility of gastric distress. If a patient swallows some of the fluoride and gastric distress ensues, he or she should be advised to discontinue the fluoride therapy.

Patients who use fluoride gel in a custom tray should be monitored so that the optimum degree of remineralization may be achieved without the risk of excessive ingestion of fluoride.

*Remineralizing rinses.* An elderly person who continually experiences new coronal or root carious lesion as a consequence of severe xerostomia can be helped to maintain his or her teeth through the use of a remineralizing solution that replaces calcium and phosphate lost from enamel or cementum during the caries process. This solution is most effective when used with topical fluoride (gel in custom trays and dentifrice), meticulous plaque removal, and physical stimulation of salivary gland activity. A self-administered protocol (oral health maintenance) that employs all these factors has been shown to effectively halt coronal and root demineralization and to remineralize softened tooth structure.[33,34]

### Plaque control for the elderly with physical limitations

Many elderly persons are hampered in their efforts to effectively perform plaque-control procedures by physical disabilities that result in lack of manual dexterity or impaired range of motion of the wrist, elbow, or shoulder. Their plaque-removal efforts may be enhanced by the use of an electric device or by adaptation of manual plaque-control aids.

### Electric devices

*Electric plaque-control devices* (such as electric toothbrushes) may be preferable to manual devices for a person with compromised manual dexterity and can be invaluable aids for the elderly when used properly. These devices have enlarged handles, which may be grasped more easily than the standard manual toothbrush handle. The major advantage derives from the fact that they are motor driven, thus requiring little or no arm or wrist movement, and make consistent movements. Some of the electric plaque-removal devices are designed in such a way that the action stops if too much pressure is applied. Devices that do not have this feature are potentially damaging to both soft and hard tissues. An elderly person who has congenital heart disease or any condition affecting heart valves should be cautioned about the danger of developing subacute bacterial endocarditis secondary to soft-tissue trauma caused by improper use of electrical devices. As with any electrical device, there is also the potential for injury through electrocution or fire, and the elderly person must be instructed in the precautions that must be taken. Additionally, patients who are immunocompromised or have prostheses should also avoid the use of these devices. Cost is another factor that must be taken into account. A traditional electric toothbrush is also heavy and cannot be easily used with a person who has no strength of grip, as in rheumatoid arthritis. A rotary electric toothbrush is similar to an electric toothbrush, except that it has the advantage of being tooth specific and much lighter than the traditional electric toothbrush. It attempts to duplicate the dentist's prophy angle in a home situation. It is dispensed only by the dentist who obtains it from the manufacturer. It is essential that dental professionals who recommend the use of electric plaque-removal devices provide instruction and supervision until assured they are being used correctly.

### Adaptive aids

If an elderly person's grip is weakened by a condition such as arthritis, he or she may encounter difficulty in grasping the slender handle of the conventional toothbrush, floss holder, or other home care aid. To enable the patient to perform effective plaque removal, the handle can be enlarged or built up so that he or she can grasp it easily and comfortably (Fig. 17-1). Although it is possible to purchase a ready-made instrument from a supplier of aids for the physically disabled, it is usally preferable to customize the handle to meet the patient's unique needs. Whenever possible, enlist the patient's assistance and creativity in designing a personalized home care aid; the patient is the best judge of what works well.

The following are a few suggestions for enlarging a handle:

Wrap the handle to desired thickness with:
1. A washcloth
2. Aluminum foil
3. Thin foam sheets, such as those used as protective packaging for fragile objects.

Insert the handle into:

1. A sponge rubber ball
2. A sponge hair roller
3. A plastic bicycle handle grip

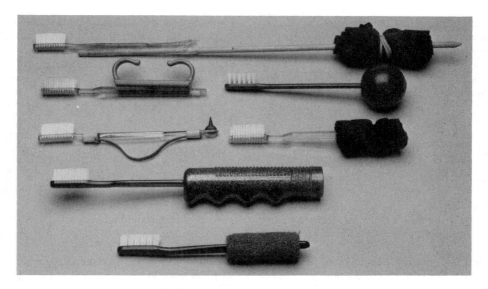

**Fig. 17-1** Adaptive aids for brushing.

If the patient is completely incapable of grasping objects with his hand, the handle of the oral home care instrument can be adapted so that it can be secured to the hand by such means as the following:

1. Attaching a Velcro strap or elastic band to the handle and then slipping it over the patient's hand
2. Attaching the handle to the curved handle of a nail brush from which the bristles have been removed and then slipping it over the fingers

If the elderly person has a limited range of motion in the shoulder, it may help to lengthen the handle of a toothbrush by attaching it to a wooden dowel. The patient can then brush without having to lift his hand to his mouth.

Although they may be very simple and seem to require little common sense, adaptations of manual home-care instruments may make a significant difference in the elderly person's ability to care for himself. At a time when a person faces potential loss of independence through diminished ability to perform simple personal tasks, enabling the patient to remain independent in one small area can greatly enhance dignity and quality of life.

## Dentures

Many edentulous elderly believe erroneously that once all their teeth have been extracted they no longer need to be concerned about oral health. It is the responsibility of the dental professional to strive to correct this misconception. The elderly who wear dentures should be taught proper home care of both dentures and tissues on which they rest as well as the need for continued professional care.

### Care of soft tissues

Since the wearing of dentures can contribute to numerous problems of the oral soft tissues, it is essential that the elderly person himself or the caregiver for the dependent patient perform certain procedures designed to ensure optimal health of the tissues upon which a denture rests.

First and most importantly, a denture must not be worn constantly. The patient should be instructed to remove it before retiring for the night. This allows for relief of compression of the soft tissues. If an elderly person refuses to sleep without a denture in place, he should be advised to remove it for significant periods of time each day—a minimum of 4 hours.

The denture wearer should be instructed to clean

and massage the tissues under a denture at least once a day. He can use a toothbrush with soft nylon bristles to clean debris from these surfaces and from the tongue, using long strokes from back to front. He can then use his thumb and forefinger (alone or covered with a clean face cloth) to massage the ridges and palate. This will increase circulation and thus enhance the health of these tissues. The patient may then wish to use a mouthrinse to freshen the mouth.

Elderly persons who wear dentures, or their caregivers, can be taught to do a simple oral examination for the purpose of observing irritated areas, lesions, or other changes that may be consequences of wearing prostheses. If there is denture-related irritation, they should be instructed to remove the denture for a few days; if the irritation persists, they should be seen by their dentist. In general, patients can be adivsed that if an oral lesion does not begin to heal within 10 days, they should consult their dentist.

### Denture care

*Cleaning dentures.* Elderly persons who wear full or partial dentures must be taught to clean these appliances in a way that is effective yet not traumatic to the denture materials. There are many reasons why maintaining the cleanliness of a denture is important, and these should be stressed with the patient:

- Stain, plaque, and calculus form on dentures just as they do on natural teeth.
- The presence of the above provide a breeding ground for bacterial and fungal organisms, which can be damaging to the oral soft tissues.
- Stained dentures not only present an esthetic problem, but also accumulate bacteria more readily.
- Offensive mouth odors may result from accumulated debris on dentures.
- A clean denture contributes to an overall sense of cleanliness and comfort.

Elderly persons will benefit from very specific *oral* and *written* instructions on how to clean a denture (see upper box on the next page).

Certain types of immersion cleaners can enhance the elderly person's efforts to clean his or her dentures and should be recommended when appropri-

ate. Immersion (soaking) cleaners are not abrasive, require little handling of the denture, and reach all parts of the denture. However, depending on the type of cleaner used, the chemicals could have a damaging effect on certain denture materials, particularly the metal clasps on a partial denture.

Another type of widely used immersion cleaner is the alkaline peroxide cleaner, an effervescent solution produced by mixing a commercial tablet or powder with water. The bubbles, signifying the release of oxygen, bombard the denture material and clean off only light debris. If used daily in combination with brushing, it may be sufficient to keep the denture clean.

The patient should be instructed to always brush and rinse the denture thoroughly before and after soaking in an immersion cleaner.

Patients should always be instructed in the care of a denture. Precautions that older adults should follow to maintain the integrity of their prosthesis are listed in the lower box on the next page.

An elderly person who has use of only one arm may find it impossible to brush a denture, a task requiring two hands. The patient can be provided with a denture brush to which suction cups have been attached. The brush can then be affixed to the back or top of a sink and the patient can move the denture against the brush. See Fig. 17-2.

*Dentures with heavy accumulation of deposits.* In the case of a chronically ill or debilitated patient, thorough cleaning of the denture may be the exception rather than the rule. The services of a dental professional may be required for a denture with tenacious stain or calculus. The dentist or hygienist may use an ultrasonic denture cleaner alone or in combination with scaling instruments.

### Denture identification

Marking an elderly person's dentures with some identification (such as name or Social Security number) is a very simple procedure that can prevent loss and costly replacement of the dentures if the patient leaves home for a stay in the hospital or other facility. In such facilities it is not uncommon that dentures are found on dinner trays by kitchen workers or in linens by laundry workers. Identification will ensure prompt return to the owner.

Dentures may be marked by the laboratory technician who fabricates them or by the dentist or

## INSTRUCTIONS FOR DENTURE CLEANING

1. Rinse your denture or dentures after each meal to remove soft debris.
2. Once a day, preferably before retiring, brush your denture according to the method described below. Then place it in a denture-cleaning solution and allow it to soak overnight or for at least a few hours. (Acrylic denture material must be kept wet at all times to prevent cracking or warping.)
3. Remove your denture from the cleaning solution and brush it thoroughly.
   a. Although an ordinary *soft* toothbrush is adequate, a specially designed denture brush may clean more effectively. (CAUTION: Acrylic denture material is softer than natural teeth and may be damaged by being brushed with very firm bristles.)
   b. Brush your denture over a sink lined with a facecloth and half-filled with water. This will prevent breakage if the denture is dropped.
   c. Hold the denture *securely* in one hand, but do not squeeze. Hold the brush in the other hand. It is not essential to use a denture paste, particularly if dentures are soaked before being brushed to soften debris. Never use a commercial tooth powder because it is abrasive and may damage the denture materials. Plain water, mild soap, or sodium bicarbonate may be used.
   d. When cleaning a *removable partial denture,* great care must be taken to remove plaque from the curved metal clasps that hook around the teeth. This can be done with a regular toothbrush or with a specially designed clasp brush.
4. After brushing, rinse your denture thoroughly and insert it into your mouth.

## TAKE CARE OF YOUR DENTURES

1. When your denture is out of your mouth, it should be stored in a water-filled container. This will prevent the denture material from drying out.
2. Place the container in a secure location where it will not be knocked onto the floor or disturbed by pets or children.
3. Never place your denture in hot water—use only cool or lukewarm.
4. Never soak dentures with metal parts in bleach.
5. Never try to adjust or repair your denture. Let an expert do it.
6. Never use abrasive powders or a hard toothbrush to clean your denture.
7. Never soak your denture in a product that contains alcohol, such as mouthwash, or clean it with regular toothpaste.
8. *ALWAYS rinse your denture thoroughly* under running water before inserting it into the mouth.

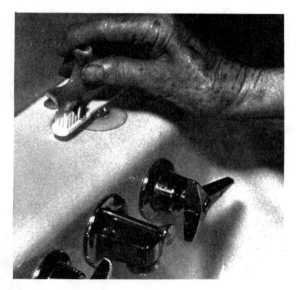

**Fig. 17-2** Patients can brush denture with just one hand.

hygienist. Some states now require that all newly fabricated oral protheses must contain a patient identifying mark. A simple procedure involves cutting a small shallow box (preferably on the flange in the posterior buccal area) with an acrylic bur, inserting a piece of onionskin paper with the identifying information (name or Social Security number) written or typed on it, and covering the box with a clear acrylic resin.

### Dependent patient

Elderly patients may be severely debilitated, physically handicapped, semiconscious, or mentally incapable of carrying out oral hygiene procedures for themselves. Nonetheless, the oral hygiene care of the dependent patient is an essential part of oral health maintenance and must be provided daily.

The debilitated patient may be at greater risk of developing oral disease than one who is healthier, for numerous reasons:

- The patient is likely to be taking medications, many of which may affect saliva production and thus compromise overall oral health.
- The debilitated patient may lack resistance to the bacterial toxins that cause periodontal disease.

- The patient may be eating soft or liquid food exclusively. If so, he lacks the stimulus for chewing, which tones the muscles of mastication, helps maintain the periodontal structures, and stimulates saliva production.
- The food, in particular the sugar in the diet, however small the amount, may remain in the mouth for long periods of time.
- With decreased immune function, increased xerostomia and frequent use of antibiotics, patients are at risk for fungal infections.

In addition to prevention of caries and periodontal disease, daily plaque removal enhances the elderly person's comfort. A clean mouth feels good and tastes good; it makes one feel better about oneself.

Daily oral home care for the dependent patient must be an integral part of the general hygiene care provided for the patient by the caregiver. In a long-term care facility this would be a nursing assistant or a nurse (Fig. 17-3). A homebound patient might be cared for by a home health aide, family member, or friend.

The person who cares for a dependent patient may not have been instructed in the technique of providing oral care for the patient or may be re-

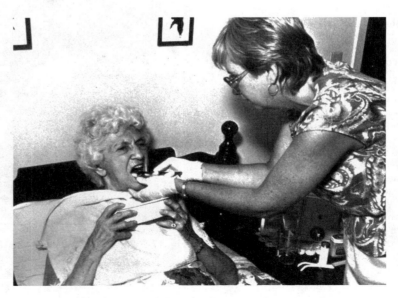

**Fig. 17-3** Bedridden patient being assisted with oral hygiene.

luctant to do so. Therefore it is essential that the dentist or hygienist train caregivers to perform these simple but essential procedures. It is equally important to motivate the caregiver to provide this service as part of overall health promotion for the dependent patient.

When instructing a caregiver in the proper way to clean the mouth of a patient with teeth, it will be helpful to have the appropriate supplies at hand. Using the proper materials and techniques can greatly simplify the task and ensure better results (Fig. 17-4). The following list includes basic supplies:

1. Disposable gloves
2. Lubricant (petroleum jelly) for lips
3. Toothbrush with soft nylon bristles
4. Toothpaste—not essential for all patients— use as indicated (do not use with an unconscious patient)
5. Dental floss (a floss holder if indicated), or an interproximal brush if there are large interdental spaces
6. 2 × 2 inch gauze squares
7. Clean towels
8. Emesis basin
9. Glass of water and straw if patient is conscious

10. Tongue blade
11. Mouth prop (for patient who cannot hold the mouth open), such as 2 or 3 tongue blades wrapped with 2 × 2 inch gauze, a folded facecloth, rubber doorstop wrapped with a facecloth, or an "Epi-stick," which is commercially available but not essential for all patients (use as indicated)
12. Enema bag or bulb syringe for lavaging mouth but not essential for all patients (use as indicated)
13. An alcohol-free mouthrinse can be used if tissues are too dry and may be irritated with an alcohol-containing mouthrinse
14. An electric or rotary toothbrush may be used, if preferred, by the caregiver

It will be helpful to give the caregiver a written list of supplies. Written instruction on the technique will serve to reinforce and clarify but not replace verbal explanation and demonstration where possible. The box on the next page lists a description that was prepared for use by home health aides, nursing assistants, and other caregivers for use in instructing caregivers in oral hygiene.

Written instructions should serve only to reinforce verbal instruction and actual demonstration

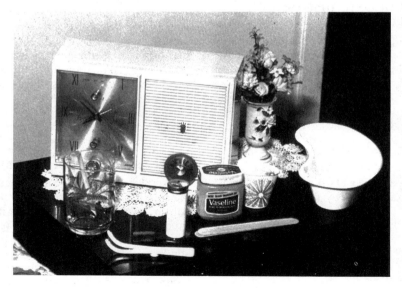

**Fig. 17-4** Supplies for oral hygiene.

---

**DENTAL CARE: INSTRUCTIONS FOR CAREGIVER**

1. If the patient is in bed, elevate his head by raising the bed or propping it with pillows and have him turn his head to face you. Place a clean towel across his chest and under his chin, and place a basin under his chin.
2. If the patient is sitting in a stationary chair or wheelchair, stand behind him and stabilize his head by placing one hand under his chin and resting his head against your body. Place a towel across his chest and over his shoulders. (It may be helpful to secure it with a safety pin.) The basin can be kept handy in the patient's lap or on a table placed in front of or at the side of the patient. A wheelchair may be positioned in front of the sink.
3. If the patient's lips are dry or cracked, apply a light coating of petroleum jelly.
4. Brush and floss the patient's teeth as you have been instructed (sulcular brushing, if possible). It may be helpful to retract the patient's lips and cheek with a tongue blade or fingers in order to see the area that is being cleaned. Use a mouth prop as needed if the patient cannot hold his mouth open. If manual flossing is too difficult, use a floss holder or interproximal brush to clean the proximal surfaces between the teeth. Use a dentifrice containing fluoride.
5. Provide the conscious patient with fluoride rinses or other rinses as indicated by the dentist or hygienist.

---

of technique. Training in the oral care of a dependent patient in a long-term care facility can be done in the context of an "in-service" presentation for home health aides or nursing assistants (in many states these are required by the licensing board for nursing homes).

## EFFECT OF CHRONIC DISEASES ON DENTAL HEALTH STATUS

Dental prevention can also mean the prevention of the medical emergency in the dental office. The next section addresses the effect of chronic diseases on oral health.[30,31,35,39,45,59]

It is rare for a person to be totally free from illness or disability throughout a lifetime. In the young and middle-aged, acute diseases prevail, whereas in the aged disease tends to be chronic. It is estimated that 86% of all aged suffer from at least one chronic disease. Most people over 65 years of age have at least two medical problems; these can be exacerbated by the medications required in the management of these problems.[24,26,38,40,55,64,65] Approximately one fourth of the elderly are dependant on prescription drugs for daily activities.[29]

### Cardiovascular disease

Cardiovascular disease is the most common cause of death in older persons and is the most prevalent

of the chronic diseases. Of these, arteriosclerotic heart disease, characterized by thickening and hardening of the arterial walls, is one of the most common cardiac problems.[3,42] Antihypertensive medications can produce mild to moderate xerostomia as a side effect (see the discussion of management of xerostomia, p. 323). Elderly persons with heart murmurs and valvular prostheses require antibiotic prophylaxis before dental treatment to prevent bacterial endocarditis. See Chapter 8 for lists of the current recommendations of the American Heart Association for antibiotic prophylaxis. Therefore cardiac patients with a history of valvular heart disorders and those taking antihypertensive medication should take particular care with oral hygiene and have frequent cleanings to prevent gingival inflammation and periodontal disease.

### Stroke (cerebrovascular accident)

Stroke is the third most common cause of death in the elderly and may be caused by thrombosis, embolism, or hemorrhage.[3] The stroke patient may experience loss of motor function (especially in the cheek and tongue), resulting in loss of chewing ability or drooling. Because there is loss of muscular activity on one side of the mouth, debris will accumulate on this side. Warfarin (Coumadin) therapy can lead to spontaneous gingival bleeding. Patients with neurologic disorders who are at risk of seizures may be placed on phenytoin, which may cause gingival hyperplasia. More frequent and effective oral cleaning is required to maintain oral health because of physiologic impairment and the medications that the patient may be taking.

## Endocrine disorders

*Diabetes mellitus and impaired glucose tolerance.* Impaired glucose tolerance is common with aging. In most cases, the elderly person is not clinically diabetic and may not require special therapy or severe dietary restrictions.[27,54] Causes of impaired glucose tolerance include:

- Obesity
- Decreased pancreatic function (beta adrenergic receptor cells)
- Altered intracellular glucose metabolism
- Reduced physical activity

Decreased resistance to infection in combination with circulatory problems seen in diabetic patients make the gingival tissues vulnerable. This results in increased gingival swelling, bleeding, and ultimately, periodontal disease. Burning tongue is frequently a presenting symptom. Candidiasis and lichen planus are more common in the diabetic patient. Effective oral home care is an important factor in preventing gingival infection.

Dental professionals must adequately assess the medical history and understand the severity of the disease and make appropriate dental treatment modification. For example, an insulin-dependent diabetic patient should be advised to decrease insulin requirement by one half the morning of the dental appointment if a stressful appointment is anticipated.

*Corticosteroid disorders.* Increased levels of corticosteroids, caused by either drug therapy or an adrenal disorder (Cushing's syndrome), will lead to increased vulnerability to infection, hot flashes, "mooning" of the face, and profound bone loss. Loss of alveolar bone can lead to periodontal disease or loss of the alveolar ridge in edentulous patients. Increased home care is necessary to prevent oral infection.

## Diseases of the nervous system

Many neurologic diseases including vascular and degenerative diseases are more prevalent in the aging population.[12]

*Trigeminal neuralgia, or tic douloureux.* This disorder is characterized by excruciating pain of the lips, gingiva, or chin, usually on one side and triggered by contact with certain areas of the face, lips, or tongue. It is seen primarily in older populations and usually does not have an assignable cause, though occasionally it may occur in patients who have multiple sclerosis or herpes zoster. Other neuralgias may occur in the tongue, pharynx, and ear.

A patient who complains of pain associated with neuralgia should be referred to an oral surgeon or physician for treatment. Trigeminal neuralgia may respond to carbamazepine (Tegretol) or phenytoin, or alcohol injection. If these therapies fail, the only option may be surgery to sever the nerve.

*Muscular dystrophy.* Muscular weakness, followed by wasting of the muscular tissue, characterizes this disorder. Patients are unable to relax muscles after contracting them and may have difficulty chewing, pursing the lips, and turning the head.[60] Since the facial muscles may become involved, it is very important to encourage and assist the patient in keeping his natural teeth because patients with muscular dystrophy may experience severe problems in keeping dentures in place. Mouth breathing, xerostomia, and edema of the oral mucous membranes attributable to medications (especially quinine) make maintenance of oral health difficult. Additionally, enlargement of the tongue because of fatty deposits and weakness of facial muscles may cause teeth to flare out. Thus effective oral hygiene and treatment of the concomitant xerostomia are necessary.

*Multiple sclerosis.* With this condition, multiple lesions caused by demyelination of long nerves may lead to paralysis of some parts of the body or the part of the body below the injury, sudden loss of vision, and diminished muscle coordination. Trigeminal paresthesia or anesthesia also may occur, and infection is common. Trigeminal neuralgia (see above) is frequently seen in patients with multiple sclerosis.

Weakness of the tongue may be the presenting symptom for multiple sclerosis. Patients with multiple sclerosis may lose upper extremity use. They may encounter difficulty in caring for natural teeth, or in both wearing and caring for a prosthesis. Effective home care is essential, especially in dentate individuals.

*Parkinson's disease.* Parkinson's disease is a slow, progressive, degenerative process of the basal ganglion of the brain and is the major cause of chronic disability in persons over 50 years of age.[66] Muscle tremors are common. In addition, muscle rigidity occurs, particularly in the face, resulting in a masklike appearance of the face. Patients have difficulty initiating a movement, and the tremor usually ceases on movement.

Loss of precision in lip, tongue, and larynx movements manifests itself in monotonous speech, a weak and feeble voice, and difficulty in articulation. Tremor and rigidity of the mouth and tongue often develop and result in difficult swallowing and drooling. Angular cheilosis, or cracks or sores at the corners of the mouth, may occur. L-Dopa is currently the most common medication used in the treatment of Parkinson's disease and may cause purposeless chewing, grinding, or tongue thrusting.[66]

Because of the moderate to severe xerostomia side effects of most antiparkinsonian medications, more frequent and effective oral home care including fluoride and mineralizing rinses for teeth become necessary. Application of petroleum jelly (Vaseline) or other emollient to the lips will help prevent cracking.

*Seizure disorders (epilepsy).* This seizure disorder of the nervous system called "epilepsy" is attributable to an intermittent, excessive, and disorderly discharge of cerebral neurons. It causes varying degrees and combinations of disturbances in sensation, consciousness, convulsive movements, and behavior. It can usually be controlled by anticonvulsant medications.

Patients who are treated with phenytoin for seizure disorders can develop enlarged gingival tissue as a side effect of the medication. There is no pain, and the gum tissue is pink and firm but may appear edematous and erythematous in the face of poor plaque control. Effective oral hygiene is important in controlling gingival hyperplasia secondary to phenytoin use.

## Oral complications of cancer therapy

Each year appproximately 1 million people in the United States develop cancer. Of these, 400,000 develop oral complications from the cancer therapy; 30,000 develop primary lesions in the head and neck areas whose treatment with radiation,

chemotherapy, or surgery almost always brings with it serious complications. They include rampant dental caries, severe inflammation of the oral mucosa (cellulitis, mucositis), dryness of the mouth (xerostomia), pain of varying intensity, osteoradionecrosis (radiologic destruction) of the jawbone, difficulty swallowing, loss of taste, and severe weight loss. In addition, damage to the mucosal barrier may lead to life-threatening septicemia.[2,13,16,20,21,23,33,46,56]

Radiation therapy to the head and neck causes xerostomia, a decrease in vascular supply, and neuronal transmission. Special precautions in oral care are very important to prevent osteoradionecrosis of the mandible, mucositis, candidiasis, viral infections, cellulitis, and trismus. These can be minimized with a rigorous preventive program.

Depending on the type of tumor and its location, one or more of the following treatments will be given:

- Radiation therapy
- Chemotherapy
- Surgery

In many cases, chemotherapy of cancerous lesions in other parts of the body also elicits several of the complications previously mentioned. Because of the high sensitivity of oral tissues and the impact of the complications on the overall nutritional status and well-being of the afflicted patients, the quality of life during and after treatment deteriorates rapidly, sometimes even causing premature death.

A central factor in the development of orally related complications in radiation therapy and chemotherapy is the effect of these treatment modalities on the salivary glands. No procedure has ever been developed to effectively shield or protect the glands during treatment. Surgery of the head and neck with or without salivary gland removal often leads to difficulties in healing, chewing, and swallowing. These problems may be further complicated by radiation therapy after surgery. The result is that salivary gland secretion diminishes greatly or ceases altogether, bringing about the dry-mouth syndrome (xerostomia) with all the adverse effects already mentioned. Several approaches have been tried to deal with these oral health problems. At Tufts University School of Dental Medicine a comprehensive oral health management system has been used since 1979.[33,34,49] Other treatment centers prescribe a fluoride rinse or daily custom fluoride tray treatments.[41]

Some of the serious oral health complications already referred to in cancer patients are also found in certain categories of noncancerous patients. The common denominator in all of these patients is decreased or lack of salivary gland function. Patients with Sjögren's syndrome suffer from dry mouth, dry eyes, and arthritis. Patients afflicted with scleroderma and autoimmune disorders, such as lupus erythematosus, Crohn's disease, primary biliary cirrhosis, polymyositis or dermatomyositis, graft-versus-host diseases, sarcoid, and autoimmune hemolytic anemia, show the same complications to varying degrees.

Furthermore, emotional states (especially fear or anxiety), drug therapies for psychoses, depression, neuroses, organic brain disorders, as well as drug therapy for other medical disorders are all known to produce dry mouth as a side effect. Some of the main medication groups are antihypertensives, antihistamines, anticonvulsants, antiparkinsonian drugs, antipsychotics, antidepressants, and antianxiety agents. In addition, salivary gland function may be diminished by obstruction of the salivary duct with a calcification (stone) upon an infection such as mumps.[23]

Malnutrition is a common result when saliva production diminishes or ceases entirely.[48] Lack of saliva can affect nutrition in several ways:

1. Chewing ability may decline because saliva is needed to moisten food.
2. The mouth may become sore and chewing painful.
3. Swallowing may be difficult because of the loss of saliva's lubricating effect and the subsequent formation of food into an easily swallowed bolus.
4. Taste perception may change, resulting in a decreased interest in eating.

In addition, saliva helps in cleaning food debris from the mouth. Without significant saliva flow, the debris remains in the mouth where bacteria produce acids and cause decay. With adequate saliva, acids are buffered and neutralized, as well as diluted. Most importantly, without the essential minerals from saliva (calcium and phosphate), the teeth will demineralize and eventually break off. No amount of restorative dentistry can prevent this from occurring. Mucositis related to xerostomia leads to constant discomfort, which affects the patient's overall quality.

Well-nourished patients are better able to undergo and recover from surgery, illness, or infection and to withstand stress and the higher doses of chemotherapy and radiation therapy. Complications of cancer therapies and some of the other ailments referred to can be eliminated or greatly diminished with appropriate oral health care.

*Xerostomia.* Salivary gland dysfunction results in xerostomia, a condition often found in the elderly. Possible causes include:

1. Medication use (At least 400 prescribed medications can cause xerostomia as a side effect.[23,61] If the xerostomia is medication induced [Fig. 17-5], the elderly person's physician should be consulted regarding the possibility of changing the medication or dose.)
2. Radiation therapy for head or neck tumors[13,33]
3. Chemotherapeutic agents used for cancer and immunosuppression therapy[50]
4. Physiologic disorders (such as fibrosis of parotid glands subsequent to mumps, blockage of salivary duct)
5. Primary or secondary Sjögren's syndrome (Fig. 17-6)

Depending on the severity of xerostomia, the patient will experience varying degrees of discomfort or dysfunction: burning sensation, difficulty in chewing or swallowing, difficulty in speaking, difficulty in retaining an upper denture, changes in taste perception with subsequent decreased interest in eating, and an increase in caries activity and tooth sensitivity.[23]

An elderly person with a natural dentition who has xerostomia can be instructed in the following home care procedures that will decrease the destructive side effects and enhance comfort:

1. Decreasing bacterial plaque through a rigorous regimen practiced twice a day (one time should be just before retiring at night). This regimen should include the use of floss

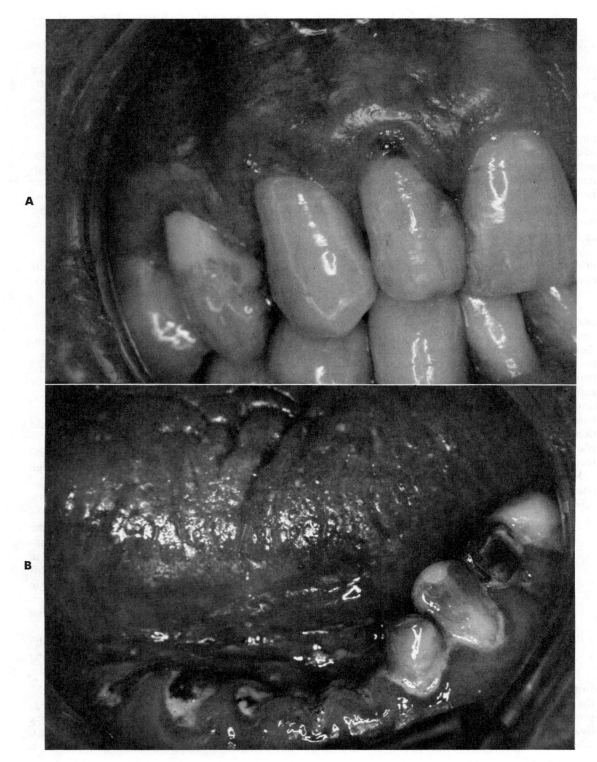

**Fig. 17-5 A,** Less obvious root caries secondary to medication-induced xerostomia. Patient had been taking antihistamines for several years. **B,** Medication-induced xerostomia. Patient had been taking belladonna for 20 years. Circumferential root caries have caused the teeth to break off.

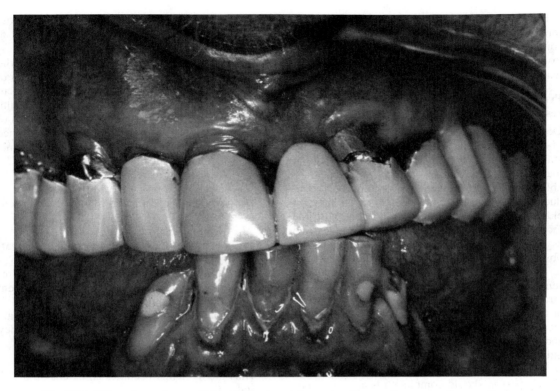

**Fig. 17-6** Sjögren's syndrome. Patient has rampant decay despite spending money for roundhouse bridge.

or other aid such as an interproximal brush, sulcular brushing, and use of cotton swabs or a rubber tip along the gingival margin for more effective plaque removal in this area.

2. Increasing remineralization of the tooth surface through the use of topical fluoride or remineralizing solutions, or both.

3. Increasing physiologic repair of the salivary glands through exercise (chewing paraffin or sugar-free inert gum. Commercial "sugarless" gum, containing a five-carbon sugar, may contribute to the caries process in patients with xerostomia.[35] Pilocarpine also has been found to be effective in the treatment of xerostomia.[23]

4. Mucositis may accompany xerostomia. The pain associated with mucositis can be alleviated through the use of a remineralizing solution (artificial saliva).[33,34]

## COMMUNITY PROGRAMS

It was stated in the beginning of this chapter that many of today's elderly have not received the benefit of preventive dentistry education and service. It was also established that there is a high prevalence of oral disease (much of it preventable) among the elderly and, further, that utilization of available dental service is low.

The reasons the elderly do not obtain oral health care are many and include the lack of perception of need or the lack of conviction of worth, reluctance to establish a relationship with a new dentist upon the retirement or death of one's former dentist, inability or reluctance to leave one's place of residence because of a physical or mental disability, and residence in a long-term care facility that does not have a functioning dental program (many facilities make provision for emergency care only). Other reasons can be cited, but these illustrate the range that exists.

How can the dental profession address the need for care in ways that are effective yet not so time consuming as to be unrealistic? A partial answer to this question can be found in community outreach programs.

### Preventive dentistry services for the elderly residing in the community

Despite certain misconceptions, the vast majority of the elderly in the United States[36] are not in institutions. One effective and enjoyable means of making initial preventive dentistry services available to those who do not seek dental care is conducting programs at senior centers, meal sites, or elderly housing units. This can be done with the local council on aging, which can provide such assistance as scheduling, publicity, and follow-up observation on referrals for care if these are made.

The program could comprise an educational presentation (excellent audiovisuals are available through the American Dental Association or state or local dental society if the dentist or dental hygienist wishes to use them), followed by a question-and-answer session; if time and personnel allow, individual screenings and consultations could also be provided. Before a screening examination, the elderly person should complete a health questionnaire. In the absence of radiographs and an extensive clinical examination the dentist can make only general recommendations for treatment.

### Preventive dentistry services for the elderly residing in long-term care institutions

A dentist and hygienist working as a team can provide comprehensive oral health care to nursing home patients. Whereas the best utilization of the dentist's time and efforts will be in diagnostic and treatment procedures (see Chapter 16 for a discussion of on-site treatment and mobile equipment), the hygienist can provide a range of preventive services.

These include:

1. In-service training of staff, including nurses, nurses' aides, occupational therapists, and dietary staff.
2. Oral health assessment of patients to assist the staff dentist in determining the priority of need for dental care among the patients.
3. Helping to determine which patients require total oral care by the nursing staff and those who might be capable of being trained to perform total or limited oral self care.
4. Providing instruction to those patients who are capable of self-care, either in groups or individually. The hygienist can train occupational therapists to conduct oral health care training sessions as part of activities of daily living (in which residents are retrained to perform basic functions such as personal hygiene, and eating).
5. Responding to requests by nursing staff to help in the oral care of difficult patients.
6. Providing identification labels for all dentures.
7. Cleaning dentures.
8. Performing prophylaxes and fluoride treatments.
9. Taking radiographs (some state requirements do not allow radiographic equipment in nursing homes).
10. Making initial assessment and appropriate consultation and referral in an emergency situation.

Thus the hygienist becomes an extension of the dental office.

## COUNSELING AND EDUCATION

Preventive dentistry counseling for the geriatric patient includes two components—education and motivation.

*Patient education* includes a discussion with the patient of the causes of current and past oral disease and the means of intervention and prevention of future disease. Discussion of etiology should be complete but appropriate to the level of understanding of the individual elderly person. The practitioner should make no assumption about a patient's level of sophistication with regard to dental knowledge. Many elderly persons are extremely well informed about health matters and will quickly lose confidence in the practitioner who talks down to them.

When one is providing instruction in home care procedures, whether teaching the elderly person himself or a caregiver, a simple yet effective model the dentist or hygienist may wish to follow is:

**Tell—show—do**

1. *Tell* or explain the procedure:
   *Why* it should be done; *when* to do it; *where* to do it; and *how* to do it.
2. *Show* or demonstrate the procedure.
   The patient's own mouth is the best visual aid for effective teaching. The patient can observe in a mirror as the dentist or hygienist demonstrates correct procedures (such as brushing, flossing, use of other plaque-removal aides, and application of fluoride)
3. Finally, the learner can *do* or practice the technique until he has mastered the skills involved in performing it effectively.
   The last step is the most important one if the learner is to develop proficiency.

If the dental practitioner intends to teach an elderly person several oral home care skills or procedures, it may be best to *partialize* the presentation rather than to attempt to present a large volume of information at one session. Doing so will decrease the risk of the elderly person being overwhelmed or intimidated by too much information. It also allows for repetition and perfection of one skill before concentrating on the next skill to be learned.

The practitioner should not expect immediate results. In many instances he will be attempting to change oral home care techniques the patient has been practicing for a lifetime. Reinforcement and encouragement should be supplied in ample doses during subsequent appointments.

When teaching new methods of oral home care, the practitioner should be careful not to convey to the elderly person the impression that what he has been doing in the past is *wrong*. He could explain that dental professionals have learned more about what causes dental disease and have developed *new* methods of *preventing* disease and *treating* the consequences of disease. It is helpful to find some aspect of the learner's technique that is correct and build on that. For example, "You are holding the toothbrush correctly, Mr. Jones. Turn your wrist slightly, and you will see how the bristles fit right under the gumline. Now, move the brush back with short strokes as you always do."

If the goal of improved home care is to be attained, both the learner and the educator must monitor and evaluate progress. In the case of plaque control, one can do this most effectively by recording periodic gingival and plaque indices and by asking the learner open-ended questions to determine whether he has understood the concepts presented (such as causes of caries and periodontal disease and home-care regimen) and is able to explain them in his own words. The learner can be encouraged to use disclosing solution at home to monitor his own progress.

The following guidelines can help the dentist or hygienist to be an effective educator:

A comfortable learning environment, both physical and emotional, will enhance the teaching and learning process.

- Teach in a clean area where there is good light.
- Be sure the patient and caregiver are comfortable.
- Eliminate distractions (such as television or radio) as much as possible.
- Be patient! Learning new skills requires practice, especially for the elderly person.
- Don't expect perfection! If you do, you will be disappointed. Motivate the learner to do the best he can, but be careful not to make him feel bad or discouraged if it is not perfect.
- *Stress the positive,* such as how good a clean mouth feels and tastes and how clean dentures look good and enhance one's smile.
- Avoid negative feedback (verbal or nonverbal); you can always find something positive to reinforce.
- Speak with authority but do not be authoritative. Encourage the learner to ask questions or express concern.

A dentist or hygienist affiliated with a long-term care institution may wish to provide oral health education to two different groups of staff:

1. Nursing assistants and nurses who provide direct care for dependent patients.
2. Occupational therapists who retrain elderly persons who have suffered loss of physical or mental ability through rehabilitative therapy. Occupational therapists conduct classes in activities of daily living in which recovering patients learn basic personal tasks such as dressing, bathing, and oral home care. By training occupational therapists, the dental practitioner can greatly extend the range of his influence and make more efficient use of

time. Occupational therapists can also devise adaptive aids for those who need them.

## Counseling and adherence

Possession of preventive knowledge and skills alone will not ensure the elderly person's attainment of the goal of preventive counseling—maintenance of optimal oral health status. The dental professional and patient must establish a therapeutic alliance whereby each party is committed to performing the activities necessary to achieve this goal.[25]

The dentist or hygienist provides both expertise (such as knowledge and diagnostic ability) and services (such as education in home-care procedures and scalings). A skillful patient educator not only will help the patient to understand the etiologic factors involved in his current oral health status, but will also help him to realize that he has control over his future oral health. The patient must be convinced that ultimately only he can help himself by adhering to the recommended preventive measures—practicing health-promoting behavior (such as plaque removal, presenting for scalings) and eliminating non–health promoting behaviors (such as frequent ingestion of fermentable carbohydrates or wearing a denture 24-hours a day).

Models for the development of health-promoting behaviors are described in Chapter 2, and you may wish to refer to these sources for a more extensive description.

In order for an elderly person to develop adherence to a prescribed regimen of oral health-promoting behaviors, he must be convinced that optimal oral health status is both worthwhile and attainable. The practitioner must work to dispel the misconception that oral disease is an inevitable consequence of aging and that, consequently, the attempt to prevent oral disease is a waste of time and effort. It may be helpful to present reasons why a healthy, well-functioning mouth is important to the elder, such as adequate nutritional intake, improved esthetics and communication, and a sense of general well-being.

If the elderly person expresses doubts about his ability to adequately perform the health-promoting behaviors that have been recommended, the dental practitioner should assure him that they will work *together* to help him develop the necessary skills.

Once the elderly person begins to see that his efforts do indeed produce positive changes (such as elimination of gingival bleeding), the satisfaction he experiences will constitute positive reinforcement, thus increasing his motivation to continue.

Another factor to consider is that aging may bring with it the diminution of certain abilities for the individual, and he may fear that he is losing control or independence. If, however, the dentist or hygienist can work with an elderly person to develop skill in performing oral home-care procedures, that person can retain control or independence in at least one aspect of his life. Although this step may seem a small success to the casual observer, it may be of great significance to the elderly person. The more a person can do for himself, the greater is his sense of dignity.

## REFERENCES

1. Banting DW, Ellen RP, and Fillery ED: Prevalence of root surface caries among institutionalized older persons, Community Dent Oral Epidemiol 8:84, 1986.
2. Beumer J, Curtis T, and Harrison RE: Radiation therapy of the oral cavity: sequelae and management, Head Neck Surg 1:301, 1979.
3. Bierman EL: Aging and atherosclerosis. In Andres R, Bierman EL, and Hazzard WR, editors: Principles of geriatric medicine, New York, 1985, McGraw-Hill Book Co.
4. Bomberg TJ and Ernst NS: Improving utilization of dental care services by the elderly, Gerodontics 2:57, 1986.
5. Bonesvoll P, Looken P, et al: Retention of chlorhexidine in the human oral cavity after mouth rinses, Arch Oral Biol 19:211, 1974.
6. Bostrom B and Weisdorf D: Mucositis and alpha-streptococcal sepsis in bone marrow transplant recipients, Lancet 1:1120, 1984 (letter).
7. Branch LG, Antczak AA, and Stason WB: Toward understanding the use of dental services by the elderly, Special Care Dent. 5(1):38, 1986.
8. Briner WW et al: Effect of chlorhexidine gluconate mouth rinse on plaque bacteria, J Periodont Res 16(suppl):44, 1986.
9. Briner WW et al: Antimicrobial profile of a chlorhexidine gluconate mouth rinse against plaque bacteria, J Dent Res 65(special issue):abstract 884, 1986.
10. Brown WE and Konig KG, editors: Cariostatic mechanisms of fluorides, Caries Res 11(suppl 1):118, 1977.
11. Burt BA, Ismail AI, and Eklund SA: Root caries in an optimally fluoridated and a high-fluoride community, J Dent Res 65:1154, 1986.
12. Calne DB: Neurological disease of the elderly. In Andres R, Bierman EL, and Hazzard WR, editors: Principles of geriatric medicine New York, 1985, McGraw-Hill Book Co.

13. Carl W: Oral complications in cancer patients, Am Fam Physician 27:161, 1983.
14. Chauncey H et al: Effects of dentition and aging on adult *restorative* needs, J Dent Res 67:356, 1988.
15. Douglass C, Gammon M, Gillings D, and Sollecito W: Estimating the market for periodontal services in the U.S., J Dent Res 63:1543, 1984.
16. Dreizen S: Oral candidiasis, Am J Med 77(suppl 4D):28, 1984.
17. Featherston J et al: Remineralization of artificial caries-like lesions in vivo by a self-administered mouth rinse or paste, Caries Res 16:235, 1982.
18. Fejerskov O et al: Rational use of fluorides in caries prevention: a concept based on the possible cariostatic mechanisms, Acta Odont Scand 39:241, 1981.
19. Ferretti G et al: Chlorhexidine for prophylaxis against oral infections and associated complications on patients receiving bone marrow transplants, J Am Dent Assoc 4:461, 1987.
20. Ferretti G et al: Effect of chlorhexidine mouthrinse on mucositis in patients receiving intensive chemotherapy, IADR Abstr no 1885, J Dent Res 66(special issue):342, 1987.
21. Ferretti GA, Raybould TP, Brown AT, et al: Chlorhexidine prophylaxis for chemotherapy and radiotherapy-induced stomatitis: a randomized clinical trial, Oral Surg Oral Med Oral Pathol 69:331, 1990.
22. Forrester DJ and Schulz EM, editors: International Workshop on Fluorides and Dental Caries Reductions, Baltimore, 1974, University of Maryland School of Dentistry.
23. Fox PC, Van der Ven PF, Sonis BC, et al: Xerostomia: evaluation of a symptom with increasing significance, J Am Dent Assoc 110:519, 1985.
24. Freedman L and Haynes S: An epidemiologic profile of the elderly. In Phillips MT and Gaylord SA, editors: Aging and public health, New York, 1987, Springer-Verlag.
25. Geboy MJ: Communication and behavior management in dentistry, Baltimore, 1985, Williams & Wilkins.
26. Gilman AG and Goodman CS, editors: Goodman and Gilman's the pharmacological basis of therapeutics ed 6, New York, 1980, MacMillan Publishing Co, p 1357.
27. Goldberg AP, Andres R, and Bierman EL: Metabolic disorders: diabetes mellitus in the elderly. In Andres R, Bierman EL, and Hazzard WR, editors: Principles of geriatric medicine, New York, 1985, McGraw-Hill Book Co.
28. Glass RL, Alman JE, and Chauncey HH: A 10-year longitudinal study of caries incidence rates in a sample of male adults in the USA, Caries Res 21:360, 1987.
29. Guttman D: A study of drug-taking behaviors of older Americans. In Beber CR and Lamy PP, editors: Medication management and education of the elderly, Amsterdam, 1978, Excerpta Medica, p 18.
30. Holm-Pedersen P and Löe H, editors: Geriatric dentistry: a textbook of oral gerontology, St. Louis, 1986, The CV Mosby Co, p 183.
31. Irvine PW: Disease in the elderly with implications for oral status and dental therapy. In Holm-Pedersen P and Löe H, editors: Geriatric dentistry: a textbook of oral gerontology, St. Louis, 1986, The CV Mosby Co, p 179.
32. Jenkins AN: Recent advances in work on fluorides and the teeth, Br Med Bull 31:192, 1975.
33. Johansen E and Olsen TO: Topical fluorides in the prevention and arrest of dental caries. In Johansen E, Taves DR, and Olsen TO: Continuing evaluation of the use of fluorides, American Association for the Advancement of Science Selected Symposium, Boulder, Col, 1979, Westview Press.
34. Johansen E, Papas A, et al: Remineralization of carious lesions in elderly patients, Gerodontics 3:47, 1987.
35. Kalfas S, Svensäter G, Birkhed D, and Edwardsson D: Sorbitol adaptation of dental plaque in people with low and normal salivary-secretion rates, J Dent Res 69(2):442, 1990.
36. Kamen S: Delivery of oral health care for the institutionalized aged and dental management of the elderly with systemic diseases. In Chauncey HH, Epstein S, Rose CL, and Hefferren JJ, editors: Clinical geriatric dentistry: biomedical and psychosocial aspects, Chicago, 1985, American Dental Association.
37. Koulourides T, Feagin F, and Pigman W: Remineralization of dental enamel by saliva in vitro, Ann NY Acad Sci 131:751, 1965.
38. Long DM: Management of pain in the elderly. In Andres R, Bierman EL, and Hazzard WR, editors: Principles of geriatric medicine, New York, 1985, McGraw-Hill Book Co.
39. Lynch MA, Brightman VJ, and Greenberg MS: Burket's oral medicine: diagnosis and treatment, ed 8, Philadelphia, 1984, JB Lippincott Co.
40. Maloney SK, Fallon B, and Wittenberg CK: Executive summary: aging and health promotion: market research for public education, Washington, DC, May 1984, SRA Technologies, Inc, and Needham Porter Novelli, Office of Disease Prevention and Health Promotion, DHHS, PHS.
41. McClure D, Barker G, Barber B, and Feil P: Oral management of the cancer patient. Part I, Oral complications of chemotherapy, Compendium 8(1):41-50, 1987.
42. Murphy ES and DeMots H: Cardiology. In Cassel CK and Walsh JR, editors: Geriatric medicine, vol 1, Medical, psychiatric and pharmacological topics, New York, 1984, Springer-Verlag.
43. National Center for Health Statistics: Edentulous persons, DHEW Publ no (HRA) 74-1516, Washington, DC, 1974, US Government Printing Office.
44. Newman MG et al: Effect of 0.12% chlorhexidine on bacterial recolonization following periodontal surgery, J Dent Res 66(special issue):280, 1987; IADR Abstr no 1384.
45. Nizel A and Papas A, editors: Nutrition in clinical dentistry, Philadelphia, 1989, WB Saunders Co.
46. Oral complications of cancer therapies: diagnosis, prevention and treatment, NIH Consensus Development Conference statement, vol 7, no 7, April 17-19, 1989.
47. Oral health of United States adults, the National Survey of Oral Health in U.S. Employed Adults and Seniors: 1985-1986, NIH publ no 87-2868, 1987.
48. Palmer C, Cassidy M, and Larson C: Nutrition, diet and dental health: concepts and methods, Chicago, 1981, American Dental Association.
49. Papas A, Johansen E, Sobel S, and Olsen T: Effects of preventive regimen on oral mucositis, J Dent Res 63(special issue):311, 1984.

50. Peterson D and Sonis S, editors: Oral complications of cancer chemotherapies, The Hague, 1983, Martinus Nijhoff.

51. Pigman W, Cueto H, and Baugh D: Conditions affecting rehardening of softened enamel, J Dent Res 43:1187, 1964.

52. Proceedings of a Joint IADR/ORCA International Symposium on Fluorides: Mechanisms of action and recommendations for use, March 21-24, 1989, J Dent Res 69(special issue), 1990.

53. Ravald N and Hamp SE: Prediction of root surface caries in patients treated for advanced periodontal disease, J Clin Periodontol 8:400, 1981.

54. Riddle MC: Diabetes mellitus. In Cassel CK and Walsh JR, editors: Geriatric medicine, vol 1, Medical, psychiatric and pharmacological topics, New York, 1984, Springer-Verlag.

55. Roe DA, editor: Drugs and nutrition in the geriatric patient, New York, 1984, Churchill Livingstone.

56. Rothwell B and Spektor WS: Palliation of radiation-related mucositis, Special Care Dentist 10(1):21, 1990.

57. Sanz M et al: A comparison of the effect of 0.12% chlorhexidine gluconate mouthrinse and placebo on postperiodontal surgical therapy, J Dent Res 66(special issue):280, 1987; IADR Abstr No 1385.

58. Scholtaus JD and Arends J: Influence of fluoridating varnishes on dentine in vitro, Caries Res 20:65, 1986.

59. Shaver RO: Dentistry for the homebound, institutionalized and elderly: a handbook for dentists, dental hygienists and nursing home administrators, p 91, Lakewood, Col, 1982, Portable Dentistry.

60. Shields RW: Diseases of striated muscle, In Andres R, Bierman EL, and Hazzard WR, editors: Principles of geriatric medicine, New York, 1985, McGraw-Hill Book Co.

61. Sreebny LM, editor: The salivary system, Boca Raton, Fla, 1987, CRC Press, Inc.

62. Stamm JW and Banting DW: Comparison of root caries prevalence in adults with lifelong residence in fluoridated and non-fluoridated communities, J Dent Res 59(special issue A):405, 1980; IADR Abstr no 52.

63. Stockey G: Topical fluoride therapy. In Harris N and Christen AG, editors: Primary preventive dentistry, Norwalk, CT, 1987, Appleton & Lange.

64. Wantz MS and Gay JE: The aging process: a health perspective, Cambridge Mass, 1981, Winthrop Publishers, Inc, p 194.

65. Wyngaarden JB and Smith LH, editors: Cecil's textbook of medicine, Philadelphia, 1985, WB Saunders Co, p 2070.

66. Yahr MD: The parkinsonian syndrome. In Beeson P, McDermott W, and Wyngaarden J, editors: Cecil's textbook of medicine, ed 15, XI, Disorders of the nervous system and behavior, section II, The extrapyramidal disorders, Philadelphia, 1979, WB Saunders Co, p 752.

# 18

# The Geriatric Population as a Target Market for Dentists

*David Schwab*
*Cathy A. Pavlatos*

## CURRENT SIZE AND PROJECTED GROWTH

The geriatric population, referred to as the "mature market" by marketing experts, presents a tremendous opportunity for dentists who know how to read the trends and reach these consumers.

As a result of advances in preventive health care and the treatment of illness, 27 years have been added to human life expectancy since the turn of the century. Today, the average American can expect to live more than 75 years.[10] People over 55—some 56 million Americans—account for one out of every five persons in this country. Their numbers are growing at a rate three times faster than the rest of the population.[2] Experts predict that by the year 2010, because of the maturation of the baby boom, more than 25% of Americans will be 55 years of age or older. These persons will be healthier and more physically fit than their predecessors because of a lifetime of improved diet and exercise. By the year 2030, one in three persons will be at least 55 years of age.[11]

This increase in the geriatric population is good news for dentistry. Although the oral health of the aged population has improved, this population still has many unmet dental needs. Because today's elderly retain more of their natural dentition than previous generations (58% are dentate),[7] they have a greater need for restorative care than previous generations of elderly. A recent study by the National Institute of Aging projects that up to 8000 dentists with advanced training in geriatrics will be needed to meet the needs of the aging population by the year 2000.[6]

Even though the elderly have significant dental needs, they have fewer dental visits than any other age group. This anomaly is partially explained by the popular misperception among the general public that the need for professional dental care is reduced with advancing age and loss of teeth. This perceived lack of need is reinforced by a recent consumer study that noted that 57% of all consumers avoid dental visits because they do not perceive a need to go.

## MYTHS ABOUT THE GERIATRIC POPULATION

If dentists are to market their services successfully to the mature market, they must understand the changing characteristics of older Americans and separate myth from reality.

**Myth 1** The mature market is poorer than younger markets.

**Reality** Households headed by persons over 65 years of age have a median net worth of $60,266 as compared to $32,667 for the general population.[4] According to the U.S. Census Bureau, 72% own their own homes and, of these, 75% are mortgage free. Although the American public at large has $80 million in disposable income per year, 60% of this, or about $50 million, is in the hands of the 50-65 age group.[3]

**Myth 2** The mature market is unwilling to spend money on anything other than absolute necessities.

**Reality**  Today's mature consumers not only have more money than any previous elderly generation, but they are also willing to spend it. The 50⁺ age group spends more on luxury items, including expensive cars and extended vacations, than any other single segment of society. These consumers also spend far above the national average on just about everything. For example, in 1984, households headed by persons 55 to 64 years of age spent 27% more on personal care products, 18% more on health care, 11% more on home furnishings, and 10% more on food.[9]

**Myth 3**  Even the relatively well-to-do elderly are excessively price conscious, bargain-hunting penny pinchers who throw nickels around as though they were manhole covers.

**Reality**  Surprisingly, among these consumers price has less influence on purchase decisions than previously understood. Older consumers are motivated by quality, value, and convenience more than price. *Megatrends* author John Naisbet reports that 89% of consumers 50 years or older would rather purchase a few high-quality items rather than many of lesser quality. In short, if they like a product or service, price is less important than perceived value.

**Myth 4**  The mature market has a poor self-image. Timid, anxious, and unable to cope with advancing technology, these individuals live out their remaining years passively, longing for the "good old days."

**Reality**  As Mark Twain said, "Age is a thing of mind over matter; if you don't mind, it doesn't matter." Although a 20 year old is likely to say that "old" begins at 63, those in their forties define it as 70 years and up.[8] Today, people in their fifties, sixties, and seventies are more likely to reject the label of "old." Both their self-image and way of living are more youthful, energetic, and forward looking.[5] They are uncomfortable with terms such as "senior citizen," "retiree," and "golden years,"[12] preferring instead to be called "mature market," "adult," and "senior."[1]

In fact, 85% of Americans over 50 years of age do not identify with people their own ages. Instead, they identify with persons younger than they are. Psychologic age, the age a person feels, and sociologic age, the age group a person feels comfortable with, fall 5 to 10 years behind a person's chronologic age.[3] This is the reason marketers typically depict people about 10 years younger in advertisements meant to appeal to the 50-and-over age group.

**Myth 5**  The mature market is composed of one large group of people—the elderly.

**Reality**  The mature market is not one homogeneous group of the nation's elderly but distinct groups of different sizes. This market can be divided into three main divisions. The youngest group, 55 to 64 years of age, variously referred to as the "new mature," the "upwardly mobile," or the "young old," accounts for nearly half of the senior market with 22 million persons. This group has more money than the others, with the highest after-tax per capita income ($15,000), partly because they were in the job market at a time when pensions became common. Almost one third of the men in this age group are retired, and 80% are married. This group is expected to grow by 7% by the year 2000.

The next segment of the mature market is made up of the 17 million adults 65 to 74 years of age. With healthier life styles and younger attitudes this group is more active and vital than their predecessors. By this time, 60% of men will have retired. Although this group represents a sizable one third of the mature market, they will experience little growth (2%) over the next 12 years, primarily because family size decreased during the Great Depression of the 1930s.

The third and most rapidly growing segment of the mature market is referred to as the "later mature," or the "oldest old," those persons 75 years of age and up. Numbering about 16 million in 1986, this group will surge to almost 24 million by the year 2000. Even so, only one in five currently lives in a nursing home.

**Myth 6**  Because women live longer than men, the over-50 market is overwhelmingly female.

**Reality**  The population of both sexes is almost equal at 55 years of age, and the gender gap in life expectancy does not appear until 65 years of age. Women do, however, make up nearly two thirds of the over-65 population. The gap widens by 85 years of age, when women outnumber men by 2½ to one. As a group, women tend to have more chronic ailments associated with old age and make up 73% of nursing home residents, simply because they live longer and there are more of them.

**Myth 7** Unlike "yuppies," the "matures" are often poorly educated and easily swayed by advertising gimmicks.

**Reality** Matures are more informed consumers than their parents and grandparents were. They are better educated, and they expect high quality in goods and services. They dislike condescending TV ads and were particularly put off by Clara Peller's memorable "Where's the beef?" performance. Although this television commercial was well-received by the public at large, older Americans felt that it fostered images of old people as cantankerous, idiosyncratic, and intellectually impaired.[12]

**Myth 8** Other than increasing in size, the mature market will not change significantly in years to come.

**Reality** The 77 million "baby boomers" born between 1946 and 1964 may be referred to as the "Good Times" or "Me" generation. When the first wave of baby boomers reach 65 years of age in the year 2011, they will be a new class of elderly, the first to grow up with television, automobiles, and more discretionary income. One in four will have a college education. They will be the best informed group of elderly consumers in history. Continuing a trend already in evidence, this group will be very interested in all aspects of health care, including both treatment and prevention.

## TARGET MARKETING

Dentists should determine which direction to channel their marketing efforts based on the potential patient yield of the surrounding community and the representation of the local demographics within the practice. If, for example, over 40% of the surrounding community is 55 to 64 years of age but only 15% of the patients of record in the practice fit this description, then this practice is not getting its fair share of this consumer market. Practitioners also need to identify which segment of the mature market will be the focus of their marketing activities. Because the needs and expectations of the youngest matures will not coincide with those of the oldest matures, the marketing approach to each of these groups should be modified to best suit the target group.

## MARKETING MIX FOR THE GERIATRIC POPULATION

There are five components of the dental marketing mix—product, price, place, promotion, and people.

*Product.* In dentistry, the product is a professional service. Every interaction between the patient and the practice affects the patient's purchasing decisions. As a group, matures expect highly personalized service. Even if they are retired, they frequently lead active lives. They dislike waiting as much as any other segment of society.

*Price.* The price component of the marketing mix includes the fee level, payment terms, and collection policies of the practice. Matures appreciate and even expect discounts for their age group. Having reached an age and income level that invites them to pamper themselves somewhat, they may make purchase decisions based on the cosmetic rather than the clinical value of a dental procedure. If they can afford recommended treatment, they will say it is "too expensive" only if they do not perceive it as being a good value. However, they are willing to spend money for perceived high-quality dentistry.

*Place.* The appearance of the dental office provides the patient with the first visual impression of the practice and the quality of service offered. The office image selected depends on which segment of the mature market the dentist wishes to target. If for example, dentists seek to expand their patient base with matures 65 years of age and over, they will have to consider some of the possible physical limitations of this age group. The office building should be accessible to the physically handicapped, the seating in the reception area should be comfortable and easy to rise from, there should be handrails in the restrooms, the restrooms and operatory should be able to accommodate a wheelchair patient, and printed matter in the reception area should contain large type. This kind of office environment would not be appropriate, however, for the dentist who elects to target upscale individuals in the 50 to 60 age group. These individuals may arrive in expensive cars, they may exercise regularly at fitness clubs, and they probably will think of themselves as anything but "old."

*Promotion.* In recent years dentists have recognized that newsletters can be a good way to remind patients of record of all the services that the practice provides. Mature consumers enjoy receiving newsletters, and they are loyal readers. Dentists who target the mature market should include articles of interest to this segment of the population, and they should also invite letters to the editor. Matures take the time to write, and they enjoy being afforded a forum for their questions and opinions.

With regard to external marketing, nursing homes, senior centers, and other community groups are possible sources of new patients. Practitioners may offer to give a brief presentation on the cost benefits of preventive dentistry, since the two major concerns of the mature market are finances and health. Participation in a dental health screening or a denture identification program will heighten community visibility and generate goodwill.

*People.* One of the most important elements of any dental practice is the dental team. The dental team must be aware of the special needs of the mature market and respond to and satisfy those needs appropriately. Some banks train tellers to provide service to the mature elderly by simulating physical impairments in the trainees. For example, trainees are required to wear eyeglasses smeared with Vaseline, use earplugs, and wear ill-fitting gloves and then attempt to fill out deposit slips and communicate with bank personnel. The goal is to give trainees an appreciation of how difficult simple tasks can be for those with visual and hearing problems and with motor skill impairment caused by arthritis. This type of sensitivity training may be valuable for members of the dental team to learn how activities in the dental office are experienced by the later matures. It is equally important, however, that the dental team learn to assess each mature patient as an individual and avoid stereotyping.

When the dental team understands the mature market and makes efforts to respond to their individual needs, the result is a high-quality service product. If the dental team works well together and the practice is committed to the concept of total customer service, mature patients will place a high value on the services provided.

## A GLIMPSE OF THE FUTURE

The future has already started to arrive in the form of a growing mature market. Dentists who appreciate the characteristics of this market will be able to position themselves as providers of quality dental services to meet their needs.

## REFERENCES

1. Perspectives, New York, March 1988, Dunn & Bradstreet, Inc.
2. The 50-Plus Market Update Newsletter 5(2): Sept-Oct 1988 (New Choices Magazine, 28 W. 23rd St New York, NY 10010; [212] 366-8800).
3. Hotchkiss, G, publisher of New Choices Magazine (formerly 50-Plus), panelist remarks: Distribution: lessons from experience, American Society on Aging Conference, Washington, DC, Sept 29, 1988.
4. Household wealth and asset ownership: 1984, US Bureau of the Census, series P-70, no 7, 1986.
5. Langer, J: The 50-plus market: "Who says I'm old?" a qualititative report prepared by Judith Langer Associates, Inc., New York, 1981, p 3.
6. Borski, RA: The importance of adequate health care for old persons [citing National Institute on Aging, Washington, DC], Special Care in Dentistry, p 250, Nov-Dec 1988.
7. National Institute of Dental Research: National Survey of Oral Health in U.S. Employed Adults and Seniors, 1985-1986.
8. Redefinition of aging: Research Alert 5(15):4, Jan 8, 1988, Alert Publishing, Inc, Long Island, NY.
9. US Bureau of Labor Statistics, Consumer Expenditure Study: As reported in American Demographics and reprinted in The 50-Plus Market Update Newsletter 5(2): Sept-Oct 1988 (New Choices Magazine, 28 W. 23rd St New York, NY 10010; [212] 366-8800).
10. US Department of Health and Human Services, National Center for Health Statistics: Monthly vital statistics report 35(6):suppl 2, Sept 26, 1986.
11. US Senate Special Committee on Aging: 1988—Aging America: trends and projections, LR 3377(1880) D 12198, Washington DC, 1988, US Department of Health and Human Services, p 10.
12. Wolfe, B: The ageless market, American Demographics, July 1987, Lifestyles and Values of Older Adults study, as commissioned by the National Association of Senior Living Industries, Annapolis, Md.

# Index